T0226540

The Pancreas Revisited

Editor

AVRAM M. COOPERMAN

SURGICAL CLINICS
OF NORTH AMERICA

www.surgical.theclinics.com

Consulting Editor
RONALD F. MARTIN

February 2018 • Volume 98 • Number 1

ELSEVIER

1600 John F. Kennedy Boulevard • Suite 1800 • Philadelphia, Pennsylvania, 19103-2899

http://www.surgical.theclinics.com

SURGICAL CLINICS OF NORTH AMERICA Volume 98, Number 1
February 2018 ISSN 0039–6109, ISBN-13: 978-0-323-57002-2

Editor: John Vassallo, j.vassallo@elsevier.com

Developmental Editor: Meredith Madeira

Surgical Clinics of North America (ISSN 0039–6109) is published bimonthly by Elsevier Inc., 360 Park Avenue South, New York, NY 10010-1710. Months of publication are February, April, June, August, October, and December. Business and Editorial Offices: 1600 John F. Kennedy Blvd., Suite 1800, Philadelphia, PA 19103-2899. Periodicals postage paid at New York, NY and additional mailing offices. Subscription prices are $350.00 per year for US individuals, $802.00 per year for US institutions, $100.00 per year for US students and residents, $420.00 per year for Canadian individuals, $1015.00 per year for Canadian institutions, $475.00 for international individuals, $1015.00 per year for international institutions and $225.00 per year for Canadian and foreign students/residents. To receive student/resident rate, orders must be accompanied by name of affiliated institution, date of term, and the *signature* of program/residency coordinator on institution letterhead. Orders will be billed at individual rate until proof of status is received. Foreign air speed delivery is included in all *Clinics* subscription prices. All prices are subject to change without notice. POSTMASTER: Send address changes to *Surgical Clinics*, Elsevier Health Sciences Division, Subscription Customer Service, 3251 Riverport Lane, Maryland Heights, MO 63043. **Customer Service (orders, claims, online, change of address): Telephone: 1-800-654-2452 (U.S. and Canada); 314-447-8871 (outside U.S. and Canada). Fax: 314-447-8029. E-mail: journalscustomerservice-usa@elsevier.com (for print support); journalsonlinesupport-usa@elsevier.com (for online support).**

Reprints. For copies of 100 or more, of articles in this publication, please contact the Commercial Reprints Department, Elsevier Inc., 360 Park Avenue South, New York, New York 10010-1710. Tel. 212-633-3874, Fax: 212-633-3820, E-mail: reprints@elsevier.com.

The Surgical Clinics of North America is also published in Spanish by McGraw-Hill Interamericana Editores S.A., P.O. Box 5-237 06500 Mexico D.F. Mexico; and in Portuguese by Interlivros Edicoes Ltda., Rua Comandante Coelho 1085, CEP 21250, Rio de Janeiro, Brazil; and in Greek by Paschalidis Medical Publications, Athens Greece.

The Surgical Clinics of North America is covered in *MEDLINE/PubMed (Index Medicus)*, *EMBASE/Excerpta Medica*, *Current Contents/Clinical Medicine*, *Current Contents/Life Sciences*, *Science Citation Index*, and *ISI/BIOMED*.

Contributors

CONSULTING EDITOR

RONALD F. MARTIN, MD, FACS
Colonel (ret.), United States Army Reserve, Department of Surgery, York Hospital, York, Maine, USA

EDITOR

AVRAM M. COOPERMAN, MD, FACS
The Pancreas, Biliary and Advanced Laparoscopy Center of New York, New York, New York, USA

AUTHORS

MAHMOUD AHMAD, MD, MBA
General Surgery Resident, Department of General Surgery, Aventura Hospital and Medical Center, Aventura, Florida, USA

HORACIO J. ASBUN, MD, FACS
Department of Surgery, Mayo Clinic, Jacksonville, Florida, USA

MURRAY F. BRENNAN, MD
International Center, Memorial Sloan Kettering Cancer Center, New York, New York, USA

HOWARD BRUCKNER, MD
The Center for Pancreatic, Biliary and Advanced Minimally Invasive Surgery of New York, New York, New York, USA

CARLO CATALANO, MD
Professor of Radiology, Department of Radiological Sciences, Sapienza University of Rome, Rome, Italy

SETH COHEN, MD
Attending, Division of Digestive Diseases, The Center for Pancreatic, Biliary and Advanced Minimally Invasive Surgery of New York, Mount Sinai Beth Israel, New York, New York, USA

AVRAM M. COOPERMAN, MD, FACS
The Pancreas, Biliary and Advanced Laparoscopy Center of New York, New York, New York, USA

SUSAN DABABOU, MD
Department of Radiological Sciences, Sapienza University of Rome, Rome, Italy

ALEXANDER T. EL GAMMAL, MD
Departments of General, Visceral and Thoracic Surgery and Experimental Oncology, University Medical Center Hamburg-Eppendorf, Hamburg, Germany

ANDREW FADER, MD
The Center for Pancreatic, Biliary and Advanced Minimally Invasive Surgery of New York, New York, New York, USA

MICHAEL FELD, MD
The Center for Pancreatic, Biliary and Advanced Minimally Invasive Surgery of New York, New York, New York, USA

SEPIDEH GHOLAMI, MD
UC Davis Comprehensive Cancer Center, Department of Surgery, Sacramento, California, USA

FRANK GOLIER, MD
The Center for Pancreatic, Biliary and Advanced Minimally Invasive Surgery of New York, New York, New York, USA

MARINA GORELIK, DO
General Surgery Resident, Department of General Surgery, Aventura Hospital and Medical Center, Aventura, Florida, USA

DAVID GROSSMAN, MD
Associate Program Director of Surgical Residency Program, Department of General Surgery, Aventura Hospital and Medical Center, Aventura, Florida, USA

MARTIN GROSSMAN, MD
General Surgeon, Department of General Surgery, Aventura Hospital and Medical Center, Aventura, Florida, USA

HILLEL HAMMERMAN, MD
The Center for Pancreatic, Biliary and Advanced Minimally Invasive Surgery of New York, New York, New York, USA

MAZEN E. ISKANDAR, MD
Assistant Professor, Department of Surgery, Division of Surgical Oncology, Mount Sinai Beth Israel, Icahn School of Medicine at Mount Sinai, Mount Sinai St Luke's and Mount Sinai West, New York, New York, USA

JAKOB R. IZBICKI, FACS, FRCS ed. Hon, MD
Department of General, Visceral and Thoracic Surgery, Center for Operative Medicine, Clinic and Polyclinic for General, Visceral and Thoracic Surgery, Hamburg, Germany

ALEXANDER C. KAGEN, MD
Associate Professor, Site Chair, Department of Radiology, Mount Sinai St Luke's and Mount Sinai West, Icahn School of Medicine at Mount Sinai, New York, New York, USA

SHALOM KALNICKI, MD, FACRO
Radiation Oncology, Montefiore Medical Park, Bronx, New York, USA

FRANKLIN KASMIN, MD
The Center for Pancreatic, Biliary and Advanced Minimally Invasive Surgery of New York, New York, New York, USA

TOMOAKI KATO, MD, MBA
Department of Surgery, Columbia University Medical Center, New York, New York, USA

MATHEW H.G. KATZ, MD, FACS
Chief, Pancreatic Surgery Service, Associate Professor of Surgical Oncology,
The University of Texas MD Anderson Cancer Center, Houston, Texas, USA

EVAN LANDAU, MD
21st Century Oncology, Ft. Lauderdale, Florida, USA

NATASHA LEIGH, MD
Department of Surgery, Mount Sinai St Luke's and Mount Sinai West, New York,
New York, USA

PETER LIOU, MD
Department of Surgery, Columbia University Medical Center, New York, New York, USA

THINZAR M. LWIN, MS, MD
Department of Surgery, UC San Diego, San Diego, California, USA; Department of
Surgery, Mount Sinai Beth Israel, New York, New York, USA

CRISTINA MARROCCHIO, MD
Department of Radiological Sciences, Sapienza University of Rome, Rome, Italy

ALESSANDRO NAPOLI, MD, PhD
Aggregate Professor of Radiology, Department of Radiological Sciences, Sapienza
University of Rome, Rome, Italy

TOM RUSH, MD
The Center for Pancreatic, Biliary and Advanced Minimally Invasive Surgery of New York,
New York, New York, USA

RICHARD D. SCHULICK, MD, MBA, FACS
The Aragón/Gonzalez-Gíustí Chair, Department of Surgery, University of Colorado,
Aurora, Colorado, USA

JEROME SIEGAL, MD
The Center for Pancreatic, Biliary and Advanced Minimally Invasive Surgery of New York,
New York, New York, USA

HARRY SNADY, MD
The Center for Pancreatic, Biliary and Advanced Minimally Invasive Surgery of New York,
New York, New York, USA

JOHN A. STAUFFER, MD, FACS
Department of Surgery, Mayo Clinic, Jacksonville, Florida, USA

JUSTIN G. STEELE, MD
The Pancreas, Biliary and Advanced Laparoscopy Center of New York, New York,
New York, USA

ROBERT J. TORPHY, MD
General Surgery Resident, Department of Surgery, University of Colorado, Aurora,
Colorado, USA

TIMOTHY J. VREELAND, MD
Fellow, Complex General Surgical Oncology, The University of Texas MD Anderson
Cancer Center, Houston, Texas, USA

MICHAEL G. WAYNE, DO
The Pancreas, Biliary and Advanced Laparoscopy Center of New York, New York,
New York, USA

ROBERT A. WOLFF, MD
Professor of Medicine, Department of Gastrointestinal Medical Oncology, The University
of Texas MD Anderson Cancer Center, Houston, Texas, USA

Contents

> Preventing cancer has much to offer. Aside from plummeting health care
> costs, we might enjoy a healthier life free of cancer and chronic disease.
> Prevention requires the adoption of healthier choices and a moderate
> amount of exercise. The supporting evidence is observational, clinical,
> and partly common sense. Further investigations reveal several sub-
> stances in a whole-food plant-based diet that have protective effects
> and an inhibitory effect on tumor development. For pancreatic cancer,
> the basis of cure remains a century-old operation that rarely cures. With
> little to lose, prevention deserves center stage and additional studies.

> As modern abdominal imaging equipment advances, pancreatic lesion
> detection improves. Most of these lesions are incidental and present a
> conundrum to the clinician and create great anxiety to the patient until a
> final diagnosis is made. For the practicing physician, the plethora of diag-
> nostic options is overwhelming. The relevant question is, what is the most
> efficient algorithm to follow and to arrive at a timely and accurate diag-
> nosis. This article presents a logical approach to the initial evaluation of
> a pancreatic lesion to get the most information possible with the least
> amount of testing and to avoid duplicative measures.

> Family history is a significant risk factor for developing pancreatic cancer,
> and this hereditary risk can be secondary to familial cancer predisposition
> syndromes, hereditary pancreatitis, or familial pancreatic cancer. Certain
> high-risk individuals are recommended to undergo screening for pancre-
> atic cancer with endoscopic ultrasound imaging or MRI/magnetic reso-
> nance retrograde cholangiopancreatography because of the potential to
> identify and curatively resect precursor lesions. The management of sus-
> picious lesions identified on screening high-risk individuals is also
> discussed.

> Complications after pancreaticoduodenal resection (PDR) occur in at least 30% of patients. Most are a direct result of an intraoperative event, dissection, or anastomoses, which account for the most serious morbidities, sepsis, pseudoaneurysms, and hemorrhage. Rarely, complications are due to the systemic impact of the procedure even if the procedure itself was unremarkable. Rare systemic complications after PDR (transfusion-transmitted babesiosis, pituitary apoplexy, and TRALI) and a number of uncommon and unusual other complications are discussed. Pancreaticoduodenal resection is a significant operation with serious consequences. Decisions on selection of candidates and safe operations should be thoughtful and always in surgeons' minds.

> Since the advent of modern surgery for pancreatic cancer, clinicians have recognized this cancer's propensity to recur locally, metastasize, and cause death. Despite significant efforts to improve patient outcomes with better adjuvant therapy, only modest gains in survival have been observed. An alternative strategy of neoadjuvant therapy followed by surgery has the potential to improve patient selection and survival and expand the pool of patients eligible for curative surgery. This article summarizes large, randomized trials of adjuvant therapy, explains the limitations imposed by up-front surgery, and suggests neoadjuvant therapy as a rational alternative to initial surgery and adjuvant therapy.

> Pancreatic cancer is an aggressive malignancy with a poor long-term survival and only mild improvement in outcomes over the past 30 years. Local failure remains a problem, and radiation can help improve control. The role of radiation therapy has been controversial and is still evolving. This article reviews the trials of pancreatic cancer and radiation in adjuvant, neoadjuvant, and unresectable lesions. It also reviews the impact and outcomes of evolving radiation technology.

> Pancreatic cancer is a poor prognostic tumor and about 20% of patients are eligible for surgical resection at the time of diagnosis. Recently, minimally invasive procedures have provided promising results as a therapeutic option for locally advanced unresectable pancreatic cancer. In particular, high-intensity focused ultrasound is an emerging noninvasive thermally ablative procedure that may have a dominant role in the future. Although

the clinical applications of minimally invasive therapies to pancreatic cancers are still in their infancy, the results at present are promising.

Incidental cystic intrapancreatic lesions are daily findings in abdominal radiology. The discovery of incidental pancreatic lesions is increasingly common with technologic diagnostic advancements. This article provides a perspective and guideline on the clinical management of incidental intraductal papillary mucinous neoplasms and cystic or premalignant lesions of the pancreas.

Asymptomatic nonfunctioning pancreatic neuroendocrine tumors are indolent, slow-growing tumors, and surveillance is safe and reasonable. Despite consensus, size may be less important than grade and Ki-67 when making decisions regarding optimal therapy. Plans to proceed with surveillance or surgical resection require a multidisciplinary approach and a shared decision-making process with colleagues, patients, and families. Decisions should be based on tumor characteristics, patient morbidities, preferences, and risks. As molecular diagnostics evolve, preoperative acquisition of tissue samples may become even more critical in choosing between operative management and surveillance.

There are a few entities that account for most solid and cystic masses of the pancreas. The pancreas harbors a wide array of diseases, including adenocarcinoma and its variants, such as anaplastic and adenosquamous carcinoma. Other neoplasms include acinar cell carcinoma, solid pseudopapillary tumor, and sarcomas. Benign lesions include hamartomas, hemangiomas, lymphangioma, and plasmacytoma. Isolated metastases include renal cell carcinoma, melanoma, and other carcinomas. Benign inflammatory conditions, such as autoimmune pancreatitis and groove pancreatitis can also mimic solid neoplasms of the pancreas.

There are several low-grade pancreatic tumors whose biology permits the use of aggressive surgery to achieve a curative resection. Tumors that are deemed unresectable by conventional techniques owing to mesenteric vessel involvement may benefit from ex vivo tumor resection and autotransplantation to allow complete resection while minimizing ischemic organ injury. Despite the excellent oncologic outcomes when used for these neoplasms, the procedure carries substantial morbidity and a high complication rate. But for patients who were otherwise offered total enterectomy and allotransplantation or told that their tumor was unresectable, ex vivo resection may offer a hope for cure.

SURGICAL CLINICS
OF NORTH AMERICA

ISSUE OF RELATED INTEREST:

Surgical Oncology Clinics, April 2016 (Vol. 25, Issue 2)
Pancreatic Neoplasms
Nipun B. Merchant, *Editor*
Available at: www.surgonc.theclinics.com

THE CLINICS ARE AVAILABLE ONLINE!
Access your subscription at:
www.theclinics.com

Foreword

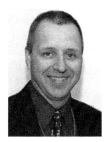

Ronald F. Martin, MD, FACS
Consulting Editor

Surgery is not synonymous with operation. Surgery is a discipline, a way of life, a state of mind, and occasionally a passion. I realize I have written this before, and probably will again, but it bears repeating because it reminds us that we as surgeons must always reflect on what we do and what we think we believe; otherwise, we lose our way.

If one studies any topic, one goes from unawareness to understanding to a feeling of proficiency, followed by a sense of mastery. That last phase is generally fairly comforting after years of living on the edge of wishing you knew just a little more; however, if one studies further and reflects even more, this sense of mastery is usually followed by the realization that there are far more errors in our thinking than we had previously wished to acknowledge. For some of us, this last step is embraced, and for some, it is eschewed. It is hard to surrender a sense of mastery.

This process is hardly unique to surgeons. The Dreyfus model describing the process of skill acquisition from novice to expert has been referred to for many years since its description in 1980 and has been modified to align with whatever goals the group using it finds useful in training its own people. In the model, experts are supposed to "'transcend reliance on rules, guidelines, and maxims,' (have) 'intuitive grasp of situations based on deep, tacit understanding,' (have) 'vision of what is possible,' (and use) 'analytical approaches' in new situations or in case of problems."[1]

Our current medical climate is, in fact, antithetical to the concept of "expertise." The idea that one could transcend rules or guidelines is an anathema to regulatory bodies and payors alike. The idea that one could "vision what is possible" is only as good as one's ability to convince the stakeholders who have a vested interest in the status quo to reconsider their position.

It is easy to understand why a medical climate such as we live in has developed. Some of the reasons are good. Not everybody who thinks he or she is an expert actually is one—probably the best reason of them all. We all have to live in a collective society so we need some rules to follow, or else there would be chaos—also a pretty good reason. In order to perform "analytical approaches," we need broader collaboration to increase our likelihood of reaching valid conclusions.

Surg Clin N Am 98 (2018) xiii–xv
https://doi.org/10.1016/j.suc.2017.10.001
0039-6109/18/© 2017 Published by Elsevier Inc.

surgical.theclinics.com

There are some less good reasons as well. The status quo always benefits somone; ergo, changing it will alter that benefit. One would like to believe that we would always try to alter the benefit in favor of the patient, or at least the community. I am not sure that always happens. We do live in a time when we are still largely compensated for doing things "to people" rather than doing things "for people." I would like to believe that we align those concepts as closely as possible, but I have been around too long to believe that is always the case.

Sometimes the emperor has no clothes. Those who worked hard to develop skills, understanding, and influence frequently become our leaders. On occasion, it is hard to let go of a concept that seemed right for such a long time—especially if one built his career on it.

How we analyze data is the era of high-speed computing has also shifted our thinking. We seem to have evolved into a place where we believe that "big data" will answer all questions. The rise in publications and presentations at regional and national meetings where "registry data" is mined and conclusions drawn seems to be rampant. Ironically, some of the presenters appear to have never been personally involved with any of the cases of which they speak. That in and of itself isn't as concerning as the concomitant rise of the following ubiquitous response to almost any question posed to the presenter, "Thank you for your excellent question. We/I cannot answer because we do not have that level of granularity since this is registry data" (roughly paraphrased from hundreds of respondents). Please do not misunderstand me, there is an absolute role for big data, especially for those things that can be measured and compared (large-population DNA sequences, large-population trends, comparing operations with narrow sets of well-defined initial conditions, eg, coronary artery bypass grafting, and so forth), but the ability to use large data sets that will inherently have large missing data values or immeasurable data values that are critical to interpreting the results (eg, the presence of occult metastatic disease, the desires of a patient, what kind of help does someone have at home) is not as useful—at least not now.

Perhaps the most concerning reason we find ourselves in a challenging medical climate is that we have a large-scale health care system that is so metastable politically, culturally, and economically that it seems too overwhelming to adopt change or perhaps too futile. Why invest significant energy changing a system that someone "in authority" will capriciously ask you to change all over again very soon? It seems a Sisyphean task.

I am not an expert on Greek mythology nor am I am expert on French absurdist writing, but Sisyphus seems like the right metaphor for us surgeons. In part because, as in the Greek myth, when we finish a task our reward and punishment is that we get to do it again. In Camus' "The Myth of Sisyphus" (please forgive my using the English translation), the story posits that Sisyphus' tragic moment is when he realizes the futility of his work. However, by acknowledging its futility (with scorn, no less), he realizes his purpose. Camus further states that because Sisyphus realizes that his purpose is to be futile we must imagine him to be happy. I am not sure I am completely convinced by the argument but it is interesting. Perhaps the most intriguing part of the story is that one observes that Sisyphus does his "realizing" on the walk down the hill. That is the time, before the boulder comes back to hit him, that he gets to reflect.

Many months ago, Dr Cooperman and I began discussions on this issue of *Surgical Clinics of North America*. We decided that we deliberately wanted to dig deeply into controversy and challenge the status quo on matters for the pancreas and pancreatic cancer to see what ideas could hold up. He and his colleagues have done an exceptional job of compiling some extremely thought-provoking articles. We are deeply indebted to them for not just their thoughtfulness but also taking on a project that is likely to force us all to look deeply at some of our foundational beliefs.

Dr Cooperman's issue should give us a chance to walk down the hill. It is a time for us to stop pushing the boulder upwards for a bit and give serious thought to what are we doing and why. It is time to think about what is real and where or how we are deluding ourselves. It is time to think of whose priorities we are really putting first and why. I wholeheartedly suggest you saunter down the hill with this information and think deeply about these things. Try to separate what is real from what is absurd. Don't worry about losing yourself in it; the boulder of work will hit you soon enough. When it does, we will go back to functioning in our confined work world, though perhaps we will be able to think about how to make the hill a better hill for the next time we need to push the boulder up.

Ronald F. Martin, MD, FACS
Colonel (ret.), United States Army Reserve
Department of Surgery
York Hospital
16 Hospital Drive, Suite A
York, ME 03909, USA

E-mail address:
rmartin@yorkhospital.com

REFERENCE

1. Dreyfus SE, Dreyfus HL. A five-stage model of the mental activities involved in directed skill acquisition. Operations Research Center. Berkeley (CA): University of California, Berkeley; 1980.

Preface

A Symposium on Pancreatic Cancer: Time for a Paradigm Shift. An Overview and Personal Reflections

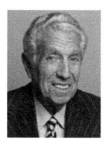

Avram M. Cooperman, MD, FACS
Editor

We can easily forgive a child who is afraid of the dark; the real tragedy of life is when men (adults) are afraid of the light.

—*Plato*

Insanity—doing the same thing over and over again and expecting a different outcome

—*Einstein*

This issue of the *Surgical Clinics of North America* is devoted to the Pancreas and Pancreatic Cancer. I previously edited a similar issue for the *Surgical Clinics of North America* in June 2002. Despite the diagnostic and therapeutic advances in medicine over the past 30 years, including significant advances in oncology, the cure rate for pancreatic cancer is dismal and unchanged for 50 years. Yet many believe the only chance for cure remains surgical resection, which has proven to be unwarranted optimism. The concept that pancreatic cancer is a systemic disease that has metastasized before the cancer is diagnosed is difficult for many surgeons to accept. This is analogous to the treatment of breast cancer before its systemic nature was accepted, a process that took many years and was hardly, but not heartily, embraced. In the 1970s, there was evidence that minimal breast procedures (ie, lumpectomy), had similar outcomes as radical procedures because both represented local control of a disease that too often was systemic at presentation. I had completed a surgical residency at the Mayo Clinic in 1970 when this concept was introduced and overlooked

Surg Clin N Am 98 (2018) xvii–xx
https://doi.org/10.1016/j.suc.2017.10.002
0039-6109/18/© 2017 Published by Elsevier Inc.

surgical.theclinics.com

by most surgeons. The rationale presented to most patients was "the best chance for breast cancer cure was with a traditional procedure" (modified radical or radical mastectomy).

After completing my military Service, I joined the Surgical Staff of the Cleveland Clinic, the home of minimal and conservative breast cancer procedures. I was never pressured to adapt this approach, but the evidence, outcomes, and patient wishes facilitated my operative choices. My senior associates, Crile, Hermann, Hoerr, and Esselstyn, were inspirational and masterful mentors. The lessons of breast cancer had come after radical surgery for thyroid cancer had been shown to be disfiguring and unnecessary and offered no better survival than a conservative approach. Somewhat sadly in both instances, the next generation of surgeons found ways to circumvent these data and has reintroduced bilateral mastectomy and total thyroidectomy using cosmesis, safe surgery, and multicentricity of microscopic tumors as substitutes for wisdom, natural history of latent tumors, experience, the published literature, and common sense.

It is no surprise that many pancreatic surgeons continue the fruitless mantra that surgery is the "first and best" approach to pancreatic cancer.

Pancreatic cancer is a lethal disease the mortality of which nearly equals its incidence. For nearly a century and continuing today, the misplaced emphasis on "first, best, and only chance of cure" has clouded the evidence that pancreatic cancer is a systemic disease, and surgery, a form of local control, could be curative. Since symptomatic patients have late-stage disease, open-minded and newer approaches are needed, and tradition and repetitive treatment patterns need be set aside. Treating a systemic disease with local therapy is in kindest terms "too little, too late," and in blunt terms absurd. The case for extending the magnitude of surgery by total pancreatectomy, vein resection, and radical node resection does not influence cure rate or survival. While these techniques are done with lower risk on patients with less advanced disease, they do not improve survival. Why do we continue this misplaced emphasis, and false optimism and security to patients, mostly elderly, who if provided the facts and likely outcome might quickly focus on the true issues: life, survival, cure, and options and alternatives to "standard of care"? This is discussed in an article on prevention or early detection. The availability of so many diagnostic tests to evaluate pancreatic disease and pancreatic masses is examined, and recommendations are made by multispecialists: gastroenterology, radiology, and surgery. Too often multiple endoscopic and imaging procedures add expense and not enlightenment. Surgeons contemplating invasive procedures may prioritize and utilize the available tests differently, plus they have an advantage of direct visualization by laparoscopy or surgery. The value and efficacy for screening pancreatic cancer in at-risk patients are critically examined, including arbitrary times between screenings.

Incidental pancreatic cystic lesions and neuroendocrine tumors in asymptomatic patients are detected with increasing frequency, often in elderly patients. Concerns for malignancy and inaccuracies in preoperative diagnosis make decision making an uncertainty. Several series have been reported, and management ranges from selective to aggressive. The rationale for each is addressed. Preoperative biliary stenting and postoperative drainage after pancreatic surgery once considered essential are being used always, selectively, and never. The rationale and results are reviewed by advocates and agnostics.

The important issue of neoadjuvant therapy and timing of surgery for pancreatic cancer is reviewed by the most experienced group, who has adapted its use. The issue of actual long-term survival is reported, addressed, and reviewed in surgical and population studies. Despite attempts to present survival in the most favorable light and bias, long-term survivors are few and even fewer in population studies. Radiation therapy is more popular in the United States than in Europe, and its many forms and timing are clarified as well as the evidence for its use in primary, adjuvant, neoadjuvant, and metastatic disease. Clarification is most welcome. The efficacy and outcomes with systemic adjuvant and neoadjuvant therapy are controversial as well. Where we are with these modalities is reviewed. Nonoperative ablation of pancreatic lesions using sound waves is finding adaption for other solid lesions, and its early use in pancreatic lesions is reviewed. Finally, applications of transplantation and vascular and pancreatic surgery for unusual lesions that invade the celiac and superior mesenteric vessels are described and unusual pancreatic lesions and their pathology reviewed.

Why procedures learned years ago in residency or fellowship continue long after outcomes indicate they need modification or elimination is unclear. In medicine and surgery, tradition is strong and common sense too often not common practice. Ineffective therapies persist because nothing better has displaced them. Frequently, the reluctance to try newer approaches requires an open-minded and objective assessment of actual data. For pancreatic cancer, that is certainly true. The suggestion that this disease may require a paradigm shift in therapy warrants closer scrutiny. Continuing ineffective therapies because nothing better or proven is available is far from a ringing endorsement of present treatments.

This issue is less how I do it and more why and what are the data, what are the actual outcomes, what are present options, and what realistically lies ahead?

The contributors are uniquely qualified, thoughtful, and experienced clinicians who address specific issues. Fresh and different viewpoints are long overdue.

To John G. Vassallo, editor, and Ronald Martin, MD, consulting editor to the *Surgical Clinics of North America*, a heartfelt thanks for their input, encouragement, and assistance in preparation of this issue, and to the development editors Meredith Madeira and Colleen Dietzler, thank you. Vignesh Viswanathan checked all references, the structure, and my editing. Thank you for your detail and accuracy.

My colleagues, Michael Wayne, Justin Steele, and Mazen Iskander, are a bright and talented group, whom I respect and admire, and who joined in ably to help this issue come together. Our staff, Jeanine Desjardins and Ruby Lau, kept tabs on the authors, deadlines, and reference articles and deserve many, many thanks.

To Howard University College of Medicine, my classmates of 1965, and its fabulous faculty, who provided an unforgettable opportunity for me and then my son, David, we are forever humbled and grateful and two of its proudest alumni!!

The Mayo Clinic provided a unique and extraordinary experience by allowing me to train and do a fellowship year at Rochester, Minnesota. My fellow residents and the surgical, medical, and administrative faculty were modest, thoughtful, highly skilled, and open-minded professionals. I was privileged by the opportunity, friendships, and education. The dignity and compassion that were extended to every patient was the consummate of professionalism. Donald McIlrath, MD took me under his wing and taught me much about surgery and life, and I have never forgotten his influence.

The Cleveland Clinic and its staff welcomed me warmly when I joined the surgical department. Unique individuals with varied interests, they were led by George Crile Jr. "Barney" as he was called had retired from surgery but was a visionary and an influence on world surgery. He enlightened many and was a clear, logical thinker, charismatic, and a great influence on me and many others. Bob Hermann, Stan Hoerr, and Caldwell "Essy" Esselstyn were great influences, friends, more experienced colleagues, and mentors. They each had a unique viewpoint on so many issues, and my good fortune was to be a colleague to each. I continue the close friendship and counsel with Essy—an ongoing benefit of the Cleveland Clinic.

I am a person of faith who was blessed by the things that really matter. How else to explain my odyssey from Brooklyn and Laurelton, New York? My late parents, Philip and Lillian, and their families were extraordinary and ideal for me and my brother, Gerald, and sister, Amy. They loved and taught us much. Their shoulders, upon which we sat and stood, provided us a deeper view and understanding of ethics, values, respect, kindness, and love of family, learning, friends, and work. My children, Jeff, David, and Beth (and Nick), continue this and are passing it on to their progeny, Lilly, Leo and Holden, Oliver, Griffin, and Laurel.

During the preparation of this issue, my brother and closest friend, Gerald, died suddenly. I dedicate this to him, the many patients I have been privileged to treat and care for, and the patients and families afflicted with Pancreatic Cancer, who suffer greatly, and the fortunate and lucky few who survive.

Avram M. Cooperman, MD, FACS
The Pancreas, Biliary and Advanced Laparoscopy Center of New York
305 Second Avenue
New York, NY 10003, USA

E-mail address:
Avram.cooperman@gmail.com

Prevention and Early Detection of Pancreatic Cancer

Avram M. Cooperman, MD[a],*, Mazen E. Iskandar, MD[b],
Michael G. Wayne, DO[a], Justin G. Steele, MD[a]

KEYWORDS

- Cancer of the pancreas (CaP) • Whole-food plant-based diet (WFPBD)
- Western illness • Latent/indolent disease

KEY POINTS

- Screening for early detection of high-risk patients is based on axial imaging, which detects premalignant lesions much more often than malignant ones.
- Interval cancers that become apparent between screens are aggressive, poor prognostic lesions.
- Prevention of cancer of the pancreas (CaP) involves mimicking food and lifestyle choices of populations where these diseases are uncommon.
- Whole-food plant-based diets (WFPBDs) with abundant fruits, supplemented with exercise and natural active movements significantly lower the risk of cancer and CaP.

An ounce of prevention is worth a pound of cure.

Benjamin Franklin[1]

Let food be thy medicine and medicine thy food. Walking is man's best medicine.

Hippocrates[2,3]

INTRODUCTION

Franklin's[1] wise adage emphasized preventing rather than extinguishing fires, whereas medicine emphasizes extinguishing rather than preventing illness. When Hippocrates of Kos (460–370 BC) 2084 years ago stated food and lifestyle were the mainstay of health, the diseases of today were inconceivable. Imagine his thoughts about big pharma and the food industry. Because the lifestyle that prevents chronic disease, heart disease, and cancer is similar, what is applicable to prevent cancer of the

---

Disclosure Statement: The authors have nothing to disclose.
[a] The Pancreas, Biliary and Advanced Laparoscopy Center of New York, 305 Second Avenue, New York, NY 10003, USA; [b] Department of Surgery, Mount Sinai Beth Israel, Icahn School of Medicine, Mount Sinai West, New York, NY, USA
* Corresponding author.
E-mail address: avram.cooperman@gmail.com

Surg Clin N Am 98 (2018) 1–12
https://doi.org/10.1016/j.suc.2017.09.001
0039-6109/18/© 2017 Elsevier Inc. All rights reserved.

pancreas (CaP) is equally effective for chronic and other malignant diseases.[4] Besides, the side effects of a healthy lifestyle are more pleasant than those of drugs/chemotherapy and much less expensive.

DEFINITION

A healthy lifestyle is one which optimizes and maintains health.[5] This lifestyle includes a whole-food plant-based diet (WFPBD) consisting of fruits, grains, legumes, and vegetables augmented by exercise and active lives and avoiding processed foods, salt, sugar, and animal protein.[6]

PREVENTION: WHY NOT?

Prevention of cancer, particularly CaP, draws scant attention for several reasons: (1) CaP takes 10 to 20 years to develop during which time it has undergone several mutations, developed its own blood supply (angiogenesis), avoided sufficient cell death (apoptosis), and possibly metastasized.[7–10] CaPs do not form de novo but progress from benign precursor lesions to invasive and metastatic lesions.[10] (2) The chances of an individual developing a CaP are small; but once established, it is likely fatal. (3) Unhealthy lifestyles are pervasive; many act as if they are immune from chronic disease and cancer. (4) CaP and many cancers present when symptomatic, a time prevention has long past and when the emphasis is on the too-little-too-late treatments. (5) Perhaps the most compelling reason to emphasize prevention is that treatment is directed at symptoms and not cause. By neglecting the cause, latent cancer can progress and new lesions develop. (6) Prevention is "pretreatment directed at causation whose goals are to maximize health, keep indolent disease dormant, and prevention of new cancers."[11,12] Prevention requires active participation, whereas early detection is physician directed and allows for passive patients. Too often, early detection is neither early nor curative.

PROOF OF CONCEPT

The association between diet and cancer is suggested by the wide international incidence of cancer and the study of migrants. Asians living in Asia have a 25 times lower incidence of prostate cancer and a 10 times lower incidence of breast cancer than migrant Asians[13–16] Monozygotic twins who share all genes do not share 85% to 90% of cancers that develop in one twin.[16] Less than 10% of cancers are genetic or familial.[17–19] Genes upregulate and mutate many times before cancer is initiated.[19] A sedentary lifestyle, smoking, animal protein, processed food, sugar, and obesity contribute to many chronic diseases and cancers, including CaP.[20–22] In 1907 a front page article in *The New York Times* noted an increased incidence of cancer in Chicago immigrants who were omnivores but not in immigrant vegetarians.[23] The relationship between diet and cancer is better understood today.[12,24–28]

Western illness including cancer has been rare in native Africans.[29–32] There was only 1 small healed myocardial infarct and 3 healed peptic ulcers. Cholecystitis, appendicitis, diverticulitis, cancer, and other Western illnesses were not evident. This finding affirmed the importance of diet, fiber, and lifestyle.

Burkitt,[30] an English surgeon in sub-Saharan South Africa, noted the native population was free of Western illnesses, that is, obesity, hypertension, appendicitis, cholecystitis, cancer, cardiac or vascular disease, and hiatal hernia, including CaP. High dietary fiber and low animal protein were thought to be important factors. This finding was not so for those who provided supportive services. They developed the common surgical and medical diseases.[30-32]

Nathan Pritikin[33], an inventor and engineer who had a myocardial infarct as a young man, researched the subject and noted two-thirds of the world's population had no coronary disease. He lived and advocated a healthy lifestyle, including a WFPBD.[33] Postmortem studies of his heart revealed soft pliable coronary arteries suggesting disease reversal.[34] This finding antedated the clinical studies of Ornish[35] and Esselstyn,[36] who independently demonstrated coronary artery disease reversal and relief of cardiovascular symptoms (angina, claudication, impotence, hypertension) in patients who adopt a WFPBD.

A 4- to 5-hour period of vasoconstriction and decrease in brachial artery flow occurs after eating fast, fried fatty foods. The resulting endothelial cell injury caused a 40% to 50% flow decrease in both healthy volunteers and cardiac patients suggesting diet can injure or maintain healthy endothelial cells.[37,38]

PREVENTING CANCER AND PANCREATIC CANCER

The studies on lifestyle and cancer are no less convincing. Several risk factors have been associated with CaP. A landmark study by Doll and Peto[13] in 1981 reviewed environmental and nutritional risks for cancer in the United States. They estimated that lung cancer deaths were tobacco related in 91% of 71,000 deaths in men and in 77% of 24,000 deaths in women. Forty-three percent and 15% of all cancer deaths in men and women were tobacco related.[13] Blot and Tarone[39] in 2015 noted that 23% of men and 19% of women smoked, and it was causal in 80%+ of lung cancers. The current estimates are that 30%+ of CaPs are tobacco related; when smoking is stopped, the cancer incidence decreases.[39] Early estimates were guesstimates, because the epidemiologic methodology was evolving. The original suggestion was 35% of cancers were diet related (range 10%–90%). Site associations were 90% for the stomach and colon; 50% for the endometrium, gallbladder, pancreas, and breast; and 20% for the lung, upper digestive tract, and cervix. Willett[11] confirmed the diet-cancer causal relationship and thought studies had underestimated the cancer risk twofold. The physiologic benefits of physical exercise are through the release of myokines, which kill cancer cells.[40] The microbiome is vital in determining health or disease through the breakdown of ingested food and release of injurious or beneficial substances. This process is directed by the myriad of gut flora.[41] The release of insulin growth factor−1 stimulated by a suboptimal diet promotes cancer growth.[42] All of the preceding favor fruits, vegetables, legumes, and grains as healthier choices and protective against pancreatic and other cancers and chronic illness.

Three large studies confirmed that red meat (animal protein) increased the risk of dying of cancer and heart disease and shortened life span.[27,43,44] The studies controlled for risk factors: alcohol, exercise, smoking, family history, caloric intake, and a WFPBD. Deaths due to meat were accelerated by heterocyclic amines, aromatic hydrocarbons, and perhaps heme iron, found in meat but not vegetables. A meta-analysis of diet and cancer prevention by Belliveau and Gingras[12] from 1980 to 2006 showed 75% of abdominal cancers could be prevented or favorably influenced by a WFPBD.

A World Cancer Research Fund Report from 1997 noted that 144 human studies have shown a statistically significant benefit of fruits and vegetables on cancer, whereas no study has confirmed any protective benefit of animal-based foods.[45] Campbell and Jacobsen[46] think a full complement of WFPB nutrients acting in synergy promotes the protective effects.

Other factors that increase the risk of CaP are obesity, excessive alcohol consumption, and ingestion of animal protein (meat, fish, fowl, or eggs).[11,29,43,44] Great concern exists about the carcinogenic potential of poultry viruses by direct contact or consumption.[47] Thirty thousand poultry workers were studied; those who slaughtered chickens had a 9 times greater risk of developing CaP and liver cancer, a risk far greater than smoking for 50 years. The risk of eating chicken and developing CaP was 72% greater when daily consumption was 50 g (<2 oz or one-quarter of a chicken breast) or more.[48]

CLINICAL STUDIES
Prostate Cancer Studies

Ornish and colleagues[49] studied 93 volunteers with early prostate cancer who were randomized to a control or healthy lifestyle group (plant-based diet, 30 minutes of walking 6 times per week, and meditation). At 1 year, the control group had a mean prostate-specific antigen (PSA) increase of 6% (several required the treatment of progressive disease), whereas in the treated group's PSA decreased 4%. A year after the study ended, 10% of the control patients required radical prostatectomy but none in the healthier group.[49]

Another prostate study showed that decreasing animal protein and increasing vegetables slowed the increase of PSA and the rate of cancer growth. Even though subjects with a healthy lifestyle ate animal protein, the 1:1 animal to vegetable ratio slowed the doubling of PSA from 21 to 58 months.[50]

Curcumin Studies

Turmeric or curcumin prevents DNA mutations and impedes tumor growth and spread. Urine from patients with lung cancer (smokers) and nonsmokers was plated on bacteria in petri dishes. There were fewer DNA mutations in the bacteria of nonsmokers. After smokers were given turmeric (8 g/d), the DNA mutation rate dropped 38%.[51] Additional in vitro studies have shown curcumin kills cancer cells and prevents the disabling of death cell receptors on cancer cells.[52]

At the MD Anderson Cancer Center, curcumin in large oral doses (8 g/d) was given to 21 patients with advanced CaP. There were 2 responders: in one a 73% tumor reduction later recurred, whereas the second had progressive improvement over 18 months. When curcumin was stopped, tumor markers increased but decreased after resumption. The 10% response rate is similar to chemotherapy outcomes.[53]

EARLY DETECTION? AND SCREENING FOR CANCER/PANCREATIC CANCER

Indolent asymptomatic microtumors and circulating cancer cells are not uncommon in healthy individuals.[54] Autopsies show 40% to 50% of men and 30% to 50% of women aged 40 to 50 years have foci of CaP or early breast cancer and 98% have microthyroid cancers.[12,54] How these cells remain latent and viable for long time periods and do not metastasize is important. Host immunity, and natural killer cells, which are influenced by inhibitory and activating receptors, and altered gene signaling pathways influence latent cell metastases and growth.[12,55] Shed cancer cell metabolites may be detected in the serum of 40% of healthy people.[55] These lesions and cells should not warrant screens or treatment. They are cancer in name but are held in check by a healthy immune system.

Early detection of cancer is a popular concept; patients and families think that treating such lesions, absent symptoms, equals a cure. Early detection places the onus on the physician and screening process. Because the behavior of individual tumors is unique, outcomes are often unpredictable. Early detection implies curability, and curability implies effective treatment. The optimism holds for many prostate, breast, and colon cancers. For nearly all CaPs and many brain and lung tumors, incurability is the rule no matter when discovered. Favorable tumor biology must be present for any lesion to be curable.[54]

Cancers are sporadic (90%–95%) or familial (5%–10%).[18,19,56] Familial cancers are genetically linked, but the pathway is undefined in most. The number of affected first-degree family members predicts the relative risk for other family members. For example, the relative risk of developing CaP is increased by a factor of 2, 6, and 30 with 1, 2, or 3 affected family members.[56]

Our better understanding of CaP has not yet improved the cure. The two precursor lesions for CaP are intraductal papillary mucinous neoplasia (IPMN) and pancreatic intraepithelial neoplasms (PanIN).[19,57]

Screening for sporadic CaP is impractical and expensive and has a low yield because CaP is uncommon, affecting 12 of 100,000.[58] Risk factors include tobacco, *Helicobacter pylori*, diabetes of recent onset (<4 years), chronic pancreatitis, obesity, and age (>55 years); but each minimally increases the screening yield.[59,60] Two-thirds of the causal factors are modifiable, adaptable, and would reduce the incidence of disease. Fruit and folate were favorable influences.

A meta-analyses of 36 studies of recent-onset diabetes (<5 years) showed a 50% greater risk of CaP than in diabetic patients of greater than 5 years. Approximately 11,000 of 1.9 million patients with newly discovered type 2 diabetes have CaP, but the risk increases by 0.58%.[61] Surgeons find the diabetes-CaP association not uncommon and the subject of several studies.[62–64]

Screening for familial CaP and its syndromes is the subject of ongoing studies and is reviewed in Robert J. Torphy and Richard D. Schulick's article, "Screening of Patients at Risk for Familial Pancreatic Cancer: What is Beneficial?" in this issue. Even when families genetically predisposed to CaP are followed, the detection of a precursor lesion is serendipitous.[56,65]

Several institutions follow high-risk individuals (HRIs) to asses screening. HRIs include a strong family history and several polyposis syndromes.[17–19,56,65] The number screened was from 38 to 216, and the positive yield was from 1.3% to 45.0%. The lesions seen on MRI are further evaluated by endoscopic ultrasound (EUS) and biopsy. IPMN, PanIN, and mucinous cystic neoplasms (MCNs) are premalignant. If the screen is further narrowed to men older than 65 years (the highest risk), the incidence increases to 16%. At present, most lesions excised are atypical and premalignant.[56,65,66] These are the target lesions, as the outcome of treated premalignant lesions is cure while for CaP the outcome are poor. The operative risk for premalignant lesions must be near zero to justify a prophylactic resection.

PATIENT (MIS)PERCEPTIONS ABOUT SCREENING

Patients raise few concerns about the value and pitfalls of screening.[67] Patients overestimate the benefits and underestimate overdiagnosis, false positives, and the implications.[68–70] Most screening information is derived from 3 malignancies (colorectal, prostate, and breast) whose incidence is higher and survival better than for CaP (**Table 1**).

Most patients anticipate a screen will be normal or show an asymptomatic and curable lesion. The concept that indolent tumors can be observed, whereas interval tumors (detected between screens) are aggressive and of poor prognosis is underemphasized.[67] Patients overestimate screening benefits by 70% to 95% and

Table 1		
Annual incidence and mortality of 4 common malignancies		
Lesion	No. Ann Dx	No. Deaths
Pancreas	43,000	40,000
Colorectal	136,119	56,813
Prostate	176,450	27,681
Breast	230,815	40,800

underestimate the downside by 70%.[68–70] The number of lives saved and incidents prevented per 5000 patients screened annually for 10 years are few; 2 to 15 breast cancers, 5 to 10 colon cancers, 75 to 85 cardiovascular events, and 50 hip fractures.[67,68] The benefits were overestimated by 90% for breast cancer screening, 82% for medicine to prevent hip fractures, 69% for cardiac medicine, and 94% for colon cancer screening. An overestimation of the benefit and an underestimation of the risk obfuscates choices particularly when surgery is involved.[69] Overestimating the benefits of lipid-lowering and antihypertensive medication has been noted as well.[71,72]

SCREENING WITH IMAGES

In the last 20 years, great refinements in imaging allow the detection of more asymptomatic pancreatic lesions.[56,66,67] The increase in imaging has uncovered many lesions, mostly pancreatic cystic lesions (PCLs). Pathologic classifications of cystic lesions are complex.[73] The common lesions include the benign serous cystadenoma, MCNs, IPMN, and its subtypes branch duct (BD), main duct (MD), or combined duct (CD). Malignant IPMNs are better behaved than most CaPs, and the cell type predicts the behavior. Of the subtypes (gastric, intestinal, oncocytic, and pancreatobiliary), pancreatobiliary is the most aggressive. PCLs are best defined by EUS, biopsy, and aspiration.[58] PCLs increase with the frequency of abdominal scans and sonograms. PCLs range from 2% to 27%; but in at-risk patients, it is 45% to 48%.[56,58,67] Canto and colleagues[56] compared the accuracy of PCL detection by EUS (45%), MRI (33%), and computed tomography (CT) (11%). MRI is more sensitive for small cysts (1 cm) and for main duct involvement. CT and MRI are useful after surgery and during chemotherapy to follow the disease. The choice (MRI, CT) depends on local practice and expertise.[74] The detection of incidental lesions does not imply a cure. Prognosis is determined by tumor biology. Newly detected lesions have likely been present for years. The diagnostic inaccuracies of PCL have been emphasized by Correa-Gallego and colleagues[75] who reviewed 136 of 330 excised asymptomatic PCLs. The preoperative diagnostic accuracy for BD lesions was 64%, and 29% had MD involvement. The diagnostic accuracy for MCN was 60%. The final pathology report included 6 invasive cancers (2 BD, 3 MD, and 1 MCN) and 19 cancer in situ (8 MD, 8 cystic endocrine lesions, and 3 unspecified lesions). Because the correct diagnosis is only made after excision, an accurate preoperative diagnosis is problematic and following lesions has a high degree of uncertainty.

SERUM MARKERS AND BIOLOGICAL MARKERS

Save for CaP, the mortality for other cancers has decreased. For CaP, there has been no change in mortality for 50 years.[4] Even if a specific and sensitive biological marker of 90% accuracy was available, 83 false-positive diagnoses would be raised for every correct diagnosis. As Kaur and colleagues[76] have said "The specific and sensitive markers for early diagnosis of pancreatic cancer remain a distant dream."

Serum markers are ideal, as they are easily obtained. The antigens in the blood stream are diluted by other proteins lessening their accuracy. CA19-9 is the only approved marker to follow CaP. It was found as a colon tumor antigen that reacted better with monoclonal antibody N19.9 in CaP and biliary cancer than colon cancer. Ca19-9 has several drawbacks, including a moderate sensitivity (69%–98%) and specificity (46%–98%), and is not expressed in 5% to 10% who are Lewis a/b negative.[77] Ca19-9 is elevated in benign and malignant conditions, including pancreatitis, cirrhosis, bile duct obstruction, and gastric, uterine, colorectal, and urologic cancers. Only two-thirds of patients with resectable PC have elevated Ca19-9. It is best used to follow patients after surgery or during chemotherapy to evaluate treatment.[78]

Other markers are being developed but are not commercially available or are of limited use. They include autoantibodies, cytokines, messenger RNA, circulating tumor cells, and mononuclear cells in blood and gene mutations.[78]

WHY CAUSATION IS IMPORTANT

Treating symptoms and lesions provides relief and may correct abnormal laboratory tests but does not correct the cause. Reversing coronary artery disease relieves symptoms and corrects the cause when done by a WFPBD as opposed to surgery or a coronary stent. If the cause is not corrected, the disease can recur or progress. For cancer, removing a target lesion does not change the soil that allowed a lesion to develop or recur. Treating breast or colon cancer by local therapy (surgery) does not prevent new or metastatic lesions. Surgically treating chronic pancreatitis by removing a segment of pancreas does not prevent cancer developing in the remaining gland. Observing an IPMN, a precursor lesion of CaP, does not limit the progression of the disease. La Femina and colleagues[79] followed 157 patients with IPMNs, 97 (62%) underwent surgery and 18 (11%) were cancer (4 were away from the IPMN). Of the 153 patients followed, 56 (20%) developed another IPMN and 3 had an invasive cancer.[80]

The two precursor lesions of CaP are ductal: PanIN and IPMN. PanINs progress from low to high grade to invasive cancer.[9,10] The low-grade lesions are present in normal pancreata, whereas high-grade lesions are found near CaP or in nontumor areas in familial syndromes.[56] Ninety percent plus of PanINs have a KRAS mutations. Tumor suppressor genes are also found in PanIN 2 and 3. KRAS is a marker of poor prognosis and is needed to sustain tumor growth.[19,78,80,81] Loss of KRAS results in tumor shrinkage. KRAS promotes the acquisition of cell nutrients, including glucose, lipids, and protein, directly and by autophagy, a way of recycling organelles and protein to sustain tumors. Inhibiting autophagy inhibits tumor growth. Other suppresser genes include SMAD4, p53, and CDKN2A.[19] A case report of KRAS recovered from pancreatic juice during endoscopic retrograde cholangiopancreatography suggest an occult malignancy.[82] Absent a visible lesion the patient was followed until a lesion was detected and treated. For CaP, this is less than ideal. Most genetic markers require tissue analyses, which for the pancreas is impractical.

EARLY DETECTION OF CANCER

An ideal test for early detection would include a sensitive, accurate serum marker to detect asymptomatic cancers that are clinically, and radiographically undetectable. Additionally, the marker should allow isolation of the organ involved and since the lesion is too small to detect be able to be treated with natural products to prevent growth and for the marker to become undetectable.[57]

Such a possibility exists with ecto nicotinamide adenine dinucleotide oxidase disulfide-thiol exchanger 2 (ENOX2), a surface protein shed by cancer cells that is then analyzed by electrophoresis to determine the site of origin. It is then treated with a capsule of decaffeinated green tea and capsicum. Of 110 healthy and apparently cancer-free volunteers, aged 40 to 84 years, 40% had ENOX2 cells detected. The cancers diagnosed were non–small cell lung (20%), breast (16%), colorectal (9%), and blood cell, ovarian, prostate, and cervix (each at 7%). Twelve patients were not retested, and in 5 retesting was done at 1 year. After 3 to 17 months of treatment, ENOX2 was not detected in 94% of patients. In 2 patients, a non–small cell lung cancer and lymphoma were diagnosed; but the patients declined treatment, and the diseases became manifest at 36 and 10 months. As opposed to detection by imaging when billions of tumor cells are present and lesions are larger, ENOX2 is detected when lesions are pinpoint (only 2 million cells).[57]

Whether this will be confirmed in further testing is unknown, but tests like this combine the earliest detection with natural plant nutrients to prevent tumor growth and detection. This practice combines prevention and true early detection.

SUMMARY

Preventing cancer has much to offer. Aside from plummeting health care costs, we might enjoy a healthier life free of cancer and chronic disease. Prevention requires the adoption of healthier choices and a moderate amount of exercise. The supporting evidence is observational, clinical, and partly common sense. Further investigations reveal several substances in WFPBD that have protective affects as well as an inhibitory effect on tumor development.[83–85] For CaP, the basis of cure remains a century old operation that rarely cures. Data notwithstanding, surgeons continue the effort to cure by resection and oncologists pursue a never-ending combination of drugs, while patients languish and suffer before the inevitable sad outcome. With little to lose, prevention deserves center stage and additional studies. Because the ever-increasing health care budget is not sustainable, emphasizing a healthy lifestyle and observing its impact on chronic disease and cancers would take years not decades to determine its efficacy.

REFERENCES

1. Franklin B. PennsyPatentia gazette Feb 4, 1735.
2. Hippocrates quotes Goodreads. Available at: http//wwwgoodreads.com/authors. 248774.
3. Hippocrates. Available at: https://brainyquote.com/quotes. 38008.
4. Cooperman AM. Cancer of the pancreas (CaP) new thoughts, new approaches for the new year pancreatic disorders and therapy. ISSN 2165-7092. January 11, 2017.
5. Healthy lifestyle. Available at: https://simple.wikipedia.org/wiki/healthy-lifestyle.
6. Cooperman AM. Longevity: some food for thought and ingestion. Healing Our World 2016;35(4):18–20.
7. Yachida S, Jones S, Bozic I, et al. Distant metastases occurs late during the genetic evolution of pancreatic cancer. Nature 2010;467:1114–7.
8. Hong SM, Park JY, Hruban R. Molecular signatures of pancreatic cancer. Arch Pathol Lab Med 2011;135(6):716–27.

9. Brat DJ, Lillemoe KD, Yeo CJ. Progression of atypical ductal hyperplasia/carcinoma in situ of the pancreas to invasive ductal carcinoma. Am J Surg Pathol 1998;22:163–9.
10. Hruban R, Wilent Z, Goggins M. Pathology of incipient cancer. Ann Oncol 1999; 10:s9–11.
11. Willett WC. Diet, nutrition, and avoidable cancer. Environ Health Perspect 1995; 103:165–70.
12. Belliveau R, Gingras D. Role of nutrition in preventing cancer. Can Fam Physician 2007;53:1905–11.
13. Doll R, Peto R. The causes of cancer: quantitative estimates of avoidable risks of cancer in the United States today. J Natl Cancer Inst 1981;66:1191–308.
14. Amer Institute for Cancer Research World Cancer Research Fund Food. Nutrition and the prevention of cancer; a global perspective. Washington, DC: Amer Inst Cancer Research; 1997.
15. Willett WC. Diet and cancer. Oncologist 2002;5:393–404.
16. Lichtenstein P, Holm NV, Verkasalo PK, et al. Environmental and heritable factors in the causation of cancer-analyses of twins from Sweden, Denmark and Finland. N Engl J Med 2000;343:78–85.
17. Klein AP, Brune KA, Petersen GM, et al. Prospective risk of pancreatic cancer in familial pancreatic cancer kindreds. Cancer Res 2004;64:2634–8.
18. Jacobs EJ, Chance SJ, Fuchs CS, et al. Family history of cancer and risk of pancreatic cancer; a pooled analyses from the pancreatic cancer cohort consortium (Pan Scan). Int J Cancer 2010;127:1421–8.
19. Ryan DP, Hong T, Bandessy N. Pancreatic adenocarcinoma. N Engl J Med 2014; 371(11):1039–49.
20. Thomson CA, LeWinn K, Newton TR. Nutrition and diet in the development of gastrointestinal cancer. Curr Oncol Rep 2003;5:192.
21. Belliveau R, Gingras D. Foods that fight cancer; preventing cancer through diet. Toronto: McClelland & Stewart Ltd; 2006.
22. Ames BN, Gold LS, Willett WC. The causes and prevention of cancer. Proc Natl Acad Sci U S A 1995;92:5258–365.
23. NY Times Cancer Increasing among meat eaters. Sept 24, 1907.
24. Bossetti C, Bravi F, Turati F, et al. Nutrient based dietary patterns and pancreatic cancer risk. Ann Epidemiol 2013;23(3):124–8.
25. Lowenfels AB, Maisonneuve P. Epidemiology and prevention of pancreatic cancer. Jpn J Clin Oncol 2004;34(5):238–44.
26. Rohrman S, linseisen J, Nothling U, et al. Meat and fish consumption and risk of pancreatic cancer, results from the European Prospective Investigation into cancer and nutrition. Int J Cancer 2013;132(3):617–24.
27. McHan J, Gong Z, Holly EA, et al. Dietary patterns and risk of pancreatic cancer in a large population based case control study in the San Francisco Bay Area. Nutr Cancer 2013;65:157–64.
28. Mills PK, Beeson WL, Abbey DE, et al. Dietary habits and past medical history as related to fatal pancreas cancer risk among adventists. Cancer 1988;61: 2578–85.
29. O'Keefe SJ, Kidd M, Espitalier-Noel G, et al. Rarity of colon cancer in Africans is associated with low animal product consumption, not fiber. Am J Gastroenterol 1999;94:173–8.
30. Burkitt D. Western diseases and their emergence related to diet. S Afr Med J 1982;61:103–15.

31. Burkitt D. Are our commonest diseases medically preventable. Prev Med 1978;6: 556–9.
32. Trowel HC, Burkitt D. The development of the concept of dietary fiber. Med Aspects Med 1987;9:7–15.
33. The McDougall Newsletter Nathan Pritikin –McDougalls most important mentor. Feb 2013.
34. Los Angeles Times autopsy of Nathan Pritikin. July 4, 1985.
35. Ornish D. Preventing and reversing heart disease the physicians committee. Available at: htpp//www.pcrm.org. about. Volunteer.
36. Esselstyn CE. A way to prevent coronary artery disease. J Fam Pract 2015; 224(63):257.
37. Lithander FE, Herlihy LK, Walsh DM. Postprandial effect of dietary fat quantity and quality on arterial stiffness and wave reflection: a randomized controlled trial. Nutr J 2013;12:93.
38. Vogel RA, Corretti MC, Plotnick GD. Effect of a single high fat meal on endothelial function in healthy subjects. Am J Cardiol 1997;79:350–4.
39. Blot WJ, Tarone RE. Doll and Peto's quantitative estimates of cancer risks: holding generally true for 35 years. J Natl Cancer Inst 2015;107(4) [pii:djv044].
40. Moore SC, Lee M, Weiderpass E. Association of leisure time physical activity with risk of 26 types of cancer in 1.44 million adults. JAMA Intern Med 2016;176(6): 816–25.
41. Colleen A. 10% Human, harper publishing. 2015.
42. Yu H, Rohan T. Role of insulin like growth factor family in cancer development and progression. J Natl Cancer Inst 2000;92(18):1472–89.
43. Sinha R, Cross AJ, Graubard I, et al. Meat intake and mortality: a prospective study of over half a million people. Arch Intern Med 2009;169(6):562–7.
44. Thiebaut AC, Jiao L, Silverman DT, et al. Dietary fatty acids and pancreatic cancer in the NIH-AARP diet and health study. J Natl Cancer Inst 2009;101(14): 1001–11.
45. World Cancer Research Fund/American Institute for Cancer Research. Food, nutrition, physical activity, and the prevention of cancer: a global perspective. Washington, DC: AICR; 2007.
46. Campbell TC, Jacobson H. Whole: rethinking the science of nutrition. Dallas (TX): Benbella Books Inc; 2013.
47. Johnson ES, Zhou Y, Lillian Yau C, et al. Mortality from malignant disease update of the Baltimore union poultry cohort. Cancer Causes Control 2010;21(2):215–21.
48. Felini M, Johnson E, Preace Y, et al. A Pilot case- cohort of liver and pancreatic cancers in poultry workers. Ann Epidemiol 2011;21(10):755–66.
49. Ornish D, Weldner G, Fair WR, et al. Intensive lifestyle changes may affect the progression of prostate cancer. J Urol 2005;174(3):1065–9.
50. Carmody JF, Olendzki BC, Merriam PA, et al. A novel measure of dietary change in a prostate cancer dietary program incorporating mindfulness training. J Acad Nutr Diet 2012;112(11):1822–7.
51. Polasa K, Raghuram TC, Krishna TP, et al. Effect of turmeric on urinary mutagens in smokers. Mutagenesis 1992;7:107–9.
52. Ravindran J, Prasad S, Aggarwal BB. Curcumin and cancer cells: how many ways can curry kill tumor cells selectively? AAPS J 2009;11(3):495–510.
53. Dhillon W, Aggarwal SS, Newman RA, et al. Phase I trial of curcumin in patients with advanced pancreatic cancer. Clin Cancer Res 2008;14:4491–8.

54. Black WC, Gilbert HG. Advances in diagnostic imaging and overestimations of disease prevalence and the benefits of therapy. N Engl J Med 1993;328(17): 1237–43.

55. Hanau C, Morre DJ, Morre DM. Cancer prevention trial of a synergistic mixture of green tea concentrate plus capsicum (Capsol-T) in a random population of subjects ages 40-84. Clin Proteomics 2014;11(1):2.

56. Canto MI, Hruban RH, Fishman EK, et al. Frequent detection of pancreatic lesions in symptomatic high risk individuals. Gastroenterology 2012;142:796–804.

57. Hruban R, Goggins M, Parsons J, et al. Progression model for pancreatic cancer. Clin Cancer Res 2000;6(8):1–7.

58. Cancer stat facts: pancreas cancer seer. Available at: Cancer.gov. Accessed November 9, 2017.

59. Gold EB. Epidemiology of and risk factors for pancreatic cancer. Surg Clin North Am 1995;75:819–43.

60. Maisonneuve P, Lowenfels A. Risk factors for pancreatic cancer: a summary review of meta-analytical studies. Int J Epidemiol 2015;44(1):186.

61. Huxley R, Ansary-Moghadden A, Berrington de GA, et al. Type II diabetes and pancreatic cancer: a meta-analyses of 36 studies. Br J Cancer 2005;92(11): 2076–83, 7319: 1109-13.

62. Pannala R, Basu A, Petersen GM, et al. New-onset diabetes: a potential clue to the early diagnosis of pancreatic cancer. Lancet Oncol 2009;10(1):88.

63. Chari ST, Leibson CL, Rabe KG, et al. Pancreatic cancer- associated diabetes mellitus: prevalence and temporal association with diagnosis of cancer. Gastroenterology 2008;134(1):95–101.

64. Permert J, Ihse I, Jorfeldt L, et al. Pancreatic cancer is associated with impaired glucose metabolism. Eur J Surg 1993;159(2):101–7, 134 (1): 95-101.

65. Ludwig E, Olson SH, Bayuga S, et al. Feasibility and yield of screening in relatives from familial pancreatic cancer families. Am J Gastroenterol 2011;106:846–54.

66. Poley JW, Kluijt I, Gouma DJ, et al. The yield of first-time endoscopic ultrasonography in screening individuals at a high risk of developing pancreatic cancer. Am J Gastroenterol 2009;104(9):2175–81.

67. Begley S. The myth of early detection. Available at: http/sharonbegley.com/early-cancer-detection-fizzlesagain.

68. Hoffman TC, DelMar C. Patient's expectations of the benefits and harms of treatments, screening, and tests a systematic review. JAMA Intern Med 2015;175(2): 274–86.

69. Hudson B, Zarifeh A, Young L, et al. Patients expectations of screening and preventive treatments. Ann Fam Med 2012;10(6):495–502.

70. Metcalfe KA, Narod SA. Breast cancer risk perception among women who have undergone prophylactic bilateral mastectomy. J Natl Cancer Inst 2002;94: 1564–9.

71. Leaman H, Jackson PR. What benefit do patients expect from adding second and third antihypertensive drugs? Br J Clin Pharmacol 2002;53(1):93–9.

72. Trewby PN, Reddy AV, Trewby CS. Are preventive drugs preventive enough? A study of patients expectations of benefit from preventive drugs. Clin Med (Lond) 2002;2(6):527–33.

73. Adsay N. Cystic lesions of the pancreas. Mod Pathol 2007;20:S71–93.

74. Loos M, Michalski C. Asymptomatic pancreatic lesions: new insights and clinical implications. World J Gastroenterol 2012;18(33):4474–7.

75. Correa-Gallego C, Ferrone C, Thayer SP, et al. Incidental pancreatic cysts: do we really know what we are watching. Pancreatology 2010;10:144–50.

76. Kaur S, Baine M, Jain M, et al. Early diagnosis of pancreatic cancer: challenges and new developments. Biomark Med 2012;695:597–612.

77. Chang TH, Steplewski Z, Sears HF, et al. Detection of monoclonal antibody-defined colorectal carcinoma antigen by solid-phase binding inhibition radioimmunoassay. Hybridoma 1981;1(1):37–45.

78. Eguia V, Goda TA, Saif M. Early detection of pancreatic cancer. JOP 2012;13(2): 131–4.

79. La Femina J, Gajoux S, D'Angelica MI, et al. Malignant progression of intraductal papillary mucinous neoplasms of the pancreas: results in 157 patients selected for radiographic surveillance. J Clin Oncol 2012;30 [abstract: 152].

80. Miller JR, Meyer JE, Waters JA, et al. Outcome of the pancreas remnant following segmental pancreatectomy for non- invasive intraductal papillary mucinous neoplasm. HPB (Oxford) 2011;13:759–66.

81. Hruban RH, Maitra A, Goggins M. Update on pancreatic intraepithelial neoplasia. Int J Clin Exp Pathol 2008;1:306–16.

82. Oehl K, Hasuoka H, Mizushima T. A case of small pancreatic cancer diagnosed by serial follow-up studies promptly by a positive K-ras point mutation in pure pancreatic juice. Am J Gastroenterol 1998;93:1366–8.

83. Ornish D, Lin J, Daubnmeir J, et al. Increased telomere activity and comprehensive lifestyle. Lancet Oncol 2008;9(11):1048–57.

84. Boffetta P, Couto E, Whichmann J, et al. Fruit and vegetable intake and overall cancer risk in the European et al prospective Investigation into Cancer and Nutrition (EPIC). J Natl Cancer Inst 2010;102:529–37.

85. Turati F, Rossi M, Pellucchi C, et al. Fruit and vegetables and cancer risk: a review of southern European studies. Br J Nutr 2015;113(Suppl 2):S102–10.

Preoperative Evaluation of a Pancreas Mass
Diagnostic Options

Seth Cohen, MD[a], Alexander C. Kagen, MD[b],*

KEYWORDS

- Pancreas • Imaging • Guideline

KEY POINTS

- CT scan is the optimal modality for the initial evaluation of solid pancreatic masses, to include local and distant staging and surgical planning.
- MRI/MRCP is the preferred modality for cystic pancreatic lesion assessment, and can be used without contrast to follow up incidental lesions.
- EUS is an excellent tool for examining pancreatic lesion and can detect, sample, and assess resectability of solid pancreatic masses. EUS is also used in conjunction with MRCP in evaluating cystic lesions. It permits examination of morphology fluid analysis and FNA of any mural nodules.

INTRODUCTION

With an aging population and constantly advancing technology, the use of medical imaging will likely continue to increase, albeit at a varied pace.[1,2] As modern abdominal imaging equipment advances, pancreatic lesion detection improves. Most of these lesions are incidental, and present a conundrum to the clinician and create great anxiety to the patient until a final diagnosis is made. For the practicing physician, the plethora of diagnostic options can be overwhelming. The relevant question at hand is what is the most efficient (in terms of cost and time for the patient and health care system) algorithm to follow and to arrive at a timely and accurate diagnosis.

The diagnostic work-up of known or suspected pancreatic cancer has been well-published, most recently in an excellent review by Feldman and Gandhi.[3] It is not the purpose of this article to re-review the work-up of pancreatic malignancy, but rather to try and present a logical approach to the initial evaluation of a pancreatic

The authors have nothing to disclose.

[a] Division of Digestive Diseases, Mount Sinai Beth Israel, 305 2nd Avenue, #3, New York, NY 10003, USA; [b] Department of Radiology, Mount Sinai West and Mount Sinai St. Luke's, Icahn School of Medicine at Mount Sinai, 1000 Tenth Avenue, 4B-25, New York, NY 10019, USA
* Corresponding author.
E-mail address: alexander.kagen@mountsinai.org

lesion to get the most information possible with the least amount of testing, and to avoid duplicative measures.

IMAGING OPTIONS

Imaging tests that best depict pancreatic lesions include computed tomography (CT); ultrasound (US), transabdominal (TAUS) or endoscopic (EUS); MRI; and PET, usually in combination with CT (ie, PET-CT).

Computed Tomography

CT scanning is the workhorse for pancreatic abnormalities; it provides excellent anatomic detail, and does so consistently. Thin-slice rapid acquisition, cubic voxel resolution less than 1 mm, and uncommon artifacts contribute to its prowess as an imaging tool. In addition, the ability to easily reformat the axial-acquired images in multiple planes is favored, particularly by surgeons and interventionalists, who generally prefer coronal plane imaging. Although the benefits to CT are many, the downsides are few but not insignificant. CT scanning requires ionizing radiation, and typical pancreas protocol CT scans are three-phase studies (precontrast, arterial phase, and portal venous phase imaging).[3] In addition, iodinated intravenous contrast is required in nearly all pancreatic protocols and may be contraindicated in the setting of moderate to severe allergy or renal failure.

Ultrasound

An even more ubiquitous (and radiation free) imaging test is US, with ever-evolving applications and devices. TAUS has the potential to depict the pancreas, pancreatic duct, and associated lesions. The challenge with TAUS in pancreatic disease is the structures that the US beam must pass before it gets to the pancreas itself. Frequently, the stomach and any other bowel is filled with gas and obscures the pancreas, as can excess abdominal wall adipose tissue. Experienced sonographers and radiologists can avoid some of these pitfalls with water to distend the stomach, varied positioning, etc, but their use is limited. In addition, it is difficult to ensure that the entire gland was imaged on any given examination. If, however, there is a specific lesion that is being followed, TAUS may be the appropriate modality.

Endoscopic Ultrasound

EUS has become the primary modality to investigate patients with pancreatic lesions and clinical symptoms. It provides excellent anatomic detail and, as opposed to non-invasive radiologic imaging, it can acquire tissue, or fluid from cystic lesions, in real time. Although it is operator dependent there is a good supply of well-trained endoscopic sonographers. Although minimally invasive, EUS does require deep sedation and thus patients must be appropriately evaluated with a pre-operative medical assessment.

MRI

The most comprehensive of abdominal examinations is MRI. With its superior contrast resolution, depiction of fluid-containing structures, and lack of radiation, MRI offers a robust and complete pancreas examination, especially for younger patients. As opposed to CT, MRI obtains multiple complimentary sequences in addition to multiple phases of contrast enhancement. Diffusion-weighted imaging, a sequence that capitalizes on the decreased random motion of water molecules to depict highly cellular tumors, is helpful in detecting otherwise occult tumors (**Fig. 1**).[4]

A summary of the previously described imaging modalities is highlighted in **Table 1**.

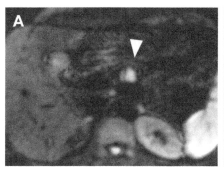
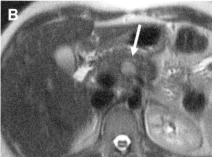

Fig. 1. A 26-year-old woman. (*A*) Single axial diffusion-weighted image demonstrating a focus of marked hyperintense signal (arrowhead), highlighting this highly cellular pancreatic neuro-endocrine tumor. (*B*) On T2-weighted images, this lesion is less well seen (*arrow*).

SYMPTOMATIC LESIONS

When deciding on management options, the first major variable is whether the patient has symptoms that are explained by a pancreatic lesion, such as weight loss, early satiety (eg, as caused by compression of the stomach), postprandial pain (eg, from a stricture or neural invasion), or new-onset diabetes. Any of these worrisome symptoms should raise concern for an abdominal malignancy, and a CT scan with and without intravenous contrast using a pancreas protocol is the next best appropriate step. CT is preferred because of its rapid acquisition, relative ubiquity in hospital and ambulatory settings, and lack of artifacts. Air within the bowel and motion can cause artifacts on MRI, but usually not for CT. Other clinical factors to consider are age older than 50, recent onset of diabetes within the last 1 to 2 years, and epigastric pain radiating to the back either constantly or worse after meals. A negative CT scan should be followed by an MRI or EUS if an occult pancreatic malignancy is suspected (**Fig. 2**).

In patients who cannot receive intravenous contrast because of a moderate or severe contrast allergy according to American College of Radiology Criteria or

Table 1			
Pancreatic imaging modalities			
Modality	**Benefits**	**Downside**	**Preferred Indications**
CT	• Rapid acquisition • Less susceptible to artifacts • High resolution	• Radiation • Need for Iodinated contrast	• Solid tumor staging
TAUS	• Low cost • Accessibility • Noninvasive	• Suboptimal pancreas visualization • User dependent	• Abdominal pain • Follow-up of a known lesion in selected patients
EUS	• High resolution • Sampling ability	• Needs intravenous sedation	• Solid lesions for tissue • Evaluate cystic lesions
MRI	• Characterize lesions based on content • Ability to depict fluid-containing structures	• Air, motion produce artifacts • High cost	• Cystic lesion assessment

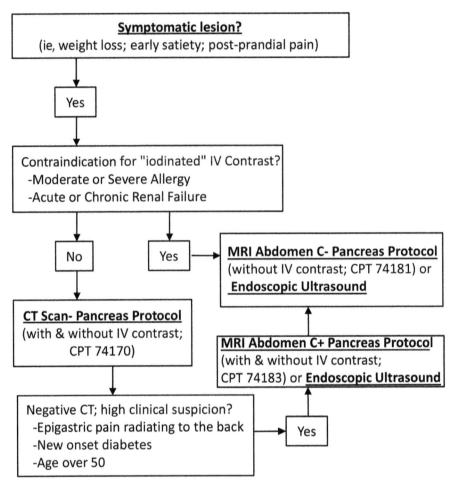

Fig. 2. Clinical algorithm for evaluation of the symptomatic pancreatic mass. IV, intravenous.

because of acute or chronic renal failure, a noncontrast CT alone adds little value.[5] However, in select cases when patients have prior cross-sectional imaging, and a suspected benign lesion is present, noncontrast CT may be adequate follow-up.

EUS is also an excellent alternative for patients who cannot get an intravenous contrast-enhanced CT scan to look for a solid or cystic pancreatic lesion and is also the most sensitive test for early chronic pancreatitis.[5]

MRI is an excellent alternate imaging test for symptomatic patients who cannot receive intravenous contrast. MRI contrast is comprised of gadolinium as opposed to CT contrast, which is iodine-based. Although there is no cross-reactivity, patients at higher risk of allergy, such as prior anaphylaxis, may be premedicated with corticosteroids.[6] Even without contrast, MRI can adequately assess the pancreas for abnormalities. A combination of acinar proteins and manganese contribute to its bright signal on T1-weighted imaging, the absence of which may herald an underlying mass or pancreatitis (**Fig. 3**).[7]

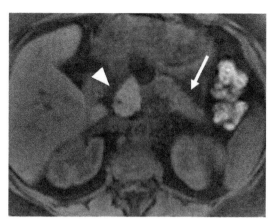

Fig. 3. A 56-year-old woman with history of chronic pancreatitis. Single axial T1-weighted MRI without intravenous contrast demonstrates low signal throughout the tail of the pancreas (*arrow*) indicating changes from chronic pancreatitis (edema, inflammation). Note the normal hyperintense signal in the head (*arrowhead*).

ASYMPTOMATIC INCIDENTAL LESIONS

In the incidental setting, techniques that optimize lesion visibility in the pancreas may not have been used, because the initial study was presumably prescribed and performed for another indication (ie, a noncontrast-enhanced chest CT for lung cancer screening). Additionally, as radiology departments expand and become more subspecialized, non-abdominal radiologists may be unaware of the most up-to-date guidelines for following abdominal lesions discovered incidentally, and may recommend excess testing. Nonetheless, these same imaging modalities can act as diagnostic tools if used appropriately.

Further diagnostic work-up of an incidental lesion should only be pursued in patients who would be medically fit for surgical resection; otherwise the additional testing does not change management.

Solid Lesions

An incidentally found solid tumor of the pancreas is certainly a more worrisome finding than that of a cystic lesion. In addition to pancreatic ductal adenocarcinoma (PDA), pancreatic neuroendocrine tumors, solid pseudopapillary epithelial neoplasm, lymphoma, and metastases are in the differential diagnosis of a solid pancreatic mass. Note should be made of the occasional benign solid pancreatic mass, such as pseudotumor (an inflammatory response that may be difficult to distinguish from PDA) and intrapancreatic splenule, which can simulate a pancreatic tail mass. The latter can be readily distinguished with MRI (because the splenule follows spleen signal on all pulse sequences) or a nuclear medicine liver-spleen scan. However, given the malignant potential (a solid pancreatic mass that overwhelmingly and unfortunately can represent PDA), CT is the best initial test (**Fig. 4**).

If a suspicious solid pancreatic tumor is seen, the question of surgery arises. Resectablility is predicted on a pancreas protocol multiphase CT scan and in conjunction with EUS, although small peritoneal implants may be occult on imaging. Some surgeons are more liberal regarding a positive preoperative diagnosis confirmed cytologically or by histology. Other surgeons favor an EUS with fine-needle aspiration (FNA)

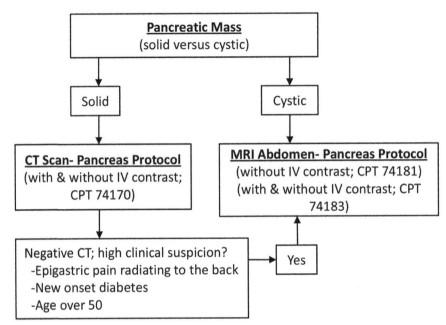

Fig. 4. Imaging work-up for solid versus cystic pancreatic mass. IV, intravenous.

for tissue diagnosis before surgery. For a solid pancreatic mass, in the absence of biliary obstruction, endoscopic retrograde pancreatography (ERCP) has no diagnostic role. EUS, for morphologic examination of the lesion, and FNA for tissue sampling, have replaced ERCP. ERCP is now solely a therapeutic procedure, such as in patients who present with a pancreatic mass and biliary obstruction. Although routine preoperative biliary stenting is controversial, many surgeons favor selective preoperative endoscopic stenting.

Cystic Lesions

There has been a marked increase in the detection of cystic lesions of the pancreas.[8] A cystic pancreatic collection should never be labeled a "pseudocyst" in the absence of a clinical history of pancreatitis. A variety of cystic lesions can arise within the pancreas: pseudocysts (in the setting of prior pancreatitis), nonneoplastic cysts (true cysts, retention cysts, mucinous nonneoplastic cysts, lymphoepithelial cysts), and pancreatic cystic neoplasms.[9] Among the pancreatic cystic neoplasms, well-established subtypes exist: serous cystadenoma, mucinous cystic neoplasm, intraductal papillary mucinous neoplasm (IPMN), in addition to solid pseudopapillary epithelial neoplasm. These all have varied malignant potential, with serous cystadenoma the least, and main duct IPMN the highest.[10–13] Preoperative imaging may not be able to distinguish with certainty between subtypes of benign or malignant lesions (**Figs. 5** and **6**). However, international consensus guidelines revamped in 2012 do provide guidance on how to approach these lesions (**Fig. 7**).

In general, any symptomatic patient (eg, with jaundice) or any measurable nodular or solid enhancing component should be considered malignant, in addition to main duct dilatation greater than 10 mm. Otherwise, a host of imaging features should guide clinical management (eg, EUS vs MRI or CT): cyst size, thickened and enhancing walls,

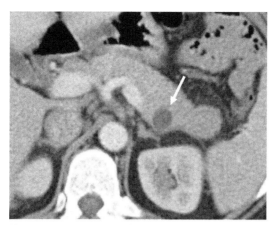

Fig. 5. A 42-year-old woman with history of pancreatitis. Single axial CT image with intravenous contrast demonstrating a unilocular homogenous hypodense cystic lesion in the tail of the pancreas (*arrow*) in this middle-aged woman. Pathology showed a benign mucinous cyst.

main duct prominence, nonenhancing mural nodules, and abrupt change in duct caliber with upstream atrophy.[14] The latter should be noted as a worrisome feature in the absence of a history of prior pancreatitis, as an occult PDA should be excluded.

Although published guidelines offer CT and MRI as equivalent follow-up imaging modalities, MRI is strongly preferred in the evaluation of cystic pancreatic masses. Heavily weighted T2 imaging, routinely used in magnetic resonance cholangiopancreatography (MRCP), can clearly outline these cystic lesions with great detail and depict intracystic anatomy without contrast. Mucin and/or proteinaceous contents can be evaluated with T1-weighted imaging.

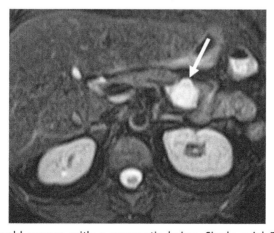

Fig. 6. A 48-year-old woman with a pancreatic lesion. Single axial T2-weighted MRI without intravenous contrast demonstrates a unilocular hyperintense rounded lesion in the tail of the pancreas (*arrow*). Pathologic examination revealed a mucinous cystic neoplasm.

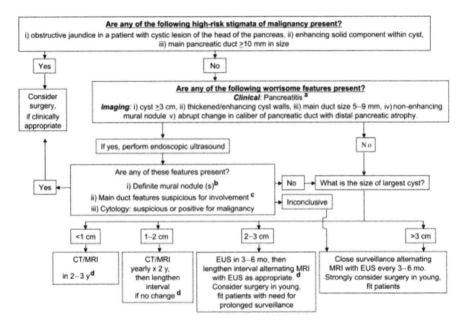

Fig. 7. Fukuoka guidelines adopted by the International Academy of Pancreatology in 2012 for the management of IPMNs. [a] Pancreatitis may be an indication for surgery for relief of symptoms. [b] Differential diagnosis includes mucin. Mucin can move with change in patient position, may be dislodged on cyst lavage and does not have Doppler flow. Features of true tumor nodule include lack of mobility, presence of Doppler flow and FNA of nodule showing tumor tisssue. [c] Presence of any one of thickened walls, intraductal mucin or mural nodules is suggestive of main duct involvement. In their absence main duct involvement is incolclusive. [d] Studies from Japan suggest that on follow-up of subjects with suspected BD-IPMN there is increased incidence of pancreatic ductal adenocarcinoma unrelated to malignant transformation of the BD-IPMN(s) being followed. However, it is unclear if imaging surveillance can detect early ductal adenocarcinoma, and, if so, at what interval surveillance imaging should be performed.

Intraductal Papillary Mucinous Neoplasm

Main duct IPMNs have the highest malignant potential of the cystic pancreatic lesions, and should be managed by a multidisciplinary team including a pancreatic surgeon, an advanced endoscopist, and an abdominal radiologist. Most patients should have an EUS with FNA of any nodular lesions. These lesions may also benefit from ERCP and intraductal pancreatoscopy with tissue and cytologic sampling. MRI/MRCP can depict main duct dilatation and can help guide the endoscopist and the surgeon (**Fig. 8**).

Side-branch IPMNs are much more prevalent,[10] and are commonly seen incidentally on cross-sectional imaging (MRI/MRCP more so than CT) (**Fig. 9**). If they are less than 10 mm without any of the previously described suspicious features, they can be followed with MRCP in 2 to 3 years.[14] This approach varies to published guidelines from American Gastroenterological Association, International Association of Pancreatology (Fukuoka guidelines), and the American College of Radiology.[15–18] As the size of the cyst increases (from 10 to 30 mm) different guidelines suggest varying degrees of conservatism toward EUS and sampling. Our practice is similar to the University of Pittsburgh Medical Center, using a 15-mm size threshold, or any worrisome features, such as thickening or a mural nodule to trigger EUS assessment.

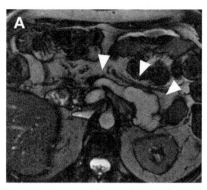
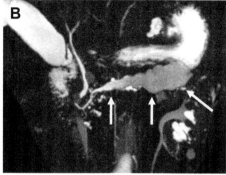

Fig. 8. A 63-year-old man. (*A*) Single axial steady state free precession image demonstrates fluid distention of the main pancreatic duct (*arrowheads*). (*B*) Coronal oblique three-dimensional MRCP images also demonstrate main duct distention (*arrows*), along with small side branch IPMNs in the head.

Serous Versus Mucinous

Cystic lesion greater than 10 mm is stratified by several different criteria: the presence or absence of symptoms; morphologically benign or suspicious findings, such as nodules or a solid mass component; and whether the cyst fluid is serous or mucinous. Serous lesions have almost no chance of malignant transformation and perhaps should not even be subject to surveillance.[19] Mucinous lesions, however, do undergo malignant transformation and should be subject to further investigation, including cyst fluid analysis. When a patient undergoes an EUS and FNA for fluid analysis the first studies are fluid carcinoembryonic antigen, fluid amylase, and cytology (**Table 2**). Pseudocysts and cystic lesions communicating with the pancreatic duct may have elevated amylases levels to 100,000 IU. Fluid carcinoembryonic antigen values greater than 200 ng/mL define the cystic lesion as "mucinous." In recent years, there has been a wider application of molecular biology. Although not accepted by consensus, DNA and molecular analysis in combination with molecular analysis of cyst fluid and clinical findings better predicted malignant potential than consensus guidelines.[20]

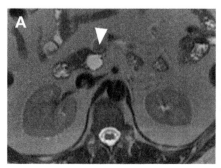
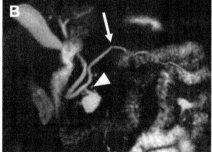

Fig. 9. A 59-year-old man. Single axial T2-weighted image demonstrates a 2.1-cm side branch IPMN in the head/uncinate process of the pancreas with a narrow connection to main pancreatic duct (*arrowheads, A, B*). Note the normal-sized pancreatic duct (*arrow, B*).

Table 2
Fluid analysis in EUS/FNA

Lesion	CEA	Amylase	Cytology/k-ras/DNA Amount/Allelic Loss of Tumor Suppressor Genes
Pseudocyst	—	Elevated (100,00 IU)	Absent
Mucinous	>200	—	Present

Abbreviation: CEA, carcinoembryonic antigen.

SUMMARY

Increased detection of pancreatic lesions may cause untoward concern for clinicians and patients alike. CT scan and MRI are powerful imaging tools for these challenging lesions. EUS is also important for diagnosis as it permits tissue sampling of solid lesions and fluid analysis in selected cystic lesions. Established guidelines, although variable, act to standardize the approach to the work-up and management of these lesions, and further research will hone and perhaps harmonize follow-up intervals and triggers for interventions.

REFERENCES

1. US Census Bureau and population clock: U.S. Government. 2017. Available at: http://www.census.gov/popclock/. Accessed May 22, 2017.
2. Levin DC, Rao VM. Factors that will determine future utilization trends in diagnostic imaging. J Am Coll Radiol 2016;13(8):904–8.
3. Feldman MK, Gandhi NS. Imaging evaluation of pancreatic cancer. Surg Clin North Am 2016;96(6):1235–56.
4. Barral M, Taouli B, Guiu B, et al. Diffusion-weighted MR imaging of the pancreas: current status and recommendations. Radiology 2015;274(1):45–63.
5. Catalano MF, Sahai A, Levy M, et al. EUS-based criteria for the diagnosis of chronic pancreatitis: the Rosemont classification. Gastrointest Endosc 2009;69:1251–61.
6. American College of Radiology. ACR manual on contrast media. Reston (VA): ACR; 2016. Available at: http://www.acr.org/Quality-Safety/Resources/Contrast-Manual. Accessed May 22, 2017.
7. Ly JN, Miller FH. MR imaging of the pancreas: a practical approach. Radiol Clin North Am 2002;40(6):1289–306.
8. Fernandez-del Castillo C, Targarona J, Thayer SP, et al. Incidental pancreatic cysts: clinicopathologic characteristics and comparison with symptomatic patients. Arch Surg 2003;138(4):427–33 [discussion: 433–4].
9. Kalb B, Sarmiento JM, Kooby DA, et al. MR imaging of cystic lesions of the pancreas. Radiographics 2009;29(6):1749–65.
10. Grutzmann R, Niedergethmann M, Pilarsky C, et al. Intraductal papillary mucinous tumors of the pancreas: biology, diagnosis, and treatment. Oncologist 2010;15(12):1294–309.
11. Zamboni G, Scarpa A, Bogina G, et al. Mucinous cystic tumors of the pancreas: clinicopathological features, prognosis, and relationship to other mucinous cystic tumors. Am J Surg Pathol 1999;23(4):410–22.

12. Reddy RP, Smyrk TC, Zapiach M, et al. Pancreatic mucinous cystic neoplasm defined by ovarian stroma: demographics, clinical features, and prevalence of cancer. Clin Gastroenterol Hepatol 2004;2(11):1026–31.

13. King JC, Ng TT, White SC, et al. Pancreatic serous cystadenocarcinoma: a case report and review of the literature. J Gastrointest Surg 2009;13(10):1864–8.

14. Tanaka M, Fernandez-del Castillo C, Adsay V, et al. International consensus guidelines 2012 for the management of IPMN and MCN of the pancreas. Pancreatology 2012;12(3):183–97.

15. Berland LL, Silverman SG, Gore RM, et al. Managing incidental findings on abdominal CT: white paper of the ACR incidental findings committee. J Am Coll Radiol 2010;7(10):754–73.

16. Singhi AD, Zeh HJ, Brand RE, et al. American Gastroenterological Association guidelines are inaccurate in detecting pancreatic cysts with advanced neoplasia: a clinicopathologic study of 225 patients with supporting molecular data. Gastrointest Endosc 2016;83(6):1107–17.e2.

17. Vege SS, Ziring B, Jain R, et al. American Gastroenterological Association institute guideline on the diagnosis and management of asymptomatic neoplastic pancreatic cysts. Gastroenterology 2015;148(4):819–22 [quiz: 12–3].

18. Lee A, Kadiyala V, Lee LS. Evaluation of AGA and Fukuoka Guidelines for EUS and surgical resection of incidental pancreatic cysts. Endosc Int Open 2017; 5(2):E116–22.

19. McGrath K. Management of incidental pancreatic cysts: which guidelines? Endosc Int Open 2017;5(3):E209–11.

20. Al-Haddad MA, Kowalski T, Siddiqui A, et al. Integrated molecular pathology accurately determines the malignant potential of pancreatic cysts. Endoscopy 2015;47:136–46.

Screening of Patients at Risk for Familial Pancreatic Cancer: What Is Beneficial?

Robert J. Torphy, MD, Richard D. Schulick, MD, MBA*

KEYWORDS

- Pancreatic cancer • Familial pancreatic cancer • High-risk individuals • Screening
- Surveillance

KEY POINTS

- Familial cancer predisposition syndromes, hereditary pancreatitis, and familial pancreatic cancer are significant risk factors for developing pancreatic cancer.
- Certain high-risk individuals should undergo screening for pancreatic cancer with EUS or MRI/magnetic resonance retrograde cholangiopancreatography.
- The goal of screening is to identify early cancer or precancerous lesions (branch-duct IPMNs, mucinous cystic neoplasms, and PanINs) that can be curatively resected.

INTRODUCTION

Pancreatic cancer is projected to be the third most deadly cancer in the United States in 2017. Despite advances in treatment, the 5-year survival remains dismal, estimated to be 8%.[1] At the time of diagnosis, only 15% to 20% of patients are candidates for surgical resection, the only potentially curable treatment, because of locoregional spread or metastatic disease. Routine screening for pancreatic cancer is not recommended because it remains a rare disease with an incidence of only 9 per 100,000 persons per year and a cumulative lifetime risk of 1.5%.[2] Identifying patients at increased risk for the development of pancreatic cancer is paramount to early diagnosis and successful treatment.

Disclosure Statement: R.J. Torphy has nothing to disclose. R.D. Schulick is a coinventor of a patent to use genetically modified *Listeria* monocytogenes to generate inflammatory response to cancer; licensed to Aduro Biotech, managed by Johns Hopkins University. He is also a coinventor of a patent to use CD112 as an immune checkpoint inhibitor; managed by University of Colorado. Dr R.D. Schulick is on the Board of Noile Immune–Tokyo (not compensated); is a consultant to Grand Rounds–Palo Alto; and provides remote second opinions for surgical oncology cases, managed by University of Colorado.
Department of Surgery, University of Colorado, 12631 East 17th Avenue, C-302, Aurora, CO 80045, USA
* Corresponding author.
E-mail address: richard.schulick@ucdenver.edu

Surg Clin N Am 98 (2018) 25–35
https://doi.org/10.1016/j.suc.2017.09.003
0039-6109/18/© 2017 Elsevier Inc. All rights reserved.

Family history is essential in identifying individuals at increased risk for developing pancreatic cancer. It is estimated that 1% to 10% of those diagnosed with pancreatic cancer have a family history of the disease.[3,4] Although environmental exposures, such as cigarette smoking, can confer some increased familial risk of developing pancreatic cancer, it is now widely accepted that this increased familial risk is largely caused by genetic inheritance.

Several different etiologies can lead to this increased inherited risk for pancreatic cancer including hereditary tumor predisposition syndromes, hereditary pancreatitis, and a growing list of newly identified mutations leading to familial pancreatic cancer (**Table 1**).[5] This growing understanding led the International Cancer of the Pancreas Screening (CAPS) Consortium to release guidelines in 2012 regarding which of these high-risk patients should undergo screening for pancreatic cancer.[6] However, there is still much uncertainty regarding the optimal screening approach and management of pancreatic lesions identified in this unique patient population.

HEREDITARY RISK FOR PANCREATIC CANCER
Hereditary Cancer Predisposition Syndromes

Known cancer predisposition syndromes account for an estimated 20% of the observed familial aggregation of pancreatic cancer.[2] Hereditary predisposition syndromes associated with pancreatic cancer include familial atypical multiple mole melanoma (FAMMM) syndrome, Peutz-Jeghers syndrome, hereditary breast-ovarian

Table 1
Hereditary risk for pancreatic cancer

	Involved Genes	Risk of Pancreatic Cancer	CAPS Screening Recommendations[6]
Hereditary Cancer Predisposition Syndromes			
Familial atypical multiple mole melanoma	CDKN2A/ p16-Leiden	17% by 75 y[8]	Yes, if one affected FDR
Peutz-Jeghers	STK11/LKB1	36% life-time risk[12]	Yes, regardless of family history
Hereditary breast-ovarian cancer	BRCA1 BRCA2	1.5%–2.1% by 70 y[14] 3.6% lifetime risk[15]	No recommendation Yes, if one affected FDR or two affected family members
Hereditary nonpolyposis colorectal carcinoma	MLH1, MSH2, MSH6	3.7% by 70 y[16]	Yes, if one affected FDR
Familial adenomatous polyposis	APC	~2% lifetime risk[17]	No recommendation
Hereditary pancreatitis	PRSS1, SPINK1, CFTR	40% by 70 y[19]	No recommendation
Familial pancreatic cancer	BRCA2, PALB2, ATM	2 affected FDRs, 8%–12% lifetime risk 3 affected FDR, 16%–30% lifetime risk[22]	Yes, if two or more affected blood relatives, with at least one affected FDR

Abbreviations: CAPS, International Cancer of the Pancreas Screening, FDR, first degree relative.

cancer (HBOC), hereditary nonpolyposis colorectal carcinoma, and familial adenomatous polyposis.

Familial atypical multiple mole melanoma

FAMMM is associated with multiple nevi, atypical nevi, and cutaneous or ocular malignant melanomas.[2] FAMMM is inherited in an autosomal-dominant manner but has a highly variable disease penetrance. At least one-quarter of patients with this syndrome have mutations in the *CDKN2A* (cyclin-dependent kinase inhibitor 2A) gene, also known as the *p16* gene.[7] Patients with a particular *CDKN2A* mutation, *p16-Leiden*, have been shown to be at increased risk for not only malignant melanoma but also pancreatic cancer. Patients with this *p16-Leiden* mutation have a significant risk of developing pancreatic cancer with an estimated cumulative risk by the age of 75 of 17% and a mean age at diagnosis of 58 years (range, 38–77 years).[8] FAMMM should be considered in patients with invasive melanoma and two or more relatives with invasive melanoma or pancreatic cancer on one side of their family, or if they have three or more primary invasive lesions.[9]

Peutz-Jeghers syndrome

Peutz-Jeghers syndrome is characterized by hamartomatous gastrointestinal polyps and mucocutaneous pigmentation with autosomal-dominant inheritance.[10] This syndrome occurs secondary to mutations in the serine/threonine kinase gene (*STK11/LKB1*), which is thought to act as a tumor suppressor gene. Patients with Peutz-Jeghers syndrome are at increased risk for gastrointestinal malignancies (gastroesophageal, small intestine, colorectal, pancreas) and breast and gynecologic malignancies with a risk of malignancy at any site by the age of 70 years of 85%. These patients have a cumulative lifetime risk of developing pancreatic cancer of 11% to 36%.[11,12]

Hereditary breast-ovarian cancer

HBOC syndrome is associated with germline mutations in *BRCA1* and *BRCA2* genes and is characterized by an increased risk for male and female breast cancer; ovarian cancer; and less commonly pancreatic cancer, prostate cancer, and melanoma.[13] *BRCA1* gene mutation carriers have been shown to have an estimated cumulative risk of developing pancreatic cancer by the age of 70 of 2.1% (male) and 1.5% (female).[14] *BRCA2* gene mutations carries are considered to be at a higher risk for developing pancreatic cancer with a cumulative age-adjusted lifetime risk of 3.6%.[15]

Hereditary nonpolyposis colorectal carcinoma

Hereditary nonpolyposis colorectal carcinoma, or Lynch syndrome, is an autosomal-dominant condition secondary to mutations in DNA mismatch repair genes: *MLH1*, *MSH2*, *MSH6*, or *PMS2*. Patients with Lynch syndrome are most susceptible to colorectal and endometrial cancers. Patients harboring these mutations have also been shown to have an increased risk for the development of pancreatic cancer with a cumulative risk by the age of 70 years of 3.68%. The median age of pancreatic cancer diagnosis in this group of patients was 51.5 years (range, 19–85).[16]

Familial adenomatous polyposis

Familial adenomatous polyposis is characterized by the formation of numerous adenomatous polyps forming in the large intestine and increased risk for developing early onset colorectal cancer caused by mutations in the *APC* gene. Although not widely studied, it is reported that these patients also have an increased risk of developing pancreatic cancer, with a relative risk of 4.5 compared with the general population.[17]

Hereditary Pancreatitis

Hereditary pancreatitis causes chronic inflammation of pancreas resulting in a predisposition to developing pancreatic adenocarcinoma. Hereditary pancreatitis is characterized by recurrent acute pancreatitis episodes and typically presents at an early age, within the first two decades of life. These patients are at risk to go on to develop chronic pancreatitis–associated risk of pancreatic fibrosis, pseudocysts, pancreatic duct strictures, exocrine insufficiency, and diabetes mellitus.[15,18] Hereditary pancreatitis is inherited in autosomal-dominant or autosomal-recessive forms and mutations to the following genes have been implicated in this disease process: *PRSS1*, *SPINK1*, and *CFTR*.

PRSS1

Mutation to the *PRSS1* gene is the most common genetic disruption leading to hereditary pancreatitis, present in 80% of cases, and is inherited in an autosomal-dominant fashion. The *PRSS1* gene encodes for the most abundant isoform of trypsin secreted by the pancreas. Many mutations in the *PRSS1* gene have been identified in patients with hereditary pancreatitis, the most common being to regions of the gene that encode regulatory domains that defend against premature activation of trypsin in the pancreas.[18]

SPINK1

SPINK1 encodes a protein that is a trypsin inhibitor found in pancreatic acinar cells and acts to inhibit prematurely activated trypsin from activating other pancreatic zymogens.[18] *SPINK1* mutations that result in hereditary pancreatitis are typically inherited in an autosomal-recessive fashion.

CFTR

Cystic fibrosis is a multiorgan disease that results secondary to a mutation in the cystic fibrosis transmembrane conductance regulatory gene (*CFTR*) causing a disruption in sodium, chloride, and bicarbonate transport. The typical presentation of cystic fibrosis with thick secretions and severe lung disease secondary to autosomal-recessive inheritance of the F508D mutation rarely causes pancreatitis. Hereditary pancreatitis secondary to *CFTR* mutations is instead more commonly associated with milder defects in *CFTR* gene and mild presentations of cystic fibrosis.[18]

Hereditary pancreatitis and risk of pancreatic cancer

Patients with hereditary pancreatitis are at increased risk for subsequently developing pancreatic adenocarcinoma. In one cohort study comparing those with hereditary pancreatitis (based on age of first episode of pancreatitis <30 years, positive family history, and no other likely cause) with population-based control subjects, patients with hereditary pancreatitis had an estimated cumulative risk of developing pancreatic cancer by the age of 70 of 40%; this cumulative risk was 75% in patients with paternal inheritance. Of the patients that went on to develop pancreatic cancer, the mean age of diagnosis was 56.9 years.[19] From analysis of data from the European Registry of Hereditary Pancreatitis and Pancreatic Cancer including 112 families from 14 countries, the cumulative risk of developing pancreatic cancer at 70 years after symptom onset was 44% with a standardized incidence ratio of 67%.[20] Furthermore, almost half of all deaths in a French cohort study of patients with hereditary pancreatitis were secondary to pancreatic cancer.[21]

Familial Pancreatic Cancer

One accepted operational definition of familial pancreatic cancer is "families with two or more first degree relatives (FDR) with pancreatic cancer that do not fulfill the criteria of any other inherited tumor syndrome," thus excluding those with cancer predisposition syndromes or hereditary pancreatitis.[5] Despite the numerous syndromes discussed previously that result in an increased risk for pancreatic cancer, familial pancreatic cancer accounts for most cases where there is an increased inherited risk of developing pancreatic cancer.

A detailed family history remains the most important clinical tool for stratifying high-risk individuals. For example, those with one, two, or three affected FDRs have a 4.6-fold, 6.4-fold, and 32-fold increased risk of developing pancreatic cancer, respectively.[22] There is also strong evidence for anticipation in familial pancreatic cancer, meaning individuals in successive generations are at risk at an earlier age than their predecessors.[23]

Recent advances in whole-genome sequencing has led to the discovery of several genes that can harbor mutations causing familial pancreatic cancer, including *BRCA2*, *PALB2*, and *ATM*. Likely more familial mutations will be identified as research into this area continues to grow.

BRCA2

BRCA2 is the most well described familial pancreatic cancer gene. Breast cancer occurs commonly in patients with *BRCA2* mutations in association with HBOC. Pancreatic cancer can develop in families with HBOC syndrome; however, pancreatic cancer has also been shown to run in families with *BRCA2* mutations in the absence of breast cancer.[24] In one study analyzing DNA from familial pancreatic cancer kindreds, who did not have another inherited tumor syndrome, 17.2% of patients had deleterious *BRCA2* mutations.[25]

PALB2

PALB2 has been shown to be a binding partner of BRCA1 and BRCA2 and that this interaction is important for DNA repair.[26] Through exome sequencing, *PALB2* mutations were shown to occur in 3.1% (4 out of 96) of patients with familial pancreatic cancer.[27] In a subsequent European study, *PALB2* mutations were identified in 3.7% of patients with familial pancreatic cancer.[28]

ATM

The *ATM* gene encodes a serine/threonine kinase involved in DNA double-strand break repair. Ataxia-telangiectasia is an autosomal-recessive syndrome that occurs in patients with homozygous mutations in *ATM* and is characterized by cerebellar ataxia; oculomotor apraxia; telangiectasias of the conjunctiva and skin; immunodeficiency; sensitivity to ionizing radiation; and an increased risk of malignancies, such as lymphoma and leukemia.[29] Genome-wide sequencing revealed that in familial pancreatic cancer kindreds with three affected family members, 4.6% carried heterozygous deleterious mutations in *ATM*.[30]

SCREENING HIGH-RISK INDIVIDUALS
Which Patients Should Be Screened?

CAPS released guidelines in 2012 regarding patient screening for pancreatic cancer.[6] They recommended against screening in the general population given the low lifetime risk of developing pancreatic cancer. The CAPS guidelines recommend screening should be considered for the following at-risk individuals:

- Those with two or more affected blood relatives, with at least one affected FDR.
- Those with Peutz-Jeghers syndrome, regardless of family history of pancreatic cancer.

- *p16* mutations carriers with one affected FDR.
- BRCA2 mutation carriers with one affected FDR, or two affected family members.
- *PALB2* mutation carriers with one affected FDR.
- Those with Lynch syndrome (mismatch repair gene mutation carriers) with one affected FDR.

At What Age Should Screening Be Initiated?

No consensus guideline has been reached on when screening should begin for high-risk individuals. The average age of diagnosis of familial pancreatic cancer is 68 years.[22] In a prospective trial screening high-risk individuals, Canto and colleagues[31] initiated screening at age 40 or 10 years younger than the youngest relative with pancreatic cancer. However, pancreatic lesions identified on screening imaging were much more common in patients greater than 50 years of age, and high-grade neoplasms were resected only in individuals older than 60 years. These results argue that screening for high-risk individuals should begin in the fifth or sixth decade of life because this produces the highest diagnostic yield. Given anticipation has been described in familial pancreatic cancer, it is reasonable to consider screening individuals 10 years before the earliest diagnosis of pancreatic cancer in their family. Patients with Peutz-Jeghers syndrome are another notable exception with a mean age of diagnosis of pancreatic cancer of 41 years, suggesting screening should begin at an earlier age in this high-risk group.[12]

How Should High-Risk Individuals Be Screened?

Endoscopic ultrasound (EUS) and MRI are the best screening modalities for high-risk individuals. Computed tomography, MRI, and EUS were compared in a multicenter prospective study screening a cohort of 216 high-risk individuals with familial pancreatic cancer, the largest study to date comparing screening modalities in high-risk individuals. Computed tomography scan only visualized 13.8% of all detectable lesions, compared with MRI/magnetic resonance retrograde cholangiopancreatography and EUS, which visualized 77% and 79% of all detectable lesions, respectively. This study also reported a diagnostic yield of first-time screening of 42.6% (pancreatic mass, cyst, or isolated dilated main pancreatic duct identified in 92 of 216 high-risk individuals).[31]

MANAGEMENT OF LESIONS IDENTIFIED IN HIGH-RISK INDIVIDUALS

The management of lesions identified when screening high-risk individuals is a challenging issue. The goal of screening this patient population is to identify early stage pancreatic cancer that can be resected with negative margins, or alternatively, to identifying precursor lesions that can be curatively resected. Known precursor lesions include pancreatic intraepithelial neoplasms (PanINs), intraductal papillary mucinous neoplasms (IPMNs), and mucinous cystic neoplasms (MCNs). It has been shown that pancreatic tissue from patients with a family history of pancreatic cancer that developed disease requiring resection have a greater number of precursor lesions, the precursor lesions were more often multifocal, and there was a higher rate of high-grade lesions when compared with nonfamilial cases.[32] Despite the known higher prevalence of microscopic precursor lesions in patients with a family history, there currently are no screening methods to accurately identify these microscopic high-risk lesions. Instead, current screening modalities, such as EUS and MRI, are sensitive at identifying small, radiographically suspicious lesions, most commonly cysts.

Branch Duct Intraductal Papillary Mucinous Neoplasms

Most cystic lesions identified on screening are branch duct IPMNs (BD-IPMNs). The updated Fukuoka International Consensus Guidelines help guide the management of sporadic BD-IPMNs. Surgical resection is considered in individuals with symptoms attributable to the suspect lesion, cysts greater than 3 cm, and cysts with mural nodules.[33] These recommendations are based on the risk of the lesions harboring or progressing to invasive disease. There is less knowledge about the risk of malignancy or progression to malignancy of BD-IPMNs identified in individuals with a family history of pancreatic cancer. A retrospective study reviewed the progression to pancreatic cancer in 300 individuals with BD-IPMNs, and evaluated a subgroup of 16 patients from this cohort with a family history of at least one first-degree relative with a history of pancreatic cancer. After controlling for age by comparing patients greater than 70 year old, they found no difference in the frequency of developing pancreatic cancer in follow-up for BD-IPMNs in patients with a family history of pancreatic cancer compared with those without.[34] A separate retrospective study also demonstrated that in resected IPMNs (including main duct, branch duct, and mixed) there was no difference in pathologic grade or invasive components of the resected IPMN when comparing those with a family history of pancreatic cancer with those without.[35]

Given these findings, the criteria for surgical resection of BD-IPMNs identified in patients with a family history of pancreatic cancer should be no different from sporadically identified BD-IPMNs. Further studies into the biologic progression of IPMNs to pancreatic cancer in the setting of known hereditary precursor mutations are needed to help better guide management of BD-IPMNs in high-risk individuals with known germline mutations. The CAPS consensus guidelines recommend repeat surveillance for BD-IPMNs without high-risk stigmata at intervals consistent with those recommended by the Fukuoka guidelines depending on lesion size.[6]

Pancreatic Intraepithelial Neoplasms

PanIN lesions arise in small pancreatic ducts, typically measure less than 0.5 cm, and are classified based on degree of dysplasia as PanIN-1, PanIN-2, or PanIN-3 (carcinoma *in situ*) lesions.[36] From genetic analysis, it is thought that PanIN lesions progressively become more dysplastic through a stepwise accumulation of mutations (*KRAS2* in PanIN-1, inactivation of *p16/CDKN2A* in PanIN-2, and inactivation of *TP53* and *MAD4/DPC4* in PanIN-3), ultimately progressing to invasive carcinoma.[37] Given this stepwise progression to invasive pancreatic cancer, identifying PanIN lesions in high-risk individuals would be an optimal opportunity for cure before progression to invasive disease in screening programs for familial pancreatic cancer. However, two complicating factors include lack of understanding of the rate of progression of early PanIN lesions to invasive disease and the limited ability to detect PanINs with current imaging techniques.

PanIN lesions have been shown to be more common in pancreatic tissue of high-risk individuals who underwent resection for suspicious lesions. Brune and colleagues[38] analyzed the histology of resected pancreas specimens from individuals screened in the CAPS 1 and CAPS 2 and identified PanIN lesions in 100% of resected specimens (eight of eight specimens). Notably, there were a mean of 34 PanIN lesions per resected specimen, as compared with a mean of 1.9 lesions in control cases. In only one specimen was PanIN-3 present. It currently is not known if PanIN lesions progress to malignancy faster in high-risk individuals than the general population, but it seems early PanIN lesions are more prevalent and multifocal. Although resection of PanIN lesions is considered a success of screening programs because of their potential for malignancy, surveillance must continue after resection because the remaining pancreatic tissue remains at risk.

Because PanIN lesions are a histologic finding without a known clinical correlate it is difficult to accurately identify these lesions with current imaging modalities, such as EUS and MRI. However, it has been demonstrated that PanIN lesions in resected specimens correlate with lobular atrophy of pancreatic parenchyma, which is detected with standard EUS, resembling chronic pancreatitis-like changes.[38] This finding on screening EUS should raise suspicion for precursor PanIN lesions and close clinical follow-up.

Mucinous Cystic Neoplasms

MCNs are a less commonly identified precursor lesion than BD-IPMNs or PanINs in high-risk individuals. MCNs are detected with traditional radiographic screening and are characterized by a well-circumscribed cystic lesion with thick septae and do not seem to communicate with the duct system.[39] In patients who underwent resection for sporadic MCNs, invasive disease was found in approximately 11% of resected specimens. Furthermore, those with no pathologic findings of invasive disease had a 5-year survival approaching 100%.[40] The underlying risk of invasive disease and the rate of progression to invasive disease in high-risk individuals with MCNs are yet to be studied. Despite this, given the potential for cure in noninvasive MCNs, current guidelines recommend considering resection for all MCNs in surgically fit patients.[33] This recommendation should hold true in high-risk individuals. Fine-needle aspiration of these lesions for cytology and tumor marker analysis is helpful in determining cyst type, because serous cystadenomas do not warrant resection.

Nonsuspicious Cysts, Duct Strictures, and Solid Lesions

The CAPS consensus guidelines recommend repeat surveillance after 6 to 12 months for nonsuspicious cysts and repeat surveillance in 3 months for pancreatic duct strictures.[6] Solid lesions are rarely encountered when screening high-risk individuals, present in only 1.4% of patients in one study.[31] Although rare, solid lesions found on screening should be considered very high risk. The decision to proceed to surgical resection for these lesions should be discussed in a multidisciplinary setting at high-volume centers. If surgical resection is not pursued, solid lesions should be surveilled within 3 months. Lesion characteristics, such as larger than 1 cm and growth on interval follow-up, should raise suspicion for progression and prompt further discussion regarding resection.

SUMMARY

Family history is a significant risk factor for developing pancreatic cancer and this hereditary risk can be secondary to familial cancer predisposition syndromes, hereditary pancreatitis, or familial pancreatic cancer. Certain high-risk individuals are recommended to undergo screening for pancreatic cancer with EUS or MRI/magnetic resonance retrograde cholangiopancreatography because of the potential to identify and curatively resect precursor lesions. To date, observational prospective studies screening patients with familial pancreatic cancer have been carried out in multiple countries with highly variable diagnostic yields (ranging from 1% to 50%).[6] Drawing conclusions about the utility of screening high-risk individuals based on these studies is difficult given their highly variable results because of underlying variation in the risk of the screened population, screening protocols used, follow-up duration, and outcomes measured. It is clear, however, that many high-risk patients have pancreatic lesions identified on screening EUS or MRI and a certain population of these individuals can undergo curative resection of premalignant lesions before they progress to pancreatic cancer. Future research should focus on developing improved screening methods and optimizing screening protocols and the management of high-risk lesions.

REFERENCES

1. Siegel RL, Miller KD, Jemal A. Cancer statistics, 2017. CA Cancer J Clin 2017; 67(1):7–30.
2. Hruban RH, Canto M, Goggins M, et al. Update on familial pancreatic cancer. Adv Surg 2010;44:293–311.
3. Schenk M, Schwartz AG, O'Neal E, et al. Familial risk of pancreatic cancer. J Natl Cancer Inst 2001;93(8):640–4.
4. Permuth-Wey J, Egan KM. Family history is a significant risk factor for pancreatic cancer: results from a systematic review and meta-analysis. Fam Cancer 2009; 8(2):109–17.
5. Bartsch DK, Gress TM, Langer P. Familial pancreatic cancer—current knowledge. Nat Rev Gastroenterol Hepatol 2012;9(8):445–53.
6. Canto MI, Harinck F, Hruban RH, et al. International cancer of the pancreas screening (caps) consortium summit on the management of patients with increased risk for familial pancreatic cancer. Gut 2013;62(3):339–47.
7. Lynch HT, Shaw TG. Familial atypical multiple mole melanoma (FAMMM) syndrome: history, genetics, and heterogeneity. Fam Cancer 2016;15(3):487–91.
8. Vasen HF, Gruis NA, Frants RR, et al. Risk of developing pancreatic cancer in families with familial atypical multiple mole melanoma associated with a specific 19 deletion of p16 (p16-Leiden). Int J Cancer 2000;87(6):809–11.
9. Soura E, Eliades P, Shannon K, et al. Hereditary melanoma: update on syndromes and management. Genetics of familial atypical multiple mole melanoma syndrome. J Am Acad Dermatol 2016;74(3):395–407.
10. Tomlinson IP, Houlston RS. Peutz-Jeghers syndrome. J Med Genet 1997;34(12): 1007–11.
11. Hearle N, Schumacher V, Menko FH, et al. Frequency and spectrum of cancers in the Peutz-Jeghers syndrome. Clin Cancer Res 2006;12(10):3209–15.
12. Giardiello FM, Brensinger JD, Tersmette AC, et al. Very high risk of cancer in familial Peutz-Jeghers syndrome. Gastroenterology 2000;119(6):1447–53.
13. Petrucelli N, Daly MB, Pal T. BRCA1- and BRCA2-associated hereditary breast and ovarian cancer. In: Pagon RA, Adam MP, Ardinger HH, et al, editors. GeneReviews(®). Seattle (WA): University of Washington; 1993. Available at: http://www.ncbi.nlm.nih.gov/books/NBK1247/. Accessed March 4, 2017.
14. Breast Cancer Linkage Consortium. Cancer risks in BRCA2 mutation carriers. J Natl Cancer Inst 1999;91(15):1310–6.
15. Brose MS, Rebbeck TR, Calzone KA, et al. Cancer risk estimates for BRCA1 mutation carriers identified in a risk evaluation program. J Natl Cancer Inst 2002; 94(18):1365–72.
16. Kastrinos F, Mukherjee B, Tayob N, et al. The risk of pancreatic cancer in families with lynch syndrome. JAMA 2009;302(16):1790–5.
17. Giardiello FM, Offerhaus GJ, Lee DH, et al. Increased risk of thyroid and pancreatic carcinoma in familial adenomatous polyposis. Gut 1993;34(10):1394–6.

18. Raphael KL, Willingham FF. Hereditary pancreatitis: current perspectives. Clin Exp Gastroenterol 2016;9:197–207.
19. Lowenfels AB, Maisonneuve P, DiMagno EP, et al. Hereditary pancreatitis and the risk of pancreatic cancer. International hereditary pancreatitis study group. J Natl Cancer Inst 1997;89(6):442–6.
20. Howes N, Lerch MM, Greenhalf W, et al. Clinical and genetic characteristics of hereditary pancreatitis in Europe. Clin Gastroenterol Hepatol 2004;2(3):252–61.
21. Rebours V, Boutron-Ruault MC, Schnee M, et al. The natural history of hereditary pancreatitis: a national series. Gut 2009;58(1):97–103.
22. Klein AP, Brune KA, Petersen GM, et al. Prospective risk of pancreatic cancer in familial pancreatic cancer kindreds. Cancer Res 2004;64(7):2634–8.
23. McFaul CD, Greenhalf W, Earl J, et al. Anticipation in familial pancreatic cancer. Gut 2006;55(2):252–8.
24. Goggins M, Schutte M, Lu J, et al. Germline BRCA2 gene mutations in patients with apparently sporadic pancreatic carcinomas. Cancer Res 1996;56(23):5360–4.
25. Murphy KM, Brune KA, Griffin C, et al. Evaluation of candidate genes MAP2K4, MADH4, ACVR1B, and BRCA2 in familial pancreatic cancer. Cancer Res 2002; 62(13):3789–93.
26. Zhang F, Ma J, Wu J, et al. PALB2 links BRCA1 and BRCA2 in the DNA-damage response. Curr Biol 2009;19(6):524–9.
27. Jones S, Hruban RH, Kamiyama M, et al. Exomic sequencing identifies PALB2 as a pancreatic cancer susceptibility gene. Science 2009;324(5924):217.
28. Slater EP, Langer P, Niemczyk E, et al. PALB2 mutations in European familial pancreatic cancer families. Clin Genet 2010;78(5):490–4.
29. Taylor AMR, Byrd PJ. Molecular pathology of ataxia telangiectasia. J Clin Pathol 2005;58(10):1009–15.
30. Roberts NJ, Jiao Y, Yu J, et al. ATM mutations in hereditary pancreatic cancer patients. Cancer Discov 2012;2(1):41–6.
31. Canto MI, Hruban RH, Fishman EK, et al. Frequent detection of pancreatic lesions in asymptomatic high-risk individuals. Gastroenterology 2012;142(4):796–804 [quiz: e14–5].
32. Shi C, Klein AP, Goggins M, et al. Increased prevalence of precursor lesions in familial pancreatic cancer patients. Clin Cancer Res 2009;15(24):7737–43.
33. Tanaka M, Fernández-del Castillo C, Adsay V, et al. International consensus guidelines 2012 for the management of IPMN and MCN of the pancreas. Pancreatology 2012;12(3):183–97.
34. Mandai K, Uno K, Yasuda K. Does a family history of pancreatic ductal adenocarcinoma and cyst size influence the follow-up strategy for intraductal papillary mucinous neoplasms of the pancreas? Pancreas 2014;43(6):917–21.
35. Nehra D, Oyarvide VM, Mino-Kenudson M, et al. Intraductal papillary mucinous neoplasms: does a family history of pancreatic cancer matter? Pancreatology 2012;12(4):358–63.
36. Hruban RH, Takaori K, Klimstra DS, et al. An illustrated consensus on the classification of pancreatic intraepithelial neoplasia and intraductal papillary mucinous neoplasms. Am J Surg Pathol 2004;28(8):977–87.
37. Hruban RH, Maitra A, Goggins M. Update on pancreatic intraepithelial neoplasia. Int J Clin Exp Pathol 2008;1(4):306–16.
38. Brune K, Abe T, Canto M, et al. Multifocal neoplastic precursor lesions associated with lobular atrophy of the pancreas in patients having a strong family history of pancreatic cancer. Am J Surg Pathol 2006;30(9):1067–76.

39. Matthaei H, Schulick RD, Hruban RH, et al. Cystic precursors to invasive pancreatic cancer. Nat Rev Gastroenterol Hepatol 2011;8(3):141–50.
40. Crippa S, Fernández-Del Castillo C, Salvia R, et al. Mucin-producing neoplasms of the pancreas: an analysis of distinguishing clinical and epidemiologic characteristics. Clin Gastroenterol Hepatol 2010;8(2):213–9.

Preoperative Stenting for Benign and Malignant Periampullary Diseases
Unnecessary if Not Harmful

Sepideh Gholami, MD[a], Murray F. Brennan, MD[b],*

KEYWORDS

- Preoperative stenting • Obstructive jaundice • Periampullary cancer
- Preoperative biliary drainage

KEY POINTS

- Preoperative biliary drainage (PBD) is often performed in patients with jaundice with the presumption that it will decrease the risk of postoperative complications.
- PBD carries its own risk of complications and, therefore, has been controversial.
- Multiple randomized controlled trials and metaanalyses have shown that PBD has significantly increased overall complications compared with surgery alone.
- The routine application of PBD should be avoided except in a subset of clinical situations.

INTRODUCTION

Although many patients are asymptomatic, among the leading symptoms at initial presentation of patients with a periampullary tumor is pruritus from icterus or obstructive jaundice. It is established that surgery in patients with jaundice can lead to coagulopathy, infection, renal dysfunction, and an increased risk of postoperative complications and worse outcomes.[1,2] Hyperbilirubinemia has been identified as a risk factor for poor outcomes in numerous studies.[3–5] It was believed that by reversing this pathophysiologic disturbance, preoperative biliary drainage (PBD) would lead to improved outcomes in patients with jaundice. Dr AO Whipple and colleagues[6] suggested that a 2-staged surgical approach, by use of a bypass to reduce preoperative hyperbilirubinemia, would improve hepatic function in patients with obstructive jaundice, whereas Brunschwig[7] at the authors' institution reported a 1-stage procedure in 1937. Currently, PBD is mostly achieved by placement of a common bile duct stent during diagnostic endoscopic

This study was supported in part by NIH/NCI P30 CA008748 (Cancer Center Support Grant).
Disclosure Statement: The authors have nothing to disclose.
[a] Department of Surgery, Memorial Sloan Kettering Cancer Center, 1275 York Avenue, C-1272, New York, NY 10065, USA; [b] Memorial Sloan Kettering Cancer Center, International Center, 1275 York Avenue, H-1203, New York, NY 10065, USA
* Corresponding author.
E-mail address: brennanm@mskcc.org

Surg Clin N Am 98 (2018) 37–47
https://doi.org/10.1016/j.suc.2017.09.005
0039-6109/18/© 2017 Elsevier Inc. All rights reserved.

surgical.theclinics.com

retrograde cholangiopancreatography or, alternatively, by percutaneous transhepatic drainage before surgical intervention.[8,9] Although initial studies showed that PBD may reduce postoperative mortality rates in jaundiced patients, more recent publications have challenged such results and presumed advantages of PBD.[10,11] This article reviews the most relevant data regarding the use of PBD in patients with benign and malignant periampullary tumors, and presents the authors' current practice and recommendations.

THE PROBLEM: INCREASED INFECTIOUS COMPLICATIONS WITH PREOPERATIVE BILIARY DRAINAGE

PBD before pancreaticoduodenectomy leads to colonization of sterile bile and consequently increases risk of infections, including surgical site infection, cholangitis, and sepsis. Numerous studies have shown that subjects undergoing PBD have higher rates of positive intraoperative bile cultures and carry higher infectious-related morbidity and mortality. In an early study from the authors' institution, Povoski and colleagues[12] reviewed 161 subjects who underwent pancreaticoduodenectomy with available intraoperative bile cultures and showed positive bile cultures in 58% of subjects and similar organism profiles of intraoperative bile cultures and associated blood cultures. On multivariate analysis, the investigators showed that PBD was associated with increased risk of postoperative infectious complications, including wound infections, intraabdominal abscess formation, and death. Together, their results suggested that PBD should be avoided due its associated complication rates.

PREOPERATIVE BILIARY DRAINAGE VERSUS EARLY SURGERY: REVIEW OF CURRENT DATA
Randomized Controlled Trials

Six randomized controlled trials (RCTs) failed to show any significant clinical benefit from routine stenting and demonstrated increased postoperative complications and poor outcome. The presumed benefits of PBD are largely theoretic.

The best designed multicenter RCT, from the Netherlands, examined 202 subjects with periampullary tumors and obstructive jaundice (bilirubin level 2.3–14.6 mg/dL) who were randomized to PBD for 4 to 6 weeks versus surgery alone within 1 week of study enrollment.[13] The primary examined outcome was the rate of severe complications during the treatment and within 120 days of randomization. A severe complication was defined as any complication related to endoscopic biliary drainage or the surgical procedure leading to additional invasive interventions and subsequent increased length of stay, readmission for disease related morbidity, or mortality. Secondary endpoints evaluated were number of invasive procedures, costs, length of hospital stay, and quality of life. PBD was successful in 94% of the subjects with a complication rate of 46%. The trial showed a lower rate of serious complications in the early surgery group compared with PBD (39% vs 74%; risk ratio [RR] = 0.54, 95% CI 0.41–0.71, $P<.001$), with equivalent postoperative surgical complication rates, mortality, and hospital stay. Based on the increased complication and morbidity, the investigators concluded that routine use of PBD in patients with obstructive jaundice was not recommended.

Similarly, other RCTs have shown that PBD is associated with equivalent or higher complication rates.[14–17] Drainage-related complication rates, hospital stay, overall morbidity, and mortality reported in these individual studies are summarized in **Table 1**.

Retrospective Studies, Metaanalysis, and Reviews

A series of retrospective studies, summarized in **Table 2**, have been published on this topic. Most of these show that PBD is associated with higher infectious

Table 1
Randomized controlled trials of preoperative biliary drainage versus direct surgery for obstructive jaundice

Study, Year	Total Number of Subjects	Treatment Group	Number of Subjects	Drainage Route	Drainage-Related Complication Rate (%)	Hospital Stay (d)	Morbidity (%)	Mortality Number (%)
Hatfield et al,[14] 1982	57	PBD	28	PTBD	>50	NA	14	4 (14)
		DS	29			NA	14	4 (14)
Lai et al,[15] 1994	87	PBD	43	Endoscopic	28	NA	37	6 (14)
		DS	44				41	6 (14)
McPherson et al,[16] 1984	65	PBD	34	PTBD	>50	40	39	11 (31)
		DS	31			23	41	6 (19)
Pitt et al,[17] 1985	75	PBD	37	PTBD	27	31	57	3 (8)
		DS	38			23	53	2 (5)
Van der Gaag et al,[13] 2010	202	PBD	102	Endoscopic	46	15	47[a]	15 (15)
		DS	96			13	37	12 (13)

Abbreviations: DS, direct surgery; NA, not available; PTBD, percutaneous transhepatic biliary drainage.
[a] Statistically significant difference with $P < .05$.

Table 2
Retrospective series of preoperative biliary stent versus no stent for obstructive jaundice

Reference, Year	N	Group	Infectious Complications (%)	Wound Infections (%)	Intraabdominal Abscess (%)	Pancreatic Leak or Fistula (%)	Morbidity (%)	Mortality (%)
Povoski et al,[12] 1999	126	Stented	41a	NA	19a	NA	55a	8a
	114	Unstented	25	NA	8	NA	39	3
Sohn et al,[18] 2000	408	Stented	32	10	4	10	35	2
	159	Unstented	22	4	6	4	30	3
Pisters et al,[19] 2001	172	Stented	37	13a	39	0	88	1
	93	Unstented	31	4	37	0	86	1
Martignoni et al,[20] 2001	99	Stented	25	5	0	1	50	2
	158	Unstented	22	6	3	3	45	3
Srivastava et al,[21] 2001	54	Stented	52a	43a	28a	20a	48	15
	67	Unstented	29	24	15	5	46	12
Sewnath et al,[22] 2002	232	Stented	37	7	16	14	50	1
	58	Unstented	31	9	16	7	55	0
Mezhir et al,[23] 2009	94	Stented	32a	20a	12a	4	51	0
	94	Unstented	13	7	3	6	41	5
Coates et al,[24] 2009	56	Stented	18	5	7	7	37	4
	34	Unstented	21	9	12	12	47	15

[a] Statistically significant difference between stented and unstented group with $P<.05$.

complications,[12,21,23] increased wound infections and intraabdominal abscesses,[12,21,23] pancreatic fistula rate,[21] and higher overall morbidity and mortality rates[12]

A metaanalysis by Sewnath and colleagues[22] showed that PBD carried no benefit and thus was not recommended to be performed routinely for malignant obstructive jaundice. Similarly, a Cochrane review published in 2008 demonstrated no clear evidence for routine drainage in this patient population.[25] Most recently, Fang and colleagues[26] reanalyzed and updated the previous metaanalysis to include the newest trial by van der Gaag and colleague.[13] This study of 520 subjects reviewed 6 randomized studies evaluating the safety and effectiveness of PBD (n = 265) versus no drainage with early surgery (n = 255). Two out of the 6 randomized trials used an endoscopic approach and 4 used a transhepatic biliary approach with a wide range of duration of drainage in 4 trials (reported mean of 7–43 days and 4–6 weeks[13]). For outcomes, they assessed rate of serious morbidity and mortality, length of hospital stay, cost, and quality of life.

The data extraction was performed by 2 independent reviewers who identified higher overall serious morbidity (grade III or IV, Clavien-Dindo classification) in the PBD group compared with early surgery (RR = 1.66; 95% CI 1.28–2.16, $P<.001$) without a significant difference in mortality (RR = 1.12; 95% CI 0.73–1.71, $P = .60$). Additionally, the investigators showed no significant difference in length of hospital stay between the 2 groups (mean difference of 4.48 days; 95% CI 1.28–11.28, $P = .12$). Quality of life and cost data were not reported in any of the trials to draw any objective conclusions about those outcomes. Based on these results, the investigators concluded that combination of PBD followed by surgery increased the rate of serious complications compared with that of surgery alone, without significant clinical advantages. Outcomes for serious complications and mortality and published forest plots are presented in **Figs. 1** and **2**, respectively.

EFFECTS ON PREOPERATIVE BILIARY DRAINAGE ON SURVIVAL

Whether PBD and the associated delay in surgery in patients with malignant pancreatic head tumors affects survival was evaluated in a multicenter trial by Eshuis and colleagues.[27] Subjects with a bilirubin of 2 to 14 mg/dL were randomized into drainage group (PBD) for 4 to 6 weeks or to proceed with early surgery (ES; <1 week). The

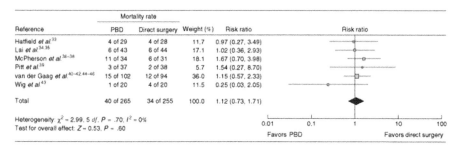

Fig. 1. Mortality rates and forest plot of randomized trials reported on PBD before surgery compared with direct surgery. A Mantel–Haenszel fixed-effect model was used for metaanalysis. RRs are shown with 95% CI. *df*, degrees of freedom. (*From* Fang Y, Gurusamy KS, Wang Q, et al. Meta-analysis of randomized clinical trials on safety and efficacy of biliary drainage before surgery for obstructive jaundice. Br J Surg 2013;100(12):1593; with permission.)

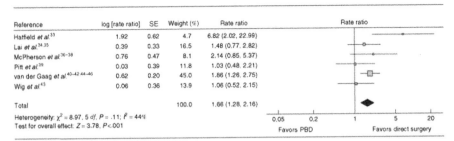

Fig. 2. Adverse events in trials that used PBD before surgery and those that did not (direct surgery). Data are shown in a logarithmic scale. An inverse-variance fixed-effect model was used for metaanalysis. Rate ratios are shown with 95% CI. (*From* Fang Y, Gurusamy KS, Wang Q, et al. Meta-analysis of randomized clinical trials on safety and efficacy of biliary drainage before surgery for obstructive jaundice. Br J Surg 2013;100(12):1593; with permission.)

investigators found that PBD and the associated delay in surgery did not affect overall survival compared with early surgery. The median survival times were comparable at 12.2 and 12.7 months in the ES and PBD group, respectively (**Fig. 3**). There was no difference in complete resection (R0) rates (73% in the ES group vs 62% in the PBD group). Univariate and multivariate analysis of predictive factors affecting overall survival of subjects who underwent surgery is shown in **Table 3**.

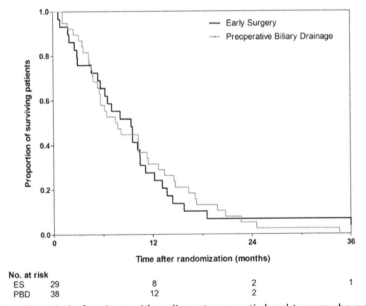

Fig. 3. Overall survival of patients with malignant pancreatic head tumors who were randomized to early surgery (ES) or PBD and underwent subsequent resection. (*From* Eshuis WJ, van der Gaag NA, Rauws EA, et al. Therapeutic delay and survival after surgery for cancer of the pancreatic head with or without preoperative biliary drainage. Ann Surg 2010;252(5):1593; with permission.)

Table 3 Univariate and multivariate analysis of predictive factors for overall survival in 180 subjects who underwent surgery for a malignant pancreatic head mass		
	Univariable, HR (95% CI)	Multivariable, HR (95%)
Time from randomization to surgery 1-wk increment	0.98 (0.92–1.05)	0.91 (0.84–0.99)[a]
Age, 1-y increment[b]	1.00 (0.98–1.02)	1.00 (0.98–1.01)
Female sex	1.06 (0.76–1.48)	1.26 (0.87–1.80)
Bilirubin at randomization (quartiles), 1 quartile increment	1.17 (1.01–1.35)[a]	1.22 (1.04–1.43)[a]
Underwent PBD	0.90 (0.65–1.24)	NA
Resection of tumor	0.32 (0.23–0.46)[c]	0.28 (0.20–0.41)[c]
Blood transfusion intraoperatively	1.10 (0.71–1.71)	1.25 (0.79–1.98)
Complications related to PBD and/or surgery	1.09 (0.79–1.51)	1.45 (1.01–2.09)[a]

Abbreviation: HR, hazard ratio.
 [a] Significant at $P<.05$ level.
 [b] At the time of surgery.
 [c] Significant at $P<.01$ level.
 From Eshuis WJ, van der Gaag NA, Rauws EA, et al. Therapeutic delay and survival after surgery for cancer of the pancreatic head with or without preoperative biliary drainage. Ann Surg 2010;252(5):845; with permission.

PLASTIC VERSUS METAL STENTS

In patients with unresectable pancreatic head tumors, metal stents are superior and preferred compared with plastic stents, whether the same is true for patients with resectable tumors when early surgery is not feasible remains an area of controversy. An attempt to answer this question was made by Crippa and colleagues[28] in a meta-analysis of 5 studies, including 1 prospective trial[29] and 4 retrospective studies,[30–33] with a total of 704 subjects (**Table 4**). The investigators evaluated the rate of endoscopic reintervention (stent failure) and overall complications as primary and secondary outcomes, respectively. They demonstrated that the rate of PBD stent failure was significantly lower in the metal stent group (3.4%) than in the plastic stent group (14.8%) (odds ratio [OR] = 0.15, 95% CI 0.05–0.46, $P = .0009$). Overall complications were lower in the metal stent group compared with the group of subjects with plastic stents (OR = 0.64, 95% CI 0.37–1.10, $P = .11$). The investigators concluded that metal stents are more effective than plastic stents and should be preferred when early surgery without PBD is not feasible. This study has several limitations, including the retrospective nature of most of the studies and lack of information regarding the specific stent type reported in most studies.

COSTS OF PREOPERATIVE BILIARY DRAINAGE

Given the increased complication rate and morbidity associated with PBD, a British group evaluated the economic implications of PBD versus direct surgery for subjects with obstructive jaundice.[34] In their model, the investigators estimated the mean costs and quality-adjusted life years per patient in the UK National Health Service over 6 months and demonstrated that PBD was more costly than surgery alone (mean cost per patient $15,616 compared with $11,914). They reported fewer quality-adjusted life years per patient in the PBD group (mean 0.337 vs 0.343). Based on their

Table 4
Summary of studies comparing plastic versus metal stents and reported rates of stent failure, overall complications, and postoperative mortality rates

Reference, Year	Study Design	Total Number of Subjects	Type of Stent (N)	Rate of Stent Failure (%)	Overall Complications Rate Related to Drainage Before Surgery (%)	Overall Pancreatic Anastomotic Leak (%)	Overall Postoperative Mortality (%)
Tol et al,[29] 2016	Prospective Multicenter	151 —	Plastic (102) Metal (49)	30 4	46 24	8 2	15 6
Haapamäki et al,[30] 2014	Retrospective —	191 —	Plastic (163) Metal (28)	7 3	3 4	15 7	0 0
Cavell et al,[31] 2013	Retrospective —	220 —	Plastic (149) Metal (71)	NA NA	NA NA	13 7	0 0
Adams et al,[32] 2012	Retrospective —	113 —	Plastic (70) Metal (43)	NA NA	21 3	NA NA	NA NA
Decker et al,[33] 2011	Retrospective —	29 —	Plastic (18) Metal (11)	39 0	NA NA	0 0	NA NA

statistical model, they calculated a cost savings of more than $3600 per patient when PBD was avoided. These results present evidence to avoid interventions that are not clinically necessary.

INDICATIONS FOR PREOPERATIVE STENTING FOR SELECTED CLINICAL SITUATION

There are several clinical circumstances in which the authors think that PBD could be beneficial. First, one should consider PBD in patients with debilitating pruritus or in cases when further extended workup is needed or a surgical intervention cannot be scheduled in a timely fashion for logistical reasons. Another group of patients in whom PBD is recommended is those who present with signs of systemic infections, such as cholangitis, and require emergent decompression. PBD is typically recommended in cases with secondary systemic organ dysfunction, most importantly compromised renal function or anticipated major vascular reconstruction, to avoid increased risks of vascular thrombosis and liver ischemia. PBD is also indicated in patients who are scheduled to receive neoadjuvant systemic therapy before surgical intervention. A metal stent should be used in these situations due to better stent patency and lower reintervention and complication rates. The level of bilirubin that should stimulate a discussion about whether to stent is unknown; because 14 mg/dL has been used as the upper limit of bilirubin level in RCTs, values above that level could be used to consider stenting.

SUMMARY AND AUTHORS' RECOMMENDATIONS

The authors do not recommend routine PBD in asymptomatic jaundiced patients with benign or malignant periampullary tumors before resection. We prefer selective PBD for patients with long-standing jaundice or cholangitis, renal impairment, severe malnutrition, neoadjuvant chemotherapy, debilitating pruritus affecting quality of life, or any special circumstance that delays a surgical procedure. We prefer the endoscopic approach for biliary drainage for periampullary tumors. Percutaneous transhepatic biliary drainage should be undertaken only in cases of failure of endoscopic approaches.

In the selected cases previously outlined, we recommend admitting the patient the night before surgery for hydration to prevent postoperative renal insufficiency. Despite the lack of benefit proven by several level 1 data, most patients are evaluated and stented before surgical evaluation. The authors stress the need for comprehensive surgical evaluation before a decision concerning to invasive biliary drainage.

REFERENCES

1. Armstrong CP, Dixon JM, Taylor TV, et al. Surgical experience of deeply jaundiced patients with bile duct obstruction. Br J Surg 1984;71:234–8.
2. Greig JD, Krukowski ZH, Matheson NA. Surgical morbidity and mortality in one hundred and twenty-nine patients with obstructive jaundice. Br J Surg 1988;75:216–9.
3. Blamey SL, Fearon KC, Gilmour WH, et al. Prediction of risk in biliary surgery. Br J Surg 1983;70:535–8.
4. Kawarada Y, Higashiguchi T, Yokoi H, et al. Preoperative biliary drainage in obstructive jaundice. Hepatogastroenterology 1995;42:300–7.
5. Dixon JM, Armstrong CP, Duffy SW, et al. Factors affecting mortality and morbidity after surgery for obstructive jaundice. Gut 1984;25:104.

6. Whipple AO, Parsons WB, Mullins CR. Treatment of carcinoma of the ampulla of Vater. Ann Surg 1935;102:763–79.

7. Brunschwig A. Resection of head of pancreas and duodenum for carcinoma pancreatoduodenectomy. Surg Gynecol Obstet 1937;65:681–4.

8. Pancreatric Section, British Society of Gastroenterology, Pancreatic Society of Great Britain and Ireland, Association of Upper Gastrointestinal Surgeons of Great Britain and Ireland, Royal College of Pathologists, Special Interest Group for Gastro-Intestinal Radiology. Guidelines for the management of patients with pancreatic cancer periampullary and ampullary carcinomas. Gut 2005; 54(Suppl 5):v1–16.

9. Glenn F, Evans JA, Mujahed Z, et al. Percutaneous transhepatic cholangiography. Ann Surg 1962;156:451–62.

10. Nakayama T, Ikeda A, Okuda K. Percutaneous transhepatic drainage of the biliary tract: technique and results in 104 cases. Gastroenterology 1978;74: 554–9.

11. Takada T, Hanyu F, Kobayashi S, et al. Percutaneous transhepatic cholangial drainage: direct approach under fluoroscopic control. J Surg Oncol 1976;8: 83–97.

12. Povoski SP, Karpeh MS, Conlon KC, et al. Association of preoperative biliary drainage with postoperative outcome following pancreaticoduodenectomy. Ann Surg 1999;230:131–42.

13. Van der Gaag NA, Rauws EA, van Eijck CH, et al. Preoperative biliary drainage for cancer of the head of the pancreas. N Engl J Med 2010;362:129–37.

14. Hatfield AR, Tobias R, Terblanche J, et al. Preoperative external biliary drainage in obstructive jaundice. A prospective controlled clinical trial. Lancet 1982;2: 896–9.

15. Lai EC, Mok FP, Fan ST, et al. Preoperative endoscopic drainage for malignant obstructive jaundice. Br J Surg 1994;81:1195–8.

16. McPherson GA, Benjamin IS, Hodgson HJ, et al. Pre-operative percutaneous transhepatic biliary drainage: the results of a controlled trial. Br J Surg 1984; 71:371–5.

17. Pitt HA, Gomes AS, Lois JF, et al. Does preoperative percutaneous biliary drainage reduce operative risk or increase hospital cost? Ann Surg 1985;201: 545–53.

18. Sohn TA, Yeo CJ, Cameron JL, et al. Pancreaticoduodenectomy: role of interventional radiologists in managing patients and complications. J Gastrointest Surg 2003;7(2):209–19.

19. Pisters PW, Hudec WA, Hess KR, et al. Effect of preoperative biliary decompression on pancreaticoduodenectomy-associated morbidity in 300 consecutive patients. Ann Surg 2001;234:47–55.

20. Martignoni ME, Wagner M, Krähenbühl L, et al. Effect of preoperative biliary drainage on surgical outcome after pancreatoduodenectomy. Am J Surg 2001; 181(1):52–9.

21. Srivastava S, Sikora SS, Kumar A, et al. Outcome following pancreaticoduodenectomy in patients undergoing preoperative biliary drainage. Dig Surg 2001; 18:381–7.

22. Sewnath ME, Karsten TM, Prins MH, et al. A meta-analysis on the efficacy of preoperative biliary drainage for tumors causing obstructive jaundice. Ann Surg 2002;236:17–27.

23. Mezhir JJ, Brennan MF, Baser RE, et al. A matched case-control study of preoperative biliary drainage in patients with pancreatic adenocarcinoma: routine drainage is not justified. J Gastrointest Surg 2009;13:2163–9.
24. Coates JM, Beal SH, Russo JE, et al. Negligible effect of selective preoperative biliary drainage on perioperative resuscitation, morbidity, and mortality in patients undergoing pancreaticoduodenectomy. Arch Surg 2009;144(9):841–7.
25. Wang Q, Gurusamy KS, Lin H, et al. Preoperative biliary drainage for obstructive jaundice. Cochrane Database Syst Rev 2008;(3):CD005444.
26. Fang Y, Gurusamy KS, Wang Q, et al. Meta-analysis of randomized clinical trials on safety and efficacy of biliary drainage before surgery for obstructive jaundice. Br J Surg 2013;100(12):1589–96.
27. Eshuis WJ, van der Gaag NA, Rauws EA, et al. Therapeutic delay and survival after surgery for cancer of the pancreatic head with or without preoperative biliary drainage. Ann Surg 2010;252(5):840–9.
28. Crippa S, Cirocchi R, Partelli S, et al. Systematic review and meta-analysis of metal versus plastic stents for preoperative biliary drainage in resectable periampullary or pancreatic head tumors. Eur J Surg Oncol 2016;42(9):1278–85.
29. Tol JAMG, van Hooft JE, Timmer R, et al. Metal or plastic stents for preoperative biliary drainage in resectable pancreatic cancer. Gut 2016;65(12):1981–7.
30. Haapamäki C, Seppanen H, Udd M, et al. Preoperative biliary decompression preceding pancreaticoduodenectomy with plastic or self- expandable metallic stent. Scand J Surg 2015;104:79–85.
31. Cavell LK, Allen PJ, Vinoya C, et al. Biliary self-expandable metal stents do not adversely affect pancreaticoduodenectomy. Am J Gastroenterol 2013;108: 1168–73.
32. Adams MA, Anderson MA, Myles JD, et al. Self-expanding metal stents (SEMS) provide superior outcomes compared to plastic stents for pancreatic cancer patients undergoing neoadjuvant therapy. J Gastrointest Oncol 2012;3:309–13.
33. Decker C, Christein JD, Phadnis MA, et al. Biliary metal stents are superior to plastic stents for preoperative biliary decompression in pancreatic cancer. Surg Endosc 2011;25:2364–7.
34. Morris S, Gurusamy KS, Sheringham J, et al. Cost-effectiveness of preoperative biliary drainage for obstructive jaundice in pancreatic and periampullary cancer. J Surg Res 2015;193(1):202–9.

A Tale of 2 Techniques
Preoperative Biliary Drainage and Routine Surgical Drainage with Pancreaticoduodenectomy

Mazen E. Iskandar, MD[a],*, Michael G. Wayne, DO[b], Justin G. Steele, MD[b], Avram M. Cooperman, MD[b]

KEYWORDS

- Pancreatectomy • Whipple procedure • Pancreatic cancer • Jaundice
- Biliary stenting • Drainage

KEY POINTS

- Deeply jaundiced patients benefit from biliary stenting with improvement of liver function, well being, immune function and nutritional status.
- Selective stenting for patients undergoing pancreaticoduodenectomy should be considered in patients with symptomatic jaundice or biliary obstruction, with biliary obstruction before neoadjuvant chemotherapy, for whom evaluation or optimization may be prolonged and therapy delayed, or with altered liver function and significant cardiac or renal disease.
- A well-placed, well-functioning drain after pancreaticoduodenectomy may not always be necessary, but it could prove invaluable and lifesaving.

INTRODUCTION

Challenging common surgical traditions is always welcome, particularly if it eliminates unnecessary practices and leads to better outcomes. Preoperative drainage of an obstructed bile duct and liver before pancreaticoduodenal resection (PDR), and placement of intraabdominal drains following pancreatic resection, have been suggested to be unnecessary and associated with a higher complication rate, although with a similar hospital stay and course, compared with a no-drain or no-stent approach. This article reviews the rationale of a 40-year evolution of understanding and practice regarding biliary stenting and postoperative drains.

Disclosure Statement: The authors have nothing to disclose.
[a] Department of Surgery, Mount Sinai Beth Israel, 10 Union Square East, Suite 2M, New York, NY 10003, USA; [b] The Pancreas, Biliary and Advanced Laparoscopy Center of New York, 305 Second Avenue, New York, NY 10003, USA
* Corresponding author.
E-mail address: mazenelia.iskandar@mountsinai.org

PREOPERATIVE BILIARY STENTING

Involvement of surgeons in treating malignant biliary obstruction came about by necessity and not design. Absent imaging, endoscopy, and nuclear medicine, surgery was a diagnostic and therapeutic modality until 40 years ago. At the end of the nineteenth century, and before resecting an ampullary tumor by segmental duodenal resection, including a wedge resection of the head of the pancreas, Halsted[1] fashioned a cholecystogastrostomy as the first of a 2-stage procedure to decompress the obstructed liver. Absent endoscopy and body imaging, the diagnosis of jaundice relied on abdominal exploration. Even when axial imaging became available, its acceptance as a preoperative predictor of tumor resectability was slow, as was acceptance of biliary endoscopy, including sonography, and stenting of obstructed bile ducts. In many centers, surgery continued as a diagnostic, palliative, and curative procedure so as not to deny cancer of the pancreas (CaP) patients the chance of cure. Though difficult to believe today, the operative mortality in patients undergoing open, palliative, biliary bypass between 1965 and 1980 averaged 29% (range 7%–50%).[2] This was a reflection of late-stage disease at presentation rather than technical issues and morbidity from the bypass itself. This was reinforced by Shapiro[3] who reported a mean operative mortality of 21% after PDR from large institutions by well-known, accomplished surgeons. Patients characteristically were jaundiced, anorectic, and had late-stage disease and limited survival regardless of therapy.

When Molnar and Stockum,[4] in Europe, and Ring and colleagues,[5] in the United States, developed percutaneous transhepatic cholangiography (PTC), it permitted preoperative visualization of the biliary tree, reduced the need for diagnostic laparotomy, and allowed external-internal drainage to decompress the obstructed liver. The ability to internalize catheters in the duodenum and exchange obstructed catheters avoided the sequela of bile loss and made patient care, catheter management, and electrolyte and fluid management more effective. This was soon supplanted by endoscopy and endoscopic retrograde cholangiopancreatograms (ERCPs), which had the added benefits of visualization of the pancreatic duct, avoidance of a percutaneous approach, and the ability to stent 1 or both ducts. It did require a repeat endoscopy and stent exchange when stents occluded. The ability of the liver to recover normal function was an important predictor of survival time. In a study of 46 consecutive jaundiced subjects (mean bilirubin 16 mg/dL) all decompressed by PTC, 17% showed no improvement in liver function or jaundice, 23% had a 50% decrease in LFTs, and the remaining 60% regained normal liver function, appetite, and well-being.[6] The inability to fully correct liver function, and the presence of hepatic metastases were important negative predictors of survival time, regardless of subsequent surgical procedures (**Table 1**). Even when LFTs returned to normal 7 out of 29 who had liver metastases died within 30 days (25%). The inability to predict responders after PTC based on presentation, and the gravity of no or partial response, and presence of hepatic metastases emphasized the necessity of stenting all jaundiced subjects and waiting until a return of normal liver function and well-being before considering resection or systemic therapy. The very limited survival of those whose livers did not clear was sobering. Additionally, fewer postoperative complications and a shorter hospital stay after resection was noted after stenting. The overall 30-day mortality of 28% was similar to the palliative surgical series and confirmed late-stage disease was the cause of the high mortality and surgery could be avoided in many. Studies and trials of preoperative biliary stenting suggest 2 complications after stenting: stent occlusion (less for covered metallic than plastic stents) and more wound infections after resection.[7] Hospital stay, fistulas, and all other complications were similar. The beneficial effects of stents are easily overlooked (relief of

Table 1				
Response of 46 subjects with malignant biliary obstruction to decompression by percutaneous transhepatic cholangiography				
Group	Bilirubin Response	Number of Subjects	Average Survival (d)	30-d Mortality (%)
I (good response)	Return to normal (average 17—> 2 mg/dL)	29 (63%)	198	10
II (intermediate response)	50% decline (average 18—>9 mg/dL)	9 (20%)	72	33
III (poor response)	No change (average 18—>17 mg/dL)	8 (17%)	12	88
	Total	46	141	28

Abbreviation: ->; decreased to.

jaundice and obstructive symptoms, improved liver function, and increased appetite and sense of well-being) because disease is detected before symptoms are present. In good measure, this represents lead time bias, the detection of lesions by axial imaging before obstructive symptoms, and an apparent longer survival but not more cures. Although the bile duct is colonized after stenting, bacteria in bile only cause symptoms after biliary obstruction. Wound infections after pancreatic surgery are multifactorial and include length of surgery, high body mass index (BMI), and cardiac disease. These may equal or outweigh the influence of stents as a causative agent.

Additional benefits of stenting are predicated on less obvious hepatic function that improved after stenting (see following sections).

Improved Overall Immunity

Biliary decompression reduces endotoxemia and cytokines, improves immune response, and decreases bacterial translocation and inflammation, which decreases cholangitis and liver failure.[8] Biliary obstruction also decreases the reticuloendothelial system function, Kupffer cell function, and endotoxin clearance. Elevation in tumor necrosis factor and interleukin-8 levels were observed in jaundiced animals.[9]

Improvement in Coagulopathy

Hemostatic derangements and hepatic dysfunction associated with jaundice include decreased production of coagulation factors and absorption of vitamin K–dependent factors II, VII, IX, and X, altering the coagulopathy and thrombophilia balance.[10]

Improvement in Renal Function

Renal failure in biliary obstruction is associated with release of atrial natriuretic peptide (ANP) causing extracellular water depletion, and increased renin and aldosterone secretion. The resulting myocardial dysfunction can cause further renal hypoperfusion, and, eventually, hepatorenal syndrome.[11–13]

Improvement in Cardiac Function

Obstructive jaundice is associated with decreased myocardial contractility, which is related to ANP elevation. ANP contributes to cardiac dysfunction by vasodilation. Padillo and colleagues[14] reported that biliary drainage decreased ANP, increased cardiac output, and restored cardiac function to normal.

Other factors that influence stenting in the jaundiced patient include referral patterns and neoadjuvant chemotherapy (see following sections).

Referral patterns

Today, decisions regarding stenting are made long before surgical consultation. Endoscopists frequently place stents when biliary and pancreatic obstruction is diagnosed for decompression. More than 50% of subjects referred for ERCP are stented, and more than 75% are stented before surgical consultation.[15]

Neoadjuvant chemotherapy

Neoadjuvant treatment was originally intended for regionally unresectable lesions and then for borderline resectable lesions. It is used increasingly for resectable lesions. It recognizes that CaP is a systemic disease and upfront treatment ensures all patients receive systemic therapy. This is important because up to 50% receive no adjuvant therapy after resection because of complications. During neoadjuvant therapy, 25% of lesions progress and reimagining shows metastases, and unnecessary surgery is avoided.[16,17] Patients who respond to systemic treatment have more favorable tumor biology and a longer survival. Considering the morbidity associated with pancreatic surgery, deliberate selection of candidates for resection is wise and necessary.

Systemic chemotherapy is far from ideal. Only a few patients derive significant benefit from chemotherapy or PDR, and both are entrenched. At the least, chemotherapy first helps select suitable candidates for resection and avoids an unnecessary operation for those who progress or remain unresectable. Surgeons who are reluctant to add biliary sepsis to the list of complications are liberal in stenting at any sign of obstruction.

To Stent or Not to Stent

The preceding laboratory and clinical evidence cites why and when biliary stenting before definitive treatment is logical and beneficial in a subset of jaundiced, obstructed, or symptomatic patients. Because pancreatic cancer is often detected incidentally by imaging and not by symptoms, stents are less necessary. The selective use of stents follows the change in presentation of disease. In medicine, the case for never stenting is almost nonexistent. The case for selective stenting is based on evolution, outcomes, experience, judgment, and evidence. The widespread use of axial imaging and endoscopy has led to the detection of asymptomatic and incidental pancreatic and periampullary lesions. Nearly half of pancreatic resections and PDRs are for nonpancreatic cancer, much different than 15 to 20 years ago when nearly all PDRs were for CaP. However, the immediate goals of surgery are unchanged: live patients with low mortality or morbidity. The issue of preoperative biliary decompression and stenting has been moot since the 1990s when endoscopists began to stent biliary obstruction, before referrals to other physicians. The authors continue to advocate and use selective stenting for:

- Symptomatic jaundiced or obstructed patients
- The obstructed patient before neoadjuvant chemotherapy
- The patient whose evaluation or optimization may be prolonged and therapy delayed
- Patients with altered liver function and significant cardiac or renal disease.

TO DRAIN OR NOT TO DRAIN THE OPERATIVE AREA

It is refreshing and laudable when traditional practices are questioned. Surgery is taught as a preceptorship whereby residents incorporate, adapt, and modify operations and procedures learned. The practice of placing drains near intraabdominal anastomoses during abdominal surgery was customary when fistulas, leaks, and collections were common. As suture materials, bowel preparation, antibiotics, and techniques improved, the use of drains was reserved for anastomoses of viscera absent serosa, where leak rates were higher (rectal, esophageal, and pancreatic anastomoses). That remains the rationale and practice for placing drains below the pancreaticojejunal anastomoses where, ideally, they should, by suction or capillarity, drain pancreatic, biliary, and enteric contents to the outside, thereby limiting infected collections, abscesses, pseudoaneurysms, and bleeding from an eroded gastroduodenal artery. As drains evolved, suction could be applied so the leakage could be collected actively, not passively. This presupposes that the drains are placed and functioning properly, and that the drain openings do not occlude with suction.

There are few papers that have examined eliminating drainage after pancreatic resection. The initial report, by Jeekel[18] in 1992, suggesting drains were not mandatory after PDR, was based on 22 PDR subjects. The initial paper from Memorial Sloan Kettering Cancer Center (MSKCC) cited no advantage to routine drainage but a higher number of fistulas and need for reintervention after drainage.[19] The initial experience was extended and also included the institutional practice of other pancreatic surgeons. The use of drains ranged from almost never, to selective, to always, depending on the individual surgeon.[20] Keeping in mind that the senior surgeons at MSKCC are very experienced, high-volume, adept surgeons, it suggested that experience and judgment strongly influence outcomes. An additional large study of nearly 400 subjects, primarily from a high-volume center in Germany, randomized 202 subjects to drainage and 193 to a control, no-drain group. Drains were passive and there was a higher incidence, 11.9% to 26.4%, of grade B and C fistulas, and fistula-related complications, in the drain group, versus 5.7% to 13% in the control group.[21] The significant open issues of this study were the 42 subjects who did not follow the assigned randomization, 40 of whom were drained, and who had a higher mortality and complication rate, than each of the 2 other groups. What would have happened had they not been drained? Drains could be removed after 2 days and drainage was passive not active. On the other hand, a US multicenter trial was designed to include 375 subjects undergoing PDR randomized to drains or no drains. This study was stopped after 136 PDRs, 68 in each group, because of 12% mortality in the no-drain group versus 3% mortality in the drained group.[22] Mortality was caused by pancreatic fistula, abscesses, and hemorrhage in the no-drain group. Prophylactic abdominal drainage after pancreatic surgery was the subject of a Cochrane database study that reviewed all pertinent studies on postoperative drainage and concluded that the studies were underpowered and the evidence was of low quality, but that early removal of drains was beneficial.[23]

What can be learned from the publications and what is the practice? Drainage after every pancreatic operation may not be mandatory, but effective drainage after some may be wise. Most complications after surgery arise from fistulas from the pancreaticojejunal anastomoses and fistula rates vary widely among surgeons. There is no substitute for experience, good judgment and technique, and accurate analyses and reporting. Minimizing fistula rates would minimize septic complications, abscesses, and hemorrhage. The authors' experience is that effective suction drainage obviates reintervention and precludes determinative errors, which is the authors' term for predicting fistulas based on patient characteristics (BMI, cardiac disease), gland texture (firm, soft), and size of the pancreatic duct.

Pending additional studies and evidence, the authors' practice pattern after PDR and distal resection is to use closed vented drains on continuous low-pressure suction, after intraoperatively ascertaining correct placement and function. The suction is discontinued when drainage is minimal (usually overnight) and the drains shortened and placed in a sealed bag on the skin. Drainage is observed for a few days and, absent a fistula, the drains are removed. Cooperman and colleagues[17] report a PDR experience in with a fistula rate of 6% and routine use of sheathed suction drains. Although pancreatic fistula rates are lower in firm glands with larger pancreatic ducts (1 cm), leaks do develop even after such anastomoses. Being uncertain which anastomoses will leak, the authors use drainage after all pancreatic resections. This has virtually eliminated the need for reoperation or interventional drainage of collections or abscesses. The pancreatic fistulas that occur have been type A and closed spontaneously.

SUMMARY

The need to question ongoing practices is laudable and a necessary part of surgery. Often initiated by experienced physicians who question the necessity of everyday routines, change is slow. Two common practices have been addressed: endoscopic or percutaneous stenting of bile ducts before pancreatic resection and postoperative drainage after pancreatic resection. The authors were early in using, studying, and advocating biliary decompression before considering PDR in jaundiced, symptomatic patients. The difference in mortality, patient well-being, activity, appetite, and recovery before surgery was dramatic and translated to fewer complications and shorter recovery time postresection. After computed tomography scans were introduced (1976) and accepted as a determinant of resectability (around 1990), the use of axial imaging became widespread and common. Jaundice and late-stage disease became less common, as did the need for stenting. Today, stenting is used on a selective basis and is not an all-or-none issue.

The authors' views on postoperative drainage are biased and based on a large pancreatic experience. Having a near-absent interventional rate for abscesses, or collections after drained PDRs, we view postoperative drains as analogous to wearing automotive seat belts. When needed, they can be lifesaving and reduce the extent and impact of injury. A well-placed, well-functioning drain after a PDR may not always be necessary but could prove invaluable and lifesaving with little to no risk.

REFERENCES

1. Halsted WS. Contributions to the surgery of the bile passages, especially of the common bile-duct. Boston Med Surg J 1899;141:645–54.
2. Sarr MG, Cameron JL. Surgical management of unresectable carcinoma of the pancreas. Surgery 1982;91(2):123–33.
3. Shapiro TM. Adenocarcinoma of the pancreas: a statistical analysis of biliary bypass vs Whipple resection in good risk patients. Ann Surg 1975;182(6): 715–21.
4. Molnar W, Stockum AE. Relief of obstructive jaundice through percutaneous transhepatic catheter–a new therapeutic method. Am J Roentgenol Radium Ther Nucl Med 1974;122(2):356–67.
5. Ring EJ, Oleaga JA, Freiman DB, et al. Therapeutic applcations of catheter cholangiography. Radiology 1978;128(2):333–8.
6. Neff RA, Fankuchen EI, Cooperman AM, et al. The radiological management of malignant biliary obstruction. Clin Radiol 1983;34(2):143–6.
7. Van der Gaag NA, Rauws EA, van Eijck CH, et al. Preoperative biliary drainage for cancer of the head of the pancreas. N Engl J Med 2010;362(2):129–37.

8. Kimmings AN, van Deventer SJ, Obertop H, et al. Endotoxin, cytokines, and endotoxin binding proteins in obstructive jaundice and after preoperative biliary drainage. Gut 2000;46(5):725–31.

9. Kuzu MA, Kale IT, Col C, et al. Obstructive jaundice promotes bacterial translocation in humans. Hepatogastroenterology 1999;46:159–64.

10. Papadopoulos V, Filippou D, Manolis E, et al. Haemostasis impairment in patients with obstructive jaundice. J Gastrointestin Liver Dis 2007;16(2):177–86.

11. Padillo FJ, Briceno J, Cruz A, et al. Randomized clinical trial of the effect of intravenous fluid administration on hormonal and renal dysfunction in patients with obstructive jaundice undergoing endoscopic drainage. Br J Surg 2005;92: 39–43, 4790.

12. Padillo FJ, Cruz A, Briceno J, et al. Multivariate analysis of factors associated with renal dysfunction in patients with obstructive jaundice. Br J Surg 2005;92: 1388–92.

13. Wadei HM, Mai ML, Ahsan N, et al. Hepatorenal syndrome: pathophysiology and management. Clin J Am Soc Nephrol 2006;1(5):1066–79.

14. Padillo J, Puente J, Gomez M, et al. Improved cardiac function in patients with obstructive jaundice after internal biliary drainage: hemodynamic and hormonal assessment. Ann Surg 2001;234:652–6.

15. Scheufele F, Schorn S, Demir IE, et al. Preoperative biliary stenting versus operation first in jaundiced patients due to malignant lesions in the pancreatic head: a meta-analysis of current literature. Surgery 2017;161(4):939–50.

16. Tzeng CWD, Tran Cao HS, Lee JE, et al. Treatment sequencing for resectable pancreatic cancer: influence of early metastases and surgical complications on multimodality therapy completion and survival. J Gastrointest Surg 2014;18: 16–25.

17. Cooperman AM, Snady H, Bruckner HW, et al. Long-term follow-up of twenty patients with adenocarcinoma of the pancreas: resection following combined modality therapy. Surg Clin North Am 2001;81(3):699.

18. Jeekel J. No abdominal drainage after Whipple's procedure. Br J Surg 1992; 79(2):182.

19. Conlon KC, Labow D, Leung D, et al. Prospective randomized clinical trial of the value of intraperitoneal drainage after pancreatic resection. Ann Surg 2001; 234(4):487–93.

20. Correa-Gallego C, Brennan MF, D'angelica M, et al. Operative drainage following pancreatic resection: analysis of 1122 patients resected over 5 years at a single institution. Ann Surg 2013;258(6):1051–8.

21. Witzigmann H, Diener MK, Kienkötter S, et al. No need for routine drainage after pancreatic head resection: the dual-center, randomized, controlled PANDRA trial (ISRCTN04937707). Ann Surg 2016;264(3):528–37.

22. Van Buren G, Bloomston M, Hughes SJ, et al. A randomized prospective multicenter trial of pancreaticoduodenectomy with and without routine intraperitoneal drainage. Ann Surg 2014;259(4):605–12.

23. Fong ZV, Ferrone CR, Thayer SP, et al. Understanding hospital readmissions after pancreaticoduodenectomy: can we prevent them?: a 10-year contemporary experience with 1,173 patients at the Massachusetts General Hospital. J Gastrointest Surg 2014;18(1):137–44 [discussion: 144–5].

Timing of Pancreatic Resection and Patient Outcomes: Is There a Difference?

Timothy J. Vreeland, MD[a], Mathew H.G. Katz, MD[b],*

KEYWORDS

- Preoperative therapy
- Pancreatic ductal adenocarcinoma
- Primary resection
- Potentially curable pancreatic cancer

KEY POINTS

- Despite improvements in chemotherapy regimens, the chance of long-term survival in patients treated for pancreatic cancer remains low.
- Failures of local control are frequent after de novo surgery for pancreatic cancer; preoperative therapy may improve the chance of an R0 resection and decrease nodal burden without prohibitive toxicity.
- Pancreatic cancer is a systemic disease and preoperative therapy ensures patients receive the systemic therapy required for optimal outcomes.
- Preoperative therapy maximizes the chance for multimodal therapy and selects for patients who benefit most from surgery.
- Although there will always be a role for primary resection in selected patients, preoperative therapy make sense for most.

INTRODUCTION

In 2016, pancreatic cancer surpassed breast cancer to become the third most common cause of cancer-related death in the United States.[1] In 2017, an estimated 53,670 new cases of pancreatic cancer will be diagnosed and 43,090 pancreatic cancer–related deaths will occur.[2] Although cancer care in general has advanced greatly with vast survival improvements, the median survival of patients with even the most favorable pancreatic cancers has remained around 2 to 2.5 years.[3–5] Although multimodal therapy is key to cure, less than 50% of patients with localized pancreatic cancer receive both surgery and chemotherapy,[6] and even fewer patients with more

Disclosure Statement: The authors have nothing to disclose.
[a] Complex General Surgical Oncology, The University of Texas MD Anderson Cancer Center, 1515 Holcombe Boulevard, Houston, TX 77030, USA; [b] Pancreatic Surgery Service, The University of Texas MD Anderson Cancer Center, 1515 Holcombe Boulevard, Houston, TX 77030, USA
* Corresponding author.
E-mail address: Mhgkatz@mdanderson.org

Surg Clin N Am 98 (2018) 57–71
https://doi.org/10.1016/j.suc.2017.09.006
0039-6109/18/© 2017 Elsevier Inc. All rights reserved.

advanced cancer do. This indicates a need for a critical reassessment of the status quo in the treatment of this disease. This article discusses the current standard of care of localized pancreatic cancer, and reviews controversies, emphasizing the effects of therapy sequence.

CURRENT STANDARD OF CARE

Current standard of care for patients with localized pancreatic cancer consists of both surgery and perioperative chemotherapy; the role of perioperative radiotherapy is uncertain. Traditionally surgery precedes chemotherapy (or radiation), but this sequence has become increasingly controversial, as demonstrated by contrasts between current National Comprehensive Cancer Network (NCCN) guidelines[7] and recently published clinical practice guidelines (CPG) from the American Society of Clinical Oncology (ASCO).[8]

National Comprehensive Cancer Network Guidelines

The NCCN guidelines describe localized pancreatic cancers as resectable, borderline resectable (BR), or locally advanced (LA) as determined by a radiographic assessment of the relationship between the tumor and adjacent mesenteric vasculature (**Table 1**).

Locally advanced, unresectable

Per NCCN guidelines, patients with LA disease should be treated with chemotherapy and/or chemoradiation as primary therapy, and patients who have a significant response to these therapies should be reassessed for resectability after induction therapy. Although conversion from an LA to technically resectable cancer has historically been rare, it is less so today,[9,10] commensurate with improvements in medical therapy that have occurred over the last decade.

Borderline resectable

Per the NCCN, BR cancers should be treated with preoperative chemotherapy and/or chemoradiotherapy (CRT), followed by restaging and consideration of resection. Patients without disease progression who have an acceptable functional status are considered for pancreatectomy.

It is noteworthy that the NCCN guidelines define BR based solely on the tumor's anatomic relationship to key vascular structures, and do not consider other clinical variables. Katz and colleagues[11] described three categories of BR pancreatic cancer: A, B, and C. Type A disease is similar to the NCCN anatomic definition (see **Table 1**). Type B describes patients with resectable or type A BR tumor anatomy, but with clinical findings suspicious, but not diagnostic, for extrapancreatic disease. Type C describes patients with marginal performance status or a severe, but potentially reversible, preexisting comorbidity profile that put them at particularly high risk for surgery.[12] Tzeng and colleagues[13] found that many patients treated for localized pancreatic cancer meet criteria for type B or C BR disease, and that these patients had markedly worse outcomes, indicating the importance of these additional categories and the need for different treatment strategies for these patients.

Resectable

The NCCN recommends surgery for patients with resectable cancers, followed by systemic chemotherapy. The role of postoperative radiation is currently being studied.[14]

Table 1
Recommended therapy: NCCN

NCCN Classification	Anatomic Criteria		Treatment Recommended
	Arterial	**Venous**	
Resectable	No contact	≤180° contact with SMV/PV	Primary resection
Borderline resectable	≤180° contact with SMA or CA or contact with CHA or >180° that allows for safe resection/ reconstruction or contact with variant arterial anatomy		Preoperative therapy
		>180° contact with SMV/PV; suitable vein for reconstruction or ≤180° contact with SMV/PV with contour irregularity; suitable vein for reconstruction or Contact with IVC	
Unresectable	>180° contact with SMA or CA, or contact with first jejunal branch of SMA		Medical therapy; possible reassessment for resectability
		Contact with proximal draining jejunal branch of SMV or Unreconstructable SMV/PV caused by tumor involvement	
Metastatic	Distant metastatic disease (including nonregional lymph node mets)		Palliative therapy

Abbreviations: CA, celiac artery; CHA, common hepatic artery; PV, portal vein; SMA, superior mesenteric artery; SMV, superior mesenteric vein.

American Society of Clinical Oncology Clinical Practice Guidelines for Potentially Curable Pancreatic Cancer

A comparison between the previously mentioned guidelines and recent ASCO CPG (**Table 2**) highlights the growing uncertainty and controversy surrounding treatment of nonmetastatic pancreatic cancer. The ASCO guidelines provide management algorithms for patients with "potentially curable pancreatic cancer"[8] (as opposed to patients with "LA, unresectable pancreatic cancer," who are discussed in a separate set of guidelines in Ref.[15]) and specifically avoid the anatomic distinction between

Table 2
Recommended therapy: ASCO CPG

Anatomic Criteria		Additional Criteria	Treatment Recommended
Arterial	Venous		
No contact	No contact	CA19-9 suggestive of potentially curable disease, no evidence of disseminated disease Performance status/comorbidity profile appropriate for major abdominal operation	Primary resection or preoperative therapy
Any contact Any of the above	Any contact		Preoperative therapy
		Radiographic findings suspicious for, or CA19-9 level suggestive of, disseminated disease	
Any of the above		Marginal performance status/comorbidity profile not appropriate (but potentially reversible)	
Distant metastatic disease			Palliative therapy

resectable and BR cancers (although the guideline committee did recognize the need for these classifications for the purpose of clinical trials).

Primary resection
Primary resection is recommended for patients with no clinical evidence of metastatic disease, an appropriate performance status and comorbidity profile, no radiographic interface between tumor and mesenteric vasculature on high-definition cross-sectional imaging, and an acceptable CA 19-9 level.

Preoperative therapy
The ASCO CPG recommend that preoperative therapy should be offered as an alternate strategy for patients who meet the previously mentioned criteria. These guidelines directly recommend preoperative therapy for patients who have clinical findings suspicious of extrapancreatic disease, have a performance status or comorbidity profile not currently appropriate (but potentially reversible), any radiographic interface between the tumor and mesenteric vasculature, or an elevated serum CA 19-9 level suggestive of disseminated disease.

The ASCO guidelines clearly break from the NCCN because they suggest a role for the administration of preoperative therapy to a broader group of patients with localized cancer. Indeed, the ASCO CPG directly recommend that preoperative therapy be administered to patients with indications of extrapancreatic disease and those with poor performance status, whereas the NCCN guidelines do not directly address these clinical variables, and instead focus on tumor anatomy.

NEED FOR MULTIMODAL THERAPY

Although there is controversy regarding the sequencing of therapies for pancreatic cancer, there is none regarding the benefits of multimodal therapy.[16] A review of adjuvant therapy is beyond the scope of this article, but is found (see R.A. Wolff's article, "Adjuvant or neoadjuvant therapy in the treatment in pancreatic malignancies: Where are we?" in this issue). It is noteworthy, however, that the CONKO-001 trial, which randomized patients after successful gross complete resection (R0 or R1) of a pancreatic cancer to 6 cycles of gemcitabine or observation, showed a median disease-free survival of 13.4 months in the chemotherapy arm compared with only 6.7 months in the observation arm ($P<.001$) and improved overall survival (OS) (22.8 months vs 20.2 months; $P = 01$).[5] This clearly demonstrated the dismal prognosis of patients treated with surgery alone and the beneficial role of postoperative chemotherapy. More recently, the ESPAC-4 trial established a new standard of care for postoperative chemotherapy when patients undergo primary resection. In this trial, patients who fully recovered within 12 weeks of a complete macroscopic resection of pancreatic ductal adenocarcinoma (PDAC) were randomized to gemcitabine alone or gemcitabine plus capecitabine. A survival benefit was associated with the combination therapy arm (median OS, 28.0 months vs 25.5 months; $P = 0.032$).[3]

Although patients with localized cancer who undergo pancreatectomy clearly benefit from postoperative therapy, improvements in survival over the past three decades of trials have been only modest and incremental. Additionally, although newer regimens (eg, nanoparticle-albumin bound paclitaxel[17] and FOLFIRINOX, a combination of 5-FU, oxaliplatin, leucovorin, and irinotecan[18]) will likely be used in the perioperative setting in the future based on their promising results in the metastatic setting, it is unlikely that they will improve survival dramatically when delivered following surgery (discussed later). Therefore, although a combination of surgery and chemotherapy has been established as necessary, there is a real need to re-examine how and when these therapies are delivered.

SEQUENCING OF THERAPY

Although preoperative chemotherapy and/or radiation therapy is becoming increasingly common, most patients with resectable pancreatic cancer still undergo pancreatectomy *de novo*.[19] Although this strategy is reasonable for the few patients who are fit and present with minimal tumor volume, for most patients with pancreatic cancer, it runs contrary to everything learned about the biology of the disease and the physiology of most patients stricken with it.

Good Surgery is Not Good Enough: Preoperative Therapy Makes Good Surgery Better

Although the benefits of perioperative chemotherapy are well-recognized, complete surgical resection is still needed to cure pancreatic cancer. Given the location of most pancreatic cancers (head or uncinate process) and the proclivity for infiltration into perineural and lymphatic tissues, positive margins and local recurrence remain common, with microscopically (R1) or macroscopically (R2) positive resection margins ranging from 33% to 85%.[20–22] Moreover, recent studies using rigorous histologic protocols have found cancer cells in at least one margin in 90% of pancreatoduodenectomy specimens, suggesting that previously reported low R1 rates may reflect less exact histologic techniques.[21,23] Part of the difficulty in achieving an R0 resection is failure of preoperative staging to appreciate the full extent of disease: even when a tumor has been deemed resectable according to current standards, resection may fail, in part because computed tomography has been shown to overestimate the margin between tumor and the superior mesenteric artery in almost 80% of patients.[24]

Regardless, these high rates of R1 resection are commensurate with high rates of locoregional recurrence observed in clinical practice. A seminal autopsy study showed that 80% of patients who underwent resection for early stage pancreatic cancer developed locoregional cancer recurrence before death.[25] Clearly, surgery, even followed by chemotherapy, is too often insufficient for durable local control.

Given the failures of preoperative staging and curative resection, the opportunity to sterilize surgical margins before surgery has great appeal. Preoperative therapy followed by resection is associated with remarkably high R0 resection rates.[26–28] A retrospective review from the University of Texas MD Anderson Cancer Center (MDACC) indicated that patients treated with preoperative CRT had a significantly lower R1 resection rate and a longer median distance between their cancers and the inked superior mesenteric artery (retroperitoneal) margin than those who underwent *de novo* pancreatectomy.[24] This finding was despite that patients in the preoperative treatment group had larger, more aggressive tumors. Other retrospective reviews have similarly demonstrated low rates of positive margins following preoperative therapy,[27] even in BR disease, where the anticipated rates of R1 resection would be high with primary resection.

There is evidence that the addition of radiotherapy to a preoperative regimen may improve local control by its activity at the surgical margins. Cloyd and colleagues[26] showed in a retrospective review of 472 patients treated for PDAC with preoperative therapy that patients treated with chemotherapy alone had more than twice the risk of local recurrence when compared with patients who received CRT. This effect was seen despite no significant difference in rates of R0 resection between the groups, indicating that neoadjuvant CRT sterilizes the tumor bed in ways not accounted for by examining margin status alone. This may in part be explained by the ability of preoperative therapy to reduce cancer burden in regional lymphatics, because Cloyd and colleagues also found a significant decrease in nodal burden in patients receiving CRT. Although not designed to parse out the effects of radiotherapy specifically, other retrospective reviews have shown that preoperative CRT improves node-negative rates.[29–31]

Despite this evidence, adoption rates outside of large academic centers remain low.[32] Critics of this therapy have raised concerns that treatment before resection may increase morbidity and impair wound healing. Notwithstanding these concerns, the preoperative setting is ideal radiotherapy, allowing for maximum efficacy of radiation therapy to a well-oxygenated tumor and minimizing toxicity to adjacent normal tissues. Additionally, preoperative therapy has not only been shown to be safe, but even to reduce rates of pancreatic fistula,[33] a serious and vexing complication of pancreatic surgery. Finally, in patients who do have major complications from surgery, those treated with preoperative therapy are far more likely to receive additional chemotherapy in the postoperative setting than those treated primarily with surgery.[34]

In summary, failure of local control after primary resection is unacceptably high, even when preoperative evaluation indicates a resectable tumor. Preoperative therapy sterilizes margins and decreasing nodal burden and the addition of radiotherapy seems to make this even more likely. Finally, despite initial concerns regarding toxicity, preoperative CRT is safe and even decreases certain dreaded complications of pancreatoduodenectomy.

Pancreatic Cancer is a Systemic Disease: Preoperative Therapy Treats a Systemic Disease

Although local control of pancreatic cancer is necessary for cure, it is not sufficient to cure what is ultimately a systemic disease. In a typical review of patients with pancreatic cancer who underwent primary surgical resection, less than 50% of patients remained disease free after 1 year and nearly 80% had recurred by 2 years.[35] Another analysis showed that 90% of recurrences within 6 months of surgery are distant.[19] Thus, even when locoregional therapy is maximally effective, early failure still frequently occurs in the form of metastases.

Early distant recurrences reflect another failure of the algorithms used to stage pancreatic cancer, which are based solely on a tumor's local anatomic relationships.

This antiquated staging method is ineffectual for the purposes of prospectively determining which patients will truly benefit from surgical resection because it specifically fails to account for the ubiquitous presence of radiographically occult metastatic disease. In reality, macroscopic metastases are encountered at surgery in 20% of "resectable" cases.[36] Additionally, Glant and colleagues[36] showed a linear relationship between the time from diagnosis to resection and the chance of unanticipated metastatic disease. Patients with any interval greater than 20 days had an increased risk of having metastatic disease found at surgery. This rapid development of metastases suggests the presence evolving metastatic disease that already exists at the time of diagnosis. Indeed, Rhim and colleagues[37] showed in a mouse model that systemic dissemination of cancer cells precedes the development of a clinically detectable primary tumor.

Although resection may contribute to local control, it does little to address the occult metastatic disease that exists in essentially all patients. This problem is compounded by the delay that patients require following surgery before starting postoperative chemotherapy. Haeno and colleagues[38] used computational modeling based on a large autopsy study and validated through a large cohort of patients with pancreatic cancer to predict the kinetics of metastasis. They suggest that metastatic cells often do exist at the time of diagnosis, and that these cells grow exponentially during postsurgical recovery. They also suggest preoperative therapy is the ideal treatment strategy when there is a possibility of undetected metastases.

Given the limitations of current staging strategies, investigators have sought surrogate markers of micrometastases. CA 19-9 is the most useful of such markers. Although not expressed in all patients (eg, negative in patients with Lewis-negative phenotype), it has been shown to correlate with clinical outcomes. A clear cutoff value predictive of metastatic disease has not been established, but pretreatment levels of 50 and 100 may correlate with early recurrence.[39,40] Additionally, a change in the level of CA 19-9 following surgery correlates with improved survival.[41] Although no single tumor marker or clinical parameter will ultimately determine resectability, the sum of factors informs the likelihood of occult metastatic disease.

Ultimately, pancreatic cancer is truly a systemic disease and should be treated as such from the time of diagnosis. To the extent that a tumor's biologic behavior can be predicted, patients at high risk of early recurrence and/or metastasis should avoid a *de novo* resection and instead receive preoperative therapy. This strategy is used not only to establish systemic control before surgery, but also to select for cancers with locally dominant biology where surgery may be effective as opposed to those with metastatic disease already taking root, who are not helped, and may even be hurt, by a highly morbid operation.

Postoperative Therapy is Not Guaranteed: Neoadjuvant Therapy Ensures a High Rate of Multimodal Therapy

Although a great many controversies exist surrounding the treatment of pancreatic cancer, there is consensus that chemotherapy improves survival after pancreatectomy. With this in mind, the goal should be to get as many patients as possible to complete both surgery and chemotherapy (with radiation therapy as thought to be indicated). The large studies of postoperative chemotherapy that have established this consensus, however, are somewhat idealistic in that they only enroll patients with the best performance status who have fully healed from successful surgical resection. Thus, although 99% of patients enrolled in the ESPAC-4 study received some chemotherapy and 60% of patients received all planned cycles,[3] these numbers are far lower for the average cohort of patients with pancreatic cancer. A recent review of National Cancer Database data found that only 58% of patients treated with *de novo* resection for early stage PDAC received any adjuvant therapy,[6] and a similar analysis in Australia showed that only 47% of patients received any adjuvant therapy.[42] Although some patients miss out on postoperative therapy because of early metastatic disease, many are excluded because of failure to fully recover after surgery.[43,44]

Failure to recover from a major pancreatic resection can occur for a variety of reasons. Patients afflicted with PDAC typically present in a state of physiologic and functional depression because of a combination of advanced age, biliary and/or enteric obstruction, malnutrition, cancer-related cachexia, or pre-existing comorbidities. Performance of major surgery in the setting of such adverse clinical parameters is associated with high morbidity and mortality, and a low long-term survival.[42,45–48] The combination of this preoperative baseline and a major pancreatic resection leads to a high complication rate[48] and, unfortunately, patients who suffer major complications after *de novo* surgery for PDAC have dismal survival rates, similar to when surgery is abandoned because of metastatic disease.[45] Understanding the growth kinetics of pancreatic cancer in conjunction with the immunosuppression associated with critical illness, this is not surprising. Because preoperative therapy ensures patients receive multimodal therapy even in the setting of a major surgical complication, it seems to mitigate the effects of these complications on mortality; patients having a surgical complication after preoperative therapy have been shown to have OS similar to patients suffering no complications.[34,45]

Whether directly related to complications from surgery or pre-existing comorbidities, elderly patients are less likely to receive adjuvant therapy and have poor outcomes after *de novo* surgery. Nagrial and colleagues[42] restricted their overall analysis of PDAC patients in Australia to elderly patients (≥70 years old), and found that only 29.8% of patients received chemotherapy. This is especially concerning given that pancreatic cancer is a disease of the elderly; the median age in this study was 67, and 40.5% of patients were 70 years or older. These elderly patients that did not receive adjuvant chemotherapy also had a particularly dismal prognosis, with a median OS of only 13 months.

The knowledge that patients, whether elderly or not, who present in a physiologically depressed state have poor outcomes with *de novo* resection led to the previously described BR type C classification of PDAC. In current practice, however, these patients are often still treated with primary resection. In an analysis of the National Surgical Quality Improvement Program database, Tzeng and colleagues[45] found that roughly one-third of patient who underwent *de novo* pancreatectomy between 2005 and 2010 could be considered to have type C BR pancreatic cancer. These patients had higher complication rates (*P*<.001) and nearly twice the 30-day mortality rate (*P*<.001) of patients who did not meet these criteria. These patients who present in a depressed physiologic state, whether because of complications from the cancer itself, identifiable comorbidities, or age, clearly do not benefit from a surgery from which they cannot recover.

In many of these patients, physiologic derangements are reversible. The time during which preoperative therapy is administered offers an ideal opportunity to optimize and reassess nutritional and physiologic indices. This occurs most efficiently through a structured multidisciplinary program of "prehabilitation" that uses internal medicine expertise, nutritional counseling, and physical therapy. This process has been shown to improve specific parameters of fitness in other patients with cancer,[49] and has been shown to be feasible at MDACC, although data regarding outcomes are not yet available.[50] Ideally, such a program will increase the percentage of patients undergoing pancreatic resection with a robust enough physiologic profile to allow meaningful recovery. In the end, broader adoption of this type C BR classification and appropriate selection of preoperative therapy for such patients is required to improve outcomes in this disease.

Multimodal therapy remains the cornerstone of PDAC treatment, but roughly half of patients approached with primary resection miss out on postoperative therapies. This is caused, in large part, by the inability of many patients to have a rapid, meaningful recovery because of a depressed physiologic state at the time of diagnosis. An approach including preoperative therapy allows patients to receive necessary chemotherapy, while simultaneously increasing their ability to tolerate surgery, thus ensuring the delivery of multimodality therapy to the highest possible percentage of patients and selecting for patients who will benefit most from surgery.

OUTCOMES OF PREOPERATIVE THERAPY

The challenges of treating pancreatic cancer and the advantages of preoperative therapy have been summarized. Skepticism exists, however, and there has long been hesitation to adopt this strategy, at least some of which is explained by a lack of high-level randomized, controlled studies on this issue. Two randomized studies were attempted, but failed to enroll enough patients to allow for meaningful conclusions.[51,52] Multiple centers have recently reported promising results with the use of preoperative therapy. Although these data must be interpreted with caution given they are mostly retrospective reviews from single institutions with inherent bias, they speak to the promise of this strategy.

Large retrospective reviews of the National Cancer Database have shown that neoadjuvant therapy is associated with more negative margins, less nodal disease, and improved survival, although this survival benefit is limited to patients with stage III disease.[32,53,54] Although these data are flawed (they only reflect patients who completed multimodal therapy, and not those who progressed before planned surgery) they are still encouraging. Additionally, retrospective comparisons of these treatment strategies typically are biased toward patients with more aggressive disease being treated with preoperative therapy.[53] Early experience with neoadjuvant therapy was almost all in patients with BR disease, whereas primary resection has been the treatment of choice in those with less advanced, resectable cancers. Importantly, when analysis is limited to resectable disease, retrospective data has shown that up to 87% of patients treated with preoperative therapy complete multimodal therapy,[55] whereas a much lower number of similar patients complete postoperative therapy delivered following primary resection.[56]

As more effective chemotherapy develops, more results are supporting the efficacy of preoperative therapy. A recently completed multicenter, single arm trial from the Alliance for Clinical Trials in Oncology, Trial A021101, provided initial evidence for the efficacy of preoperative FOLFIRINOX in patients with BR disease.[57] In this trial, patients were treated preoperatively with a novel and aggressive regimen of modified FOLFIRINOX, followed by radiation therapy with concurrent capecitabine, resection in appropriate surgical candidates, and finally postoperative gemcitabine. Of the 22 patients who initiated therapy, 15 (68%) underwent surgery, with 12 undergoing vascular resection and reconstruction. R0 resection was achieved in 14 of 15 (93%; 64% of 22 patients initiating therapy) patients and 10 had node-negative disease on final pathology. The median survival for the 22 patients initiating therapy was 21.7 months, with even better outcomes in the 15 patients who underwent resection (18 month OS, 67%).[57] Although this initial experience is small, it is encouraging given

Table 3
Ongoing phase III randomized trials of neoadjuvant versus adjuvant therapy

Study	Surgery First Arm	Neoadjuvant Arm	Phase	Inclusion Criteria	# Patients	Estimated Completion Date	NCT Trial #
PACT-15	Surgery 6 mo cisplatin, epirubicin, gemcitabine, capecitabine	3 mo cisplatin, epirubicin, gemcitabine, capecitabine Surgery 3 mo cisplatin, epirubicin, gemcitabine, capecitabine	II/III	Stage I-II resectable PDAC	370	June, 2017	NCT01150630
NorPACT-1	Surgery Gemcitabine + capecitabine	FOLFIRINOX Surgery Gemcitabine + oxaliplatine	II/III	Resectable PDAC of head of pancreas	90	October, 2021	NCT02891787
NEPAFOX	Surgery Gemcitabine	6 cycles FOLFIRINOX Surgery 6 cycles FOLFIRINOX	II/III	Resectable or borderline resectable PDAC	126	June, 2019	NCT02172976
	Surgery 45Gy/25 fx, then 9Gy/5 fx with 6 wk gemcitabine Maintenance gemcitabine (4 cycles)	45Gy/25 fx, then 9Gy/5 fx with 6 wk gemcitabine Surgery Maintenance gemcitabine (4 cycles)	II/III	Borderline resectable PDAC	116	December, 2017	NCT01458717
NEOPA	Surgery 6 cycles adjuvant gemcitabine	6 wk CRT with gemcitabine + 50.4Gy/28 fx Surgery 6 cycles adjuvant gemcitabine	III	Borderline resectable PDAC	410	February, 2020	NCT01900327

Data from Ref. clinicaltrials.gov.

the advanced stage of these patients. Importantly, this pilot study also accrued ahead of schedule, demonstrating the feasibility of such a trial. Based on these results, this group is currently enrolling the phase II A021501 trial comparing a similar preoperative regimen with or without radiation therapy.[58]

Finally, perhaps the most comprehensive data to date on preoperative therapy, although retrospective, were recently reported from MDACC.[31] A total of 622 patients who received chemotherapy and/or chemoradiation before pancreatectomy over a 25-year period were reviewed. The percentage of patients presenting with BR or LA tumors increased significantly over the course of this study, as did the use of vascular resection and reconstruction during pancreatectomy. Despite this obvious increase in the disease burden, there was a steady increase in survival over this 25-year period. The median OS of the most recent cohort, patients treated between 2010 and 2014, was 43 months, with zero 90-day mortalities. Additionally, patients treated in the last 10 years of the study had an impressive 5-year OS of 35%. Our group has also recently published an analysis of patients with major pathologic response to preoperative chemotherapy. Although this only occurred in 13.2% of patients, these patients had a remarkable 5-year OS rate of 58%.[59] Although these results are from a single institution, they are clearly noteworthy in the context of an average nationwide 90-day mortality rate of almost 7.4%,[60] and de novo surgery followed by adjuvant therapy currently yielding a median OS of 28 months[3] and a 5-year OS of 20.7%.[4]

In addition to these compelling retrospective data, there are multiple on-going randomized controlled trials, summarized in **Table 3**.[58] These trials may finally offer high-level data of the efficacy of neoadjuvant therapy.

SUMMARY

Although there will always be a role for primary resection of pancreatic cancer in the select group of robust patients with small tumors and no evidence of extrapancreatic disease, the new ASCO CPG reflects a much-needed shift toward more use of preoperative therapy. Preoperative therapy allows for better sterilization of tumor margins and peritumoral nodes, offers early systemic therapy for a systemic disease, ensures that all patients receive chemotherapy while selecting for patients who actually benefit from a morbid operation, and gives time for possible optimization of comorbidities in patients who predictably fare poorly following primary resection.

REFERENCES

1. Pancreatic Cancer Facts 2016. Pancreatic Cancer Action Network Web site. 2016. Available at: http://www.pancan.org. Accessed April 1, 2017.

2. Key Statistics for Pancreatic Cancer. 2017. Available at: https://www.cancer.org/cancer/pancreatic-cancer/about/key-statistics.html. Accessed April 1, 2017.

3. Neoptolemos JP, Palmer DH, Ghaneh P, et al. Comparison of adjuvant gemcitabine and capecitabine with gemcitabine monotherapy in patients with resected pancreatic cancer (ESPAC-4): a multicentre, open-label, randomised, phase 3 trial. Lancet 2017;389(10073):1011–24.

4. Oettle H, Neuhaus P, Hochhaus A, et al. Adjuvant chemotherapy with gemcitabine and long-term outcomes among patients with resected pancreatic cancer: the CONKO-001 randomized trial. JAMA 2013;310(14):1473–81.

5. Oettle H, Post S, Neuhaus P, et al. Adjuvant chemotherapy with gemcitabine vs observation in patients undergoing curative-intent resection of pancreatic cancer: a randomized controlled trial. JAMA 2007;297(3):267–77.

6. Dimou F, Sineshaw H, Parmar AD, et al. Trends in receipt and timing of multimodality therapy in early-stage pancreatic cancer. J Gastrointest Surg 2016;20(1): 93–103 [discussion: 103].

7. NCCN Clinical Practice Guidelines in Oncology: Pancreatic Adenocarcinoma. version 2.2017. 2017. Available at: https://www.nccn.org/professionals/physician_gls/pdf/pancreatic.pdf. Accessed May 1, 2017.

8. Khorana AA, Mangu PB, Berlin J, et al. Potentially curable pancreatic cancer: American Society of Clinical Oncology clinical practice guideline. J Clin Oncol 2016;34(21):2541–56.

9. Pompa TA, Morano WF, Jeurkar C, et al. Complete response after treatment with neoadjuvant chemoradiation with prolonged chemotherapy for locally advanced, unresectable adenocarcinoma of the pancreas. Case Rep Oncol Med 2017; 2017:7834702.

10. Lakatos G, Petranyi A, Szűcs A, et al. Efficacy and safety of FOLFIRINOX in locally advanced pancreatic cancer. a single center experience. Pathol Oncol Res 2017. https://doi.org/10.1007/s12253-016-0176-0.

11. Katz MH, Pisters PW, Evans DB, et al. Borderline resectable pancreatic cancer: the importance of this emerging stage of disease. J Am Coll Surg 2008;206(5): 833–46 [discussion: 846–8].

12. Schwarz L, Katz MH. Diagnosis and management of borderline resectable pancreatic adenocarcinoma. Hematol Oncol Clin North Am 2015;29(4):727–40.

13. Tzeng C-WDW, Fleming JB, Lee JE, et al. Defined clinical classifications are associated with outcome of patients with anatomically resectable pancreatic adenocarcinoma treated with neoadjuvant therapy. Ann Surg Oncol 2012;19(6): 2045–53.

14. RTOG 0848 Protocol Information. RTOG Foundation Web site. 2017. Available at: https://www.rtog.org/ClinicalTrials/ProtocolTable/StudyDetails.aspx?study=0848. Accessed March 15, 2017.

15. Balaban EP, Mangu PB, Khorana AA, et al. Locally advanced, unresectable pancreatic cancer: American Society of Clinical Oncology clinical practice guideline. J Clin Oncol 2016;34(22):2654–68.

16. Bakkevold KE, Arnesjø B, Dahl O, et al. Adjuvant combination chemotherapy (AMF) following radical resection of carcinoma of the pancreas and papilla of Vater–results of a controlled, prospective, randomised multicentre study. Eur J Cancer 1993;29A(5):698–703.

17. Von Hoff DD, Ervin T, Arena FP, et al. Increased survival in pancreatic cancer with nab-paclitaxel plus gemcitabine. N Engl J Med 2013;369(18):1691–703.

18. Conroy T, Desseigne F, Ychou M, et al. FOLFIRINOX versus gemcitabine for metastatic pancreatic cancer. N Engl J Med 2011;364(19):1817–25.

19. Groot VP, Rezaee N, Wu W, et al. Patterns, timing, and predictors of recurrence following pancreatectomy for pancreatic ductal adenocarcinoma. Ann Surg 2017. https://doi.org/10.1097/SLA.0000000000002234.

20. Butler JR, Ahmad SA, Katz MH, et al. A systematic review of the role of periadventitial dissection of the superior mesenteric artery in affecting margin status after pancreatoduodenectomy for pancreatic adenocarcinoma. HPB (Oxford) 2016;18(4):305–11.

21. Verbeke CS, Gladhaug IP. Resection margin involvement and tumour origin in pancreatic head cancer. Br J Surg 2012;99(8):1036–49.

22. Verbeke CS, Leitch D, Menon KV, et al. Redefining the R1 resection in pancreatic cancer. Br J Surg 2006;93(10):1232–7.

23. Verbeke CS. Resection margins in pancreatic cancer: are we entering a new era? HPB (Oxford) 2014;16(1):1–2.

24. Katz MH, Wang H, Balachandran A, et al. Effect of neoadjuvant chemoradiation and surgical technique on recurrence of localized pancreatic cancer. J Gastrointest Surg 2012;16(1):68–78 [discussion: 78–9].

25. Iacobuzio-Donahue CA, Fu B, Yachida S, et al. DPC4 gene status of the primary carcinoma correlates with patterns of failure in patients with pancreatic cancer. J Clin Oncol 2009;27(11):1806–13.

26. Cloyd JM, Crane CH, Koay EJ, et al. Impact of hypofractionated and standard fractionated chemoradiation before pancreatoduodenectomy for pancreatic ductal adenocarcinoma. Cancer 2016;122(17):2671–9.

27. Kharofa J, Tsai S, Kelly T, et al. Neoadjuvant chemoradiation with IMRT in resectable and borderline resectable pancreatic cancer. Radiother Oncol 2014;113(1):41–6.

28. Sho M, Akahori T, Tanaka T, et al. Pathological and clinical impact of neoadjuvant chemoradiotherapy using full-dose gemcitabine and concurrent radiation for resectable pancreatic cancer. J Hepatobiliary Pancreat Sci 2013;20(2):197–205.

29. Colbert LE, Hall WA, Nickleach D, et al. Chemoradiation therapy sequencing for resected pancreatic adenocarcinoma in the National Cancer Data Base. Cancer 2014;120(4):499–506.

30. Felice FDE, Musio D, Raffetto N, et al. Neoadjuvant strategy as initial treatment in resectable pancreatic cancer: concrete evidence of benefit. Anticancer Res 2014;34(9):4673–6.

31. Cloyd JM, Katz MH, Prakash L, et al. Preoperative therapy and pancreatoduodenectomy for pancreatic ductal adenocarcinoma: a 25-year single-institution experience. J Gastrointest Surg 2017;21(1):164–74.

32. Youngwirth LM, Nussbaum DP, Thomas S, et al. Nationwide trends and outcomes associated with neoadjuvant therapy in pancreatic cancer: an analysis of 18 243 patients. J Surg Oncol 2017. https://doi.org/10.1002/jso.24630.

33. Cooper AB, Parmar AD, Riall TS, et al. Does the use of neoadjuvant therapy for pancreatic adenocarcinoma increase postoperative morbidity and mortality rates? J Gastrointest Surg 2015;19(1):80–6 [discussion: 86–7].

34. Tzeng C-WDW, Tran Cao HS, Lee JE, et al. Treatment sequencing for resectable pancreatic cancer: influence of early metastases and surgical complications on multimodality therapy completion and survival. J Gastrointest Surg 2014;18(1):16–24 [discussion: 24–5].

35. Van den Broeck A, Sergeant G, Ectors N, et al. Patterns of recurrence after curative resection of pancreatic ductal adenocarcinoma. Eur J Surg Oncol 2009;35(6):600–4.

36. Glant J, Waters J, House M, et al. Does the interval from imaging to operation affect the rate of unanticipated metastasis encountered during operation for pancreatic adenocarcinoma? Surgery 2011;150(4):607–16.

37. Rhim AD, Mirek ET, Aiello NM, et al. EMT and dissemination precede pancreatic tumor formation. Cell 2012;148(1–2):349–61.

38. Haeno H, Gonen M, Davis M, et al. Computational modeling of pancreatic cancer reveals kinetics of metastasis suggesting optimum treatment strategies. Cell 2012;148(1–2):362–75.

39. Kang CM, Kim JY, Choi GH, et al. The use of adjusted preoperative CA 19-9 to predict the recurrence of resectable pancreatic cancer. J Surg Res 2007;140(1):31–5.

40. Ballehaninna UK, Chamberlain RS. The clinical utility of serum CA 19-9 in the diagnosis, prognosis and management of pancreatic adenocarcinoma: an evidence based appraisal. J Gastrointest Oncol 2012;3(2):105–19.
41. Ferrone CR, Finkelstein DM, Thayer SP, et al. Perioperative CA19-9 levels can predict stage and survival in patients with resectable pancreatic adenocarcinoma. J Clin Oncol 2006;24(18):2897–902.
42. Nagrial AM, Chang DK, Nguyen NQ, et al. Adjuvant chemotherapy in elderly patients with pancreatic cancer. Br J Cancer 2014;110(2):313–9.
43. Merkow R, Bentrem D, Mulcahy M, et al. Effect of postoperative complications on adjuvant chemotherapy use for stage III colon cancer. Ann Surg 2013;258(6):847.
44. Merkow RP, Bilimoria KY, Tomlinson JS, et al. Postoperative complications reduce adjuvant chemotherapy use in resectable pancreatic cancer. Ann Surg 2014; 260(2):372–7.
45. Tzeng C-WDW, Katz MH, Fleming JB, et al. Morbidity and mortality after pancreaticoduodenectomy in patients with borderline resectable type C clinical classification. J Gastrointest Surg 2014;18(1):146–55 [discussion: 155–6].
46. Davila JA, Chiao EY, Hasche JC, et al. Utilization and determinants of adjuvant therapy among older patients who receive curative surgery for pancreatic cancer. Pancreas 2009;38(1):e18–25.
47. Lahat G, Sever R, Lubezky N. Pancreatic cancer: surgery is a feasible therapeutic option for elderly patients. World J Surg Oncol 2011;9:10. Available at: https://wjso.biomedcentral.com/articles/10.1186/1477-7819-9-10.
48. Aoki S, Miyata H, Konno H, et al. Risk factors of serious postoperative complications after pancreaticoduodenectomy and risk calculators for predicting postoperative complications: a nationwide study of 17,564 patients in Japan. J Hepatobiliary Pancreat Sci 2017;24(5):243–51.
49. Huang GH, Ismail H, Murnane A, et al. Structured exercise program prior to major cancer surgery improves cardiopulmonary fitness: a retrospective cohort study. Support Care Cancer 2016;24(5):2277–85.
50. Ngo-Huang A, Parker N, Martinez VA, et al. Poster 68 feasibility of a prehabilitation program for patients with potentially resectable pancreatic cancer: pilot study. PM R 2016;8(9S):S183.
51. Casadei R, Di Marco M, Ricci C, et al. Neoadjuvant chemoradiotherapy and surgery versus surgery alone in resectable pancreatic cancer: a single-center prospective, randomized, controlled trial which failed to achieve accrual targets. J Gastrointest Surg 2015;19(10):1802–12.
52. Golcher H, Brunner TB, Witzigmann H, et al. Neoadjuvant chemoradiation therapy with gemcitabine/cisplatin and surgery versus immediate surgery in resectable pancreatic cancer: results of the first prospective randomized phase II trial. Strahlenther Onkol 2015;191(1):7–16.
53. Mirkin KA, Hollenbeak CS, Wong J. Survival impact of neoadjuvant therapy in resected pancreatic cancer: a prospective cohort study involving 18,332 patients from the National Cancer Data Base. Int J Surg 2016;34:96–102.
54. Shubert CR, Bergquist JR, Groeschl RT, et al. Overall survival is increased among stage III pancreatic adenocarcinoma patients receiving neoadjuvant chemotherapy compared to surgery first and adjuvant chemotherapy: an intention to treat analysis of the National Cancer Database. Surgery 2016;160(4):1080–96.
55. Christians KK, Heimler JW, George B, et al. Survival of patients with resectable pancreatic cancer who received neoadjuvant therapy. Surgery 2016;159(3): 893–900.

56. Labori KJ, Katz MH, Tzeng CW, et al. Impact of early disease progression and surgical complications on adjuvant chemotherapy completion rates and survival in patients undergoing the surgery first approach for resectable pancreatic ductal adenocarcinoma: a population-based cohort study. Acta Oncol 2016; 55(3):265–77.
57. Katz MH, Shi Q, Ahmad SA, et al. Preoperative modified FOLFIRINOX treatment followed by capecitabine-based chemoradiation for borderline resectable pancreatic cancer: alliance for clinical trials in oncology trial A021101. JAMA Surg 2016;151(8):e161137.
58. Multiple study pages. 2017. Available at: https://clinicaltrials.gov. Accessed June 15, 2017.
59. Cloyd JM, Wang H, Egger ME, et al. Clinical factors associated with a major pathologic response following preoperative therapy for pancreatic ductal adenocarcinoma. JAMA Surg 2017. [Epub ahead of print].
60. Swanson RS, Pezzi CM, Mallin K, et al. The 90-day mortality after pancreatectomy for cancer is double the 30-day mortality: more than 20,000 resections from the national cancer data base. Ann Surg Oncol 2014;21(13):4059–67.

Cancer of the Pancreas—Actual 5, 10, and 20+Year Survival: The Lucky and Fortunate Few

Avram M. Cooperman, MD[a],*, Howard Bruckner, MD[a],
Harry Snady, MD[a], Hillel Hammerman, MD[a], Andrew Fader, MD[a],
Michael Feld, MD[a], Frank Golier, MD[a], Tom Rush, MD[a],
Jerome Siegal, MD[a], Franklin Kasmin, MD[a], Seth Cohen, MD[a],
Michael G. Wayne, DO[a], Mazen E. Iskandar, MD[b],
Justin G. Steele, MD[a]

KEYWORDS

- Cancer of the pancreas (CaP) • Pancreaticoduodenal resection (PDR)
- 5Fluorouracil, Streptozotocin, Cis-Platinum (FSP) • Chemoradiation therapy (CRT)
- Lead time bias, Selection bias, Length bias • Actual vs actuarial survival

KEY POINTS

- Cancer of the pancreas is an abysmal disease, increasing annually worldwide, and with dismal cure rates.
- Survival notwithstanding surgery remains the basis of therapy.
- Initial systemic treatment may improve selection, lower morbidity and improve survival.
- Since metastases exist before tumors are detected initial systemic therapy is indicated, and surgery in selective responders may be a more logical approach.
- Since 1986 a shared multidisciplinary approach has included initial multidrug chemo radiationtherapy at first in borderline resectable or regionally unresectable patients, and surgery after maximum response.
- In a 10 year period (1991–2000) 80/180 PDR's were for CaP and 17 (175) survived 5 + years, 15 ten plus years+ (15%) and 3, 20+ years (3%).
- Nearly half of the long term survivors were initially unresectable and had CRT before resection.
- Nearly 80% of the PDR's were done in a 50 bed community hospital in Dobbs Ferry NY, at a Center for Pancreatic and Biliary Surgery and care was provided by a multidisciplinary dedicated team.

Disclosure Statements: The authors have nothing to disclose.
[a] The Pancreas, Biliary and Advanced Laparoscopy Center of New York, 305 Second Avenue, New York, NY 10003, USA; [b] Division of Surgical Oncology, Mount Sinai Beth Israel, New York, NY, USA
* Corresponding author.
E-mail address: avram.cooperman@gmail.com

INTRODUCTION

Cancer of the pancreas (CaP) is a dismal, uncommon, systemic malignancy. Although CaP is the twelfth most common malignancy and accounts for only 3% of all cancers, it is the 3-5th most common cause of cancer deaths worldwide and has the poorest survival of any solid cancer.[1–7] Significant gains in diagnosis by endoscopic and axial imaging, and by guided tissue sampling, facilitate accurate diagnosis. Selection of suitable candidates for resection is more objective and operative mortality has declined to less than 5%.[6,8–11] All these advances are offset by the fact that the cure rate remains dismal and unchanged for 50 years.[12–14] Systemic therapy may add 3 to 10 months to life and responses range from none to complete remission, with side effects of varying severity.[15–17] These statistics aside, a few unpredictable CaP patients are fortunate and lucky to be long-term survivors or are cured.[7–10,18–28]

This article updates an earlier experience of actual long-term survival of CaP in patients treated between 1991 to 2000, and reviewed the literature. Survival is expressed as actual, not projected, survival.[7]

UPDATED SERIES

Between May, 1991, and January 1, 2001,180 pancreaticoduodenal resections (PDRs) were performed, including 80 for carcinoma of the pancreas (CaP). Seventy eight percent of operations were done at a 50-bed community hospital 18 miles from New York City (**Table 1**).[7]

OUTCOMES

There was 1 procedure-related death (0.55%), a cardiac event on the fifth postoperative day. For all patients, mean and median operative time was 150 minutes and mean hospital stay was 8 days. Blood was transfused during hospitalization in 14 (7%) operations, and a stage A pancreatic fistula developed in 6%, which closed spontaneously in all. The selection criteria for surgery and operative technique have been described.[7,29–32]

OVERALL SURVIVAL

Seventeen patients survived 5 survived at least 5 years (21%), 15 at least ten years(19%), and 3 at least 20 years (4%) 2 of whom still survive. There were 3 groups. Group 1 had resection followed by adjuvant therapy (8), group 2 had resection and no additional therapy (1), and group 3 had chemotherapy (1) or chemoradiation therapy (7) followed by PDR (**Table 2**).

NEOADJUVANT THERAPY

Between 1984 and 1996, 346 patients with CaP were treated by 1 oncologist (HB). Of these, 168 had metastases or bulky local disease amenable to chemotherapy but not

Table 1 Demographics	
180 PDRs, 1994–2001	150 min operation time (180)
80 CaP (all adenocarcinoma), all PDR	8 d median hospitalization
62 PDR + adjuvant	7% blood tx
18 neoadjuvant + surgery	6% stage A pancreatic fistula
78% Dobb's Ferry Hospital	3 reoperations, 2 bleeding

Table 2 Current status years	
Living NED	17 4/12, 20 2/12, 23 4/12
Unknown status (NED last visit) ?	20 8/12, 14 5/12, 13 6/12, 15 1/12 13/7/12, 14 2/12.13
Died NED	12, 14 2/12, 15, 10 3/12, 11 1/12
Died of Mets	7, 9 10/12

radiation, 90 patients received adjuvant therapy after resection, and 88 unresectable patients were treated by chemoradiation therapy.[32] Unresectability was determined at surgery in 52 and by axial imaging in 36. A positive biopsy of adenocarcinoma was obtained in all and confirmed in review.[33]

CHEMORADIATION THERAPY

An initial 20 unresectable patients were part of a phase 2 study and the next 68 were included in this study. All were treated to maximum response. Chemoradiation therapy consisted of streptozotocin (350–500 mg/m2), cisplatin (100 mg/m2), and fluorouracil (1 g/m2). Radiation (5400 cGy) was split-course. The protocol was in-hospital Sunday to Friday, 1 week per month, and has been detailed.[33]

SURGERY

Surgery-first, plus adjuvant therapy, was done in 62 PDRs. Surgery-last was considered in 22 out of 68 responders to neoadjuvant therapy. In 2 treatment toxicity and frailty precluded resection. Two underwent surgery elsewhere and died after complications. An initial 2 underwent surgery-last elsewhere and died after complications. The mean and median operative times for the 18 resected neoadjuvant subjects were 3 hours and 20 minutes and 3 hours. Two operations took more than 4 hours and the median and mean hospitalization was 13 and 16 days. Four were hospitalized for more than 20 days (21, 22, 29, and 32 days), including 3 with delayed gastric emptying after pylorus preservation (**Table 1**).[7]

OVERALL RESULTS

Tables 2 and **3** summarize overall survival and patient status as of April 2017. Seventeen survived at least 5 years, 15 at least 10 years, 9 at least 15 years and 3 at least 20 years. Five died with no evidence of disease (NED) and 7 were lost to follow-up, all NED (**Table 2**). Two developed second primary tumors, a lymphoma in the twentieth year (well in year 24) and a prostate cancer, which was fatal in year 15. Two others died of metastases in the seventh, and ninth year.

RESULTS OF NEOADJUVANT THERAPY

Eight of 15 who survived at least 10 years had neoadjuvant therapy. The 8 came from 68 neoadjuvant treated patients whereas the 9 whose initial treatment was surgery came from a much larger group of whom less than 10% were resectable. The 68 reported neoadjuvant patients were compared with 91 matched PDR-adjuvant therapy patients and there was a projected survival advantage for neoadjuvant therapy (23 vs 14 months), which increased to 33 months after resection. The difference would be more striking now given the 17 additional years of follow-up. Neoadjuvant therapy continued from 5–16 months (mean 11 months), until maximum tumor response. In

Table 3
Individual patient status

Patient Initials	Date of Diagnosis (mo/y)	Date of Surgery	Status (mos)
	PDR+ ADJUVANT THERAPY		
TM	9/1994	—	D 144 NED
GM	9/1994	—	L 248 NED ?
AR	8/1996	—	L 173 NED ?
FW	7/1997	—	L 162 NED ?
RG	6/1998	—	L 181 NED ?
JR	11/1999	—	L 208 NED
RD	!2/2000	—	D 118 metastases
MH	9/2000	—	D 84 metastases
	PDR NO ADJUVANT THERAPY		
FM	6/1995	—	L 163 NED ?
JP	1/1987	—	L 241 NED ?
	NEOADJUVANT THERAPY + PDR		
NN	10/1990	5/1991	D 170 s primary
AK	9/1991	3/1992	L 170 NED ?
GS	10/1991	2/1992	L 280 NED
DD	8/1992	4/1993	L 156 NED ?
AB	7/1994	12/1994	D 180 NED
ES	11/1995	5/1996	D 123 NED
GF	2/1996	11/1996	D 133 NED
JS	2/1997	6/1998	L 242 NED

5 resected specimens, there was no residual gross or microscopic tumor, yet 3 patients died at 32, 32, and 19 months of metastases and 2 survived 10-plus years with NED.

DISCUSSION

Actual, not projected, 5 and 10 or more year survival from CaP is uncommon and the subject of several recent reports. The highest survival rates are from surgical databases and the lowest from population-based studies (**Tables 4** and **5**).[7–11,18,28,34–42] The relative 1-year survival for CaP in England and Wales, 1971 to 1975, and 2005 to 2009, was 6% and 17.4% and the 5-year survival was 2% and 3.6%, respectively.[4,21] Relative survival is the percent of patients with cancers surviving relative

Table 4
Population-based studies: CaP Patients - 5 year survival

City, Country	Number of CaP Patients	5-y Survival (Estimated) (%)
Victoria, Australia	763	1.3
Shanghai, China	11,672	4.1
Norway	21,163	<3
San Francisco, CA, USA	1954	1.3
Sweden	4321	2.8
Finland	4922	0.6

	Number of	5-y	10-y	20-y
Table 5				
Actual 5-plus–year survival literature review				
Institution	Subjects	Survival (%)	Survival (%)	Survival (%)
Manheim, Germany	53	13	8	—
Johns Hopkins	201	10	1	—
Dobbs Ferry, NY	80	21	19	4
Toronto	123	14.6	4	—
Amsterdam	160	4	—	—
Nagoya, Japan	182	4.3	—	—
Indiana University	226	4	—	—
Seoul, Korea	242	4	—	—
Mayo Clinic	357	17	6	—
France: Lyons, Nantes, and Strasbourg	302	10	3	—
Tampa, FL	149	8.5	—	—
Memorial Sloan Kettering Cancer Center, NY	618	12	5	—
MD Anderson Cancer Center	329	27	14	—
Massachusetts General Hospital, MA	499	19	10	—
Taipei, Taiwan	169	6.5	14	—
Athens, Greece	86	14	—	—
Osaka, Japan	147	12	—	—
Virginia Mason, Clinic	42	45	28	—
Madrid, Spain	128	7.0	—	—

to a healthy population. Relative 1-year survival reflects the stage of disease at diagnosis, whereas the 5-year statistics reflect survival after therapy. Although more cases were detected earlier, survival has not improved. Gudjonsson, in several publications, analyzed CaP and survival, and noted only 65 5-year survivors by 1978, 8 of whom were not resected.[43] By 1987, 5-year survivors had increased to 165, of whom 12 were not resected.[44–46] By 2016, an estimated 2800 in 433,000 (<1%) CaP patients survived 5 years.[24,26,27]

Before biliary stents were used to decompress jaundice and axial imaging was available, mortality rates exceeded 20%. Based on high mortality and morbidity rates after surgery, Crile.[47] in 1970, and Shapiro,[48] in 1975, questioned the value and wisdom of pancreatic resection. Eckstam[49] reported on a 10-year survivor in 1994 and cited 13 others in a literature review.[47]

This study is among several in the last decade of actual survival of CaP. It is derived from carefully evaluated PDR subjects with CaP.[27,30–36] The actual 5,10,and 20 year survival was 21%,19% and 4%. The overall and individual survival is summarized in **Tables 2** and **3**. Seven were lost to follow up. All were NED at 13–20 years after treatment. Two of three 20 year survivors survive NED and 2 others are in years 18, and 19 NED. The longest survivor, now in year 24 since diagnosis had a small focus of tumor left on the superior mesenteric vein (SMV) and received additional radiation therapy. He developed lymphoma in year 20 and is NED in year 24. Another developed a fatal prostate cancer and died at 14 years, 2 months. Others have noted synchronous or metachronous second primary lesions in the same or other organ sites.[50–53] This is most unusual after CaP for an obvious reason: few survive long enough to develop a second primary lesion. The authors have noted a second primary pancreatic cancer after distal resection for a primary lesion, and have reported 3 synchronous, simultaneous lesions in the head of the pancreas (2 distinct adenocarcinomas and a neuroendocrine tumor).[51] The present and overall status of each patient is summarized in **Tables 2** and **3**. The incomplete follow-up of 7 patients is due to loss of data during transfer and storage of records, and changing computer systems. We make no projections about them and simply state the last contact with them, all of whom were NED after 10 years (see **Table 2**).

The unusual features in this series include: 78% of operations were done in a 50-bed community hospital, a high number of 5-year and 10-year survivors[7,16] relative to the number of operations, a low recurrence rate after 5 years (2 out of 17), the development of second primary lesions in 2 patients, and nearly half the survivors had neoadjuvant therapy (8 out of 17, all of whom lived at least 10 years).[7,28] The neoadjuvant group, was much smaller than the surgery-first adjuvant group who came from a much larger number of referred and screened patients.

TUMOR CHARACTERISTICS

Histologic features, lymph node status, tumor size, margin status, and vein involvement are considered important survival determinants.[4,7,8,18–20,24,25,27,29] Common sense would suggest that patients with smaller, well-differentiated tumors, negative lymph nodes, and uninvolved resected margins fare better than those with large, poorly differentiated lesions with positive nodes, positive margins, and vein wall involvement. Yet these factors are irrelevant in predicting actual long-term survival.[1,6,20] Nearly half of the 5-year and 10-year survivors were initially unresectable. One subject, JP, had a difficult postoperative course marked by portal vein thromboses and ascites from which she fully recovered. One year later she developed a malignant right pleural effusion. After drainage and pleurodesis with tetracycline, she remained disease-free an additional 19-plus years. Treated in 1987, before this study, she is cited to highlight the unpredictable pattern and unusual course of individual survivors.

SURGERY

Treatment was decided by multimodality specialists after review of all physiologic and diagnostic tests, and patient and family input. Of the operations, 78% were done at a 50-bed community hospital 18 miles outside New York City, suggesting that centers of specialization are independent of institution size and academic affiliations.[7,28] The annual resectability rate for explored CaP patients was 93% to 98%. Survival for CaP should favor resected patients because of selection and lead-time bias. Smaller, less extensive, tumors; patients with fewer comorbid risk factors; and incidentally detected lesions, rather than surgery per se, may be the important survival determinants. Criteria for surgery should remain strict and selective because of the systemic nature of CaP. Four of the 17 survivors had pylorus preservation and 13 had distal gastric resection. The operative technique has constantly evolved since 1973 and now includes laparorobotic approaches.[13,30,31] These technical modifications are important but do not affect tumor biology. The mean and median operative time was 150 minutes for primary resection and 30 to 40 minutes longer in the neoadjuvant patients. Blood transfusions during surgery or hospitalization (7%), and pancreatic fistula (6%), all type A were infrequent. Two of the long-term survivors presented with complete superior mesenteric vein obstruction, which cleared with neoadjuvant therapy, suggesting vein obstruction could be caused by extrinsic compression and not tumor invasion. In both cases, the pancreas could be dissected from the vein. This began the authors' experience with skeletonization of the vein, which occurs when tumors abut the vein.[31] A recent review of vein resection for PDR indicated 50% of vein resections showed no vein involvement and deeper invasion of the vein wall or arterial involvement represented incurable disease.[54,55]

RECURRENCE AFTER TREATMENT

The low recurrence rate of 2 out of 17 subjects after 5 years may reflect a modest sample size or benefit of neoadjuvant therapy, which continued to maximum response. All 8 neoadjuvant 5-year survivors survived at least 10 years. Surgical tradition is difficult to change and neoadjuvant therapy has had a low impact on surgical practice for CaP. Surgery-last rather than surgery-first for CaP is logical. It precludes surgery when disease progresses during treatment; it ensures all patients receive systemic therapy, including the 20% to 40% whose postoperative morbidity excludes systemic therapy; it allows the results of treatment to be followed during therapy; and, most importantly, it may improve survival by killing microscopic systemic metastases.[7,9,25] Neoadjuvant therapy has been an integral part of treatment of CaP at MD Anderson Cancer Center since 1990.[9,25] From 1990 to 2002, 329 resected CaP subjects (77%) received neoadjuvant therapy and 91% received systemic therapy. Katz and colleagues[14] reported an actual 5-year and 10-year survival of 27% (88 out of 329) and 14% (20 out of 145) of eligible subjects.[9] Recurrence rates were 73% before 5 years but 8% after that. In their subsequent report survival is projected, but the use of chemotherapy-first continued in 3 out of 4 of subjects.[25] This is an important, well-formulated study with a high percentage of actual 5-year and 10-year survivors. Although vein resections were done in 1 out of 3 PDRs, the incidence of vein involvement was not stated. An updated MD Anderson experience correlated preoperative imaging and vein involvement, and indicated safe resection rates, but found that deeper vein wall involvement led to poorer survival.[55] Of 98 vein resections from 277 PDR subjects, 36% had no vein involvement and 17% had adventitial involvement. When greater than 180° vein involvement was present, tumor involvement exceeded 82% and survival was poor.[55] The senior surgeons (AMC) preference and experience supports teasing the pancreas from the lateral vein with a Freer vascular dissector and not resect the vein. "Skeletonization" of the vein has not compromised outcomes or resulted in local recurrence.[31]

LITERATURE REVIEW

Five and 10-year survival with CaP does not imply cure because of the likelihood of tumor recurrence after 5 years. A study from Memorial Sloan Kettering Cancer Center reported 75 of 618 (12%) resected CaP patients survived 5 years and 18 of 353 (5%) survived 10 or more years.[18] The recurrence rate after 5 years was 19 out of 75 (26%), all of whom died in the year 6. Most deaths occurred in low-stage cancers (1a, 1b, and 2b). Only 20% of resected subjects received adjuvant therapy. A report from The Massachusetts General Hospital cited 499 CaP patients followed at least 5 years.[18] Actual 5-year and 10-year survival was 19% (95 of 499) and 10% (33 of 329). Favorable factors included negative margins and negative nodes. However, 41% (39 out of 95) of survivors had positive nodes and 24% (23 out of 95) had positive margins. Twenty-three patients died after surviving 5 years, 12 of disease, 10 of unknown cause, and

1 unrelated to cancer. Several patients had recurrence after 10 years, 2 of whom had pulmonary resection for isolated lung metastases. Their conclusions: "prognosis is determined by tumor biology rather than clinicopathologic features."[8] Nearly 50% received adjuvant chemotherapy. Trede and colleagues[11,12] report a long experience in Manheim, Germany, with PDR and CaP dating to 1972. Of 130 PDR for CaP, there were 25 (19%) 5-year survivors. Six of 9 subjects with early cancers (<2-cm negative nodes and lymphatics) died of recurrence and the remaining 3 were well at 19, 42, and 65 months.[11,12]

EXPRESSING SURVIVAL

In the last 15 years, more reports of actual 5-year survivors have been published suggesting longer patient survival. This has not improved the cure rate.[6,13,14] Until recently, most reports were from large centers and were expressed as actuarial, not actual survival.[21,22,46] Actuarial survival is an inaccurate and misleading projection of outcomes that fall short of reality. Short follow-up and patients lost to follow-up (censored patients) lessen the denominator of the equation: number of survivors to number of operations, and overstate survival. Actuarial survival may overestimate actual survival by 3-fold to 7-fold or as much as 20%. Gudjonsson cited a study in which 11 out of 200 (5%) CaP subjects survived 5 years, whereas the actuarial survival was 22%.[21,22,27] In 1958, the actuarial method most commonly used was suggested by Kaplan and Meir[56] as a way of projecting survival when follow-up was incomplete. Today, centers have the capability to follow patients for 5, 10, and more years, longitudinal follow-ups expressing actual survival would be more accurate than multiple reports of the same patients projecting survival. Lead-time bias is an important factor that may explain the increase in actual 5-year survival but not cure. Lead-time bias favors patients with asymptomatic cancers detected earlier in development, which allows longer survival, than patients whose onset of cancer is the same but whose detection is delayed until symptomatic, which for CaP is often preterminal. This suggests the 10-year to 20-year span for pancreatic cancers from development to death provides an apparent longer survival for asymptomatic patients. Today, many CaPs are discovered in a preclinical stage, by axial imaging, in nonjaundiced patients with nonspecific symptoms. These tumors are detected earlier then 20-plus years ago, before axial scans, when jaundice and cancer cachexia (late symptoms) were common.[57] Earlier is not the same as early because latent metastases have occurred.[58] Depending on immune and defense mechanisms, metastases become evident months to years after the primary tumor is treated. Survival may seem longer for preclinical than symptomatic patients but the difference may be apparent, not real, and due to lead-time and selection bias. Because the percentage of resectable CaP cases has remained consistent at 10% to 20% for 5 decades, additional 5-year survivors represent earlier, but not early, detection.[59] This may explain the apparent increased survival but not cure.[14,58]

Survival statistics may be misleading. At best 20% of CaP are resected, or 20 of 100 CaP. A 20% 5 year survival usually refers to resected patients since 80% of CaP are unresectable and very few survive 5 years. Thus the "20% survival" figure refers to only 4 patients (20% of 20 resections) and not 20.

SYSTEMIC THERAPY

Because pancreatic cancer is a systemic disease, logic and common sense hold that systemic therapy be given first, before rather than after surgery.[7,9,25,33,60] Although the value of chemotherapy in pancreatic and other cancers has been questioned, there are significant responses, even complete resolution.[7,9,33] As personal therapy becomes available, outcomes may improve. Although the use of chemotherapy is not questioned, its benefits may be overestimated. Morgan, Ward, and Barton[15] reviewed the contribution of cytotoxic chemotherapy to 5-year survival in 22 malignancies in the United States and Australia. The estimated overall benefits were 2.3% in Australia and 2.1% in the United States. For pancreatic cancer in which 5-year survival is less than 5%, it was difficult to determine a survival benefit.

LATENT OR DORMANT DISEASE

Some CaP patients are cured or improved after chemotherapy. Because the mean age for CaP is the mid-60s, the benefits of effective therapy have natural time limits. More than 80% metastasize and are viable but dormant, until they overcome or are overcome by host defenses.[57] The latent cells have properties of stem cells, express transcription factors, and slowly proliferate and have a high initial attrition rate.[58] Monocyte transported natural killer cells kill latent tumors and the protumor and antitumor actions of the immune system determine whether tumors will remain latent or lethal. Certainly, a few CaP patients are cured. Whether the surviving patients in this report will continue disease free and possibly cured is not known. Relative to most patients with treated CaP they are part of a fortunate and lucky few.

PERSONAL THOUGHTS

This study adapted a trial of neoadjuvant multidrug chemoradiation therapy for pancreatic cancer 30 years ago, believing that the mantra that pancreatic resection offers the only chance of cure was misleading and ignored the true outcomes of CaP. Patients may be misled and uninformed by a surgery-first approach and, if aware of morbidity, survival, and cure, might be receptive to other options. If the treatment of pancreatic cancer were a business model, it would have been scraped long ago and open-minded newer alternatives sought. For CaP, these include targeted therapy, neoadjuvant therapy, and prevention, all worthy of further exploration.

SUMMARY

Cure of pancreatic cancer is unlikely. A modest series is presented and followed for more than 10 years. Although the results compare favorably to other reports of actual survivors, nearly half had neoadjuvant therapy for initially unresectable lesions, and were treated to maximum response before consideration of surgery. Fifteen of 17 5-year survivors lived 10 or more years from diagnosis and 3 surpassed 20 years, 2 of whom are alive. Similar if not more impressive outcomes are reported from MD Anderson, at which chemotherapy before surgery has become their standard of care. A century of thinking that surgery is the only chance of cure should be replaced by the more accurate aphorism, surgery has little chance of cure. If surgery-first remains a standard, or traditional, approach, little change in outcome can be anticipated. An open-minded, less repetitive and more innovative approach is long overdue. Preventing pancreatic cancer should be everyone's first choice and effective therapy a distant second.[58]

Between 1991 to 2000, the years of this study, patients were treated and followed at The Pancreas and Biliary Center at Dobbs Ferry Hospital, NY, where nearly all of the authors practiced, or consulted. Since then, physician affiliations have become more diverse and include the Mount Sinai–affiliated institutions, Lenox Hill-Northwell Hospital, Dobbs Ferry Hospital, and Albert Einstein-Montefiore Hospitals.

ACKNOWLEDGMENTS

The authors acknowledge Ted Casper, MD and Charles Fishman, MD who provided expert critical and pulmonary care in the latter years of the study, and the extraordinary nursing staff at Dobbs Ferry Hospital who provided compassionate and superb care.

REFERENCES

1. Howlader N, Noone AM, Krapcho M, et al. SEER cancer statistics review 975-2010 NCI, Bethesda (MD).
2. Beger HG, Bettina R, Gansauge F, et al. Pancreatic cancer low survival rates. Dtsch Arztebl Int 2008;105:255–62.
3. Carpelan- Holmstrom M, Nording S, Pukkala E. Does anyone survive pancreatic ductal adenocarcinoma? A nationwide study reevaluating the data of the Finnish Cancer Registry. Gut 2005;54:385–7.
4. Office for national statistics, Cancer survival in England; Patients diagnosed 2005-2009 and followed up to 2010 LONDON, ONS 1959.
5. Gong Z, Holly EA, Paige M. Survival in ppopulation based pancreatic cancer patients; San Francisco Bay Area, 1995-1999. Am J Epidemiol 2011;174(12):1373–81.
6. Cooperman A. Pancreatic cancer: the bigger picture. Surg Clin North Am 2001;81:557–74.
7. Cooperman AM, Snady H, Bruckner H, et al. Long-term follow-up of twenty patients with adenocarcinoma of the pancreas: resection following combined modality therapy. Surg Clin North Am 2001;81:699–708.
8. Ferrone CR, Vanmarcke RP, Bloom JR, et al. Pancreatic ductal adenocarcinoma: long term survival does not equal cure. Surgery 2012;152:S43–9.
9. Katz MHG, Wang H, Fleming J, et al. Long term survival after multidisciplinary management of resected pancreatic adenocarcinoma. Ann Surg Oncol 2009;16:836–47.
10. Rocha F, Hashimoto Y, Traverso W, et al. Interferon-based adjuvant chemoradiation for resected pancreatic head cancer: long-term follow-up of the Virginia Mason protocol. Ann Surg 2016;263(2):376–84.
11. Trede M, Schwall G, Seeger HD. Survival after pancreaticoduodenectomy 118 consecutive resections without an operative mortality. Ann Surg 1990;211:447–58.
12. Trede M, Richter A, Wendel K. Personal observations, opinions, and approaches, to cancer of the pancreas and periampullary area. Surg Clin North Am 2001;81:595–611.
13. Cooperman A, Wayne M, Steele J. Editorial cancer of the pancreas (CaP) New thoughts, new approaches for the new year pancreatic disorders & therapy. ISSN: 2165-7992.
14. Luberice K, Downs D, Sadowitz B, et al. Has survival improved following resection for pancreatic adenocarcinoma? Am J Surg 2017;214(2):341–6.
15. Morgan GM, Ward R, Barton M. The contribution of cytotoxic chemotherapy to 5 year survival in adult malignancies. Clin Oncol 2004;16:549–69.
16. Wagman R, Grann A. Adjuvant therapy for pancreatic cancer: current treatment approaches and future challenges. Surg Clin North Am 2001;81:667–83.

17. Kozuch P, Petryk M, Evans A, et al. Therapy for regionally unresectable pancreatic cancer. Surg Clin North Am 2001;81:691–9.
18. Ferrone CR, Brennan M, Gonen M, et al. Pancreatic adenocarcinoma: the actual 5 year survivors. J Gastrointest Surg 2008;12:701–6.
19. Helm JF, Centeno BA, Coppola D, et al. Outcomes following resection of pancreatic adenocarcinoma: 20-year experience at a single institution. Cancer Control 2008;15(4):288–94.
20. Schnelldorfer T, Ware AL, Sara MG, et al. Long term survival after pancreatoduodenectomy for pancreatic adenocarcinoma: is cure possible. Ann Surg 2008;247:456–62.
21. Riall TS, Cameron JL, Lillemoe KD. Resected periampullary adenocarcinoma: 5 year survivors and their 6-10 year follow up. Surgery 2006;140:764–72.
22. Yeo CJ, Cameron JL, Lillemoe KD. Pancreaticoduodenectomy for cancer of the head of the pancreas. Ann Surg 1995;221(6):721–33.
23. Cleary SP, Gryfe R, Guindi M. Prognostic factors in resected pancreatic adenocarcinoma: analyses of actual5 year survivors. J Am Coll Surg 2004;198:722–31.
24. Perysinkas I, Avonitis S, Georgiadou D. Five-year actual survival after pancreatoduodenectomy for pancreatic head cancer. ANZ J Surg 2015;85(3):183–6.
25. Cloyd JM, Katz MH, Prakash L, et al. Pancreaticoduodenectomy for pancreatic ductal adenocarcinoma. A 25 year single institution experience. J Gastrointest Surg 2017;21(1):164–74.
26. Duran H, Lelpo B, Diaz E, et al. Real 5 year survival after radical surgery for pancreatic carcinoma: can it be predicted with the usual prognostic factors. JOP.
27. Kuhlman KFD, deCastro SMM, Wesseling SG. Surgical treatment of pancreatic adenocarcinoma; actual survival and prognostic factors in 343 patients. Eur J Cancer 2004;40(4):549–58.
28. Kure S, Kaneko T, Takeda S. Analysis of long term survivors after surgical resection for invasive pancreatic cancer. HPB (Oxford) 2005;7:129–34.
29. Cooperman AM, Schwartz E, Fader A, et al. Safey, efficacy and cost of ancreaticoduodenal resection in a specialized center based at a community hospital. Arch Surg 1997;132:744–8.
30. Cooperman AM. Pancreaticoduodenal resection pearls, perils, pitfalls. Surg Clin North Am 2001;81(3):579–93.
31. Cooperman AM, Wayne M, Iskandar M. Steele Skeletonization in lieu of portal mesenteric vein resection during pancreaticoduodenal resection J GI Research and Therapy Vil 1 ;1;2016
32. Cooperman A, Fader A, Cushin B, et al. Surgery for cancer of the pancreas: will common sense become common practice. Hematol Oncol Clin North Am 2002;16(1):81–94.
33. Snady H, Bruckner H, Cooperman AM, et al. Survival advantage of combined chemoradiotherapy compared with resection as the initial treatment of patients with regional pancreatic carcinoma; an outcomes trial. Cancer 2000;89:314–37.
34. Lambe M, Elorante S, Wigertz A, et al. Pancreatic cancer; reporting and long term survival in Sweden. Acta Oncol 2011;50(8):1220–7.
35. Soreide K, Agnes B, Moller B, et al. Epidemiology of pancreatic cancer in Norway:trends in incidence, basis of diagnosis and survival 1965-2007. Scand J Gastroenterol 2010;45:82–92.
36. Luo J, Xiao L, Wu C, et al. The incidence and survival rate of population based pancreatic cancer patients: Shanghai cancer registry 2004-2009. PLoS One 2013;8(10):e76052.

37. Coleman MP, Babb P, Damiecki P, et al. Cancer survival trends in England and Wales 1971-1995. Deprivation and National Health Service regional series SMDS 61 London ONS 1959.
38. Speer AG, Thurfield VJ, Tom-Broors Y, et al. Pancreatic cancer: surgical management and outcomes after 6 years of follow-up. Med J Aust 2012;196(8):511–5.
39. Adham M, Jack D, Le Borgne JL. Long term survival (5-20 years)after pancreatectomy for pancreatic ductal adenocarcinoma: a series of 30 patients collected from 3 institutions. Pancreas 2008;37:352–7.
40. Kimura K, Amano R, Nakata B. Clinical and pathological features of five-year survives after pancreatectomy for pancreatic adenocarcinoma. World J Surg Oncol 2014;12:350.
41. Cooperman AM, Bruckner HB, Siegal J, et al. Is pancreatic cancer curable by surgery alone? [abstract]. Gastroenterology 1994;110:4.
42. Gudjonsson BEM, Livstone EM, Spiro HM. Cancer of the pancreas diagnostic accuracy and survival statistics. Cancer 1978;42:2494–506.
43. Gudjonsson B. Cancer of the pancreas 50 years of surgery. Cancer 1987;60:2284–303.
44. Gudjonsson B. Pancreatic cancer: 80 years of surgery-percentage and repetitions. HPB Surg 2016;2016:6839687.
45. Gudjonsson B. Letter to the editor. J Am Coll Surg 1996;183:290–1.
46. Gudjonsson B. Carcinoma of the pancreas critical analyses of costs, results of resections, and the need for standardized reporting. J Am Coll Surg 1995;181(6):483–503.
47. Crile G Jr. The advantage of bypass operations over radical pancreaticoduodenectomy in the treatment of pancreatic carcinoma. Surg Gynecol Obstet 1970;130(6):1049–53.
48. Shapiro TM. Adenocarcinoma of the pancreas: a statistical analyses of biliary bypass vs Whipple resection in good risk patients. Ann Surg 1975;182(6):715–21.
49. Eckstam M. Survival 13 years after pancreatectomy for ductal adenocarcinoma of the head of the pancreas. Wis Med J 1994;93:266–9.
50. Grundman RT, Meyer F. Second primary malignancy among cancer survivorsepidemiology, prognosis and clinical relevance. Zentralbl Chir 2012;137(6):565–74 [in German].
51. Sastry A, Wayne M, Steele J, et al. Three separate synchronous, sporadic and separate periampullary and pancreatic tumors; more than a coincidence. World J Surg Oncol 2014;12:382.
52. Shen M, Boffetta P, Olsen J, et al. Pooled analysis of second primary pancreatic cancers. Am J Epidemiol 2006;163(6):502–11.
53. Akabai H, Shiomi H, Naka S. Resectable carcinoma developing in the remnant pancreas 7 years and 10 months after distal pancreatectomy for invasive ductal carcinoma of the pancreas. World J Surg Oncol 2014;12:224.
54. Barreto SG, Windsor JA. Justifying vein resection with pancreaticoduodenectomy. Lancet Oncol 2016;17:e118–24.
55. Tran C, Bao HS, Balanchander A, et al. Radiographic tumor vein interface as a predictor of intraoperative pathologic and oncologic outcomes in resected Borderline resected pancreas cancer. J Gastrointest Surg 2014;18(2):269–78.
56. Kaplan EI, Meier P. Nonparametric estimation from incomplete observations. J Am Stat Assoc 1958;457–81.
57. Pollard JW. Defining metastatic cell latency. N Engl J Med 2016;375(3):280–2.

58. Ryan DR, Hong TS, Bardea TJ. Pancreatic adenocarcinoma. N Engl J Med 2014; 371:1039–49.
59. Cooperman AM, Iskandar M, Wayne M, et al. Prevention and early detection of pancreatic cancer. Surg Clin North Am, in press.
60. Chen SC, Shyr YM, Wang SE. Long term survival after pancreaticoduodenectomy for periampullary adenocarcinomas. HPB (Oxford) 2013;15:951–7.

Rare, Uncommon, and Unusual Complications After Pancreaticoduodenal Resection

Thinzar M. Lwin, MS, MD[a,b], Natasha Leigh, MD[c],
Mazen E. Iskandar, MD[b,c], Justin G. Steele, MD[d],
Michael G. Wayne, DO[d], Avram M. Cooperman, MD[d,*]

KEYWORDS

- Pancreaticoduodenal resection • Pancreaticoduodenectomy • Whipple procedure
- Postpancreatectomy complications • Pituitary apoplexy
- Transfusion-transmitted babesiosis • Transfusion-related lung injury
- Pseudoaneurysm

KEY POINTS

- Pancreaticoduodenal resection is a complex procedure associated with several postoperative complications due to multivisceral and anastamoses.
- Nearly all complications are a direct result of the operation; others are due to the systemic impact of the procedure often on compromised patients even if the procedure was unremarkable.
- Three rare complications include babesiosis, pituitary apoplexy, and transfusion-related acute lung injury.

INTRODUCTION

The perils of pancreatic surgery, in particular pancreaticoduodenal resection (PDR), are well known to physicians, patients, and their families. Most complications are related to the operation. Vascular injuries or enterotomies usually occur during dissection. Fistulas, abscesses, and their sequelae follow anastomotic breakdown. Rarely, complications are systemic from altered immunity or changes in the cardiovascular system even when surgery was apparently uneventful for both the surgeon and the

Disclosure: The authors have nothing to disclose.
[a] Department of Surgery, University of California San Diego, 3855 Health Sciences Drive, La Jolla, CA 92093, USA; [b] Department of Surgery, Mt Sinai Beth Israel, 10 Nathan D Perlman Place, New York, NY 10003, USA; [c] Department of Surgery, Mt Sinai St Luke's-West Medical Center, 1000 10th Avenue, New York, NY 10019, USA; [d] The Pancreas, Biliary and Advanced Laparoscopy Center of New York, 305 Second Avenue, New York, NY 10003, USA
* Corresponding author.
E-mail address: avram.cooperman@gmail.com

https://doi.org/10.1016/j.suc.2017.09.015
0039-6109/18/© 2017 Elsevier Inc. All rights reserved.
surgical.theclinics.com

patient. This article reviews rare (case reports), uncommon (5%–10% incidence), and unusual (<5%) complications of PDR.

RARE COMPLICATION (CASE REPORTS)

Despite a long experience with PDR and its complications, 3 complications not technically related to PDR stand out as singularly unusual events: babesiosis, pituitary apoplexy, and transfusion-related acute lung injury (TRALI). The first 2 are discussed in detail and the case TRALI is summarized.

Babesiosis

Postoperative anemia is common in patients after PDR. Usually reflective of intraoperative blood loss or continued oozing from small vessels, it is usually self-limited and successfully treated with transfusion and correction of any coagulopathies. Post-PDR patients, however, in particular those who have undergone splenectomy, are a unique group of immunosuppressed patients susceptible to unusual blood-borne pathogens.

A 46-year-old healthy man from Macedonia underwent pancreaticoduodenectomy for pancreatic adenocarcinoma. He had a microscopically positive resection margin at the pancreatic tail and a completion total pancreatectomy with splenectomy. Postoperatively, the patient suffered from acute blood loss anemia and received a transfusion of 1 unit of packed red blood cells. He contracted mild *Clostridium difficile* diarrhea and was treated with vancomycin with resolution. He received all postsplenectomy vaccinations 2 weeks postoperatively. The patient was readmitted 6 weeks postoperatively and found to have new bilateral lower extremity deep vein thrombosis. While on anticoagulation, he developed anemia, altered mental status, fever, malaise, tachycardia, leukocytosis, and elevated transaminases. He again received a transfusion of 2 units of packed red blood cells without appropriate increase in hemoglobin levels. Blood smears demonstrated hemolysis, intraerythrocytic parasites and Maltese cross forms consistent with *Babesia microti* infection. This was confirmed with polymerase chain reaction (PCR) testing. The patient underwent urgent exchange transfusions and received antibiotics (quinidine and clindamycin) with decreasing parasitemia on subsequent blood smears. Testing of the index transfused unit of red blood cells showed *Babesia mcroti*. The donor was recalled for testing. He was clinically asymptomatic but had positive serology for the organism. The patient had a prolonged hospital course and expired 2 months postoperatively from recurrent parasitemia and vancomycin-resistant enterococcal bacteremia. This is the first report that the authors know of a patient who developed transfusion-transmitted babesiosis after pancreatectomy and splenectomy. This patient was young and previously healthy and expired within 2 months after surgery. The synergistic effects of babesiosis, asplenia, and pancreatic cancer were responsible for a fulminant process with early recurrence and death.

Babesiosis is a rare blood-borne illness caused by infection with the intraerythrocytic parasite *Babesia*. This global disease, although uncommon in the United States, is seen more frequently in parts of Europe and the developing world, where it is transmitted most commonly via tick bites.[1] Transfusion-related babesiosis is accountable for the vast minority of cases; however, it remains an underappreciated etiology with increasing incidence. Of the 150 reported cases, 75% were reported after 2000.[2] The parasite survives standard blood product processing and storage and there is currently no screening protocol for donor detection. Laboratory tests demonstrate hemolytic anemia; however, key to establishing the diagnosis are a blood smear with intraerythrocytic parasites and PCR testing. Although not necessarily clinically significant in all patients, the immunocompromised host is especially susceptible, particularly patients after splenectomy. Suspicion should be increased in immunosuppressed patients with persistent anemia and signs of hemolysis. In immunocompetent patients, symptomatology may be mild with a nonspecific febrile illness. Progression to multisystem organ failure, disseminated intravascular coagulation, and death, however, have been reported in 5% to 6.5% of immunocompromised patients.[3,4] Treatment consists of atovaquone and azithromycin or quinine and clindamycin for 7 days to 10 days.[5] Severe cases may require more prolonged courses and repeat exchange transfusions. Patients who have undergone PDR are a susceptible, immunosuppressed group who are more likely to receive blood transfusions postoperatively. Additional screening measures may need to be considered in transfusing these patients.[6–9]

Pituitary Apoplexy

A 64-year-old previously healthy woman presented for evaluation of abdominal discomfort and weight loss. Evaluation revealed a pancreatic mass suspicious for cancer, which was confirmed by biopsy. After a thorough evaluation and discussion with her and her family, she underwent a PDR for pancreatic cancer. The procedure was uneventful, with 3 hours of operative time, less than 300 mL of estimated blood loss, and no major blood pressure fluctuations. She became hypertensive in the recovery room and complained of a frontal headache. On examination, she had ophthalmoplegia with medial and lateral gaze palsies, right eye ptosis, and a right dilated nonreactive pupil. An MRI demonstrated a hypoenhancing pituitary mass with displacement of the cavernous segments of bilateral internal carotid arteries with mass effect on the optic chiasm. She underwent successful trans-sphenoidal pituitary resection the next day with complete resolution. She remains symptom-free, other than a mild proptosis 6 months later. Pathology was notable for a pituitary adenoma, gonadotroph cell–type expressing chromogranin, and leutenizing hormone. It is likely that blood pressure swing contributed to the etiology in this patient. Although there are other reports of pituitary apoplexy triggered after cardiac, orthopedic, head and neck, and laparoscopic abdominal surgeries, this is the only case report of pituitary apoplexy after pancreatic surgery.[10–14]

Pituitary apoplexy was first reported by Bailey[15] in 1898 as a cluster of symptoms, including altered mental status, headache, nausea, vomiting, and visual changes associated with hormonal dysfunction. An incidence of 0.6% to 9.1% in symptomatic patients compared with up to 25% in asymptomatic patients has been reported.[16–18] The etiology remains unclear; however, it is commonly believed that tissue expansion without increase in blood flow leads to areas with tenuous blood supply. A lack of autoregulation from the transmitted systemic and intracranial pressure fluctuations during surgery can lead to ischemia with subsequent hemorrhagic necrosis.[19–21] Pancreatic surgery is often associated with significant fluid shifts and hemodynamic changes. Although the surgery was uneventful, presumably these physiologic fluctuations led to a hemorrhagic infarct into a previously clinically silent pituitary adenoma. A high index of suspicion for pituitary apoplexy in patients with typical symptomatology facilitates expeditious diagnosis and prompt treatment to prevent permanent visual and neurologic deficits.

Transfusion-Related Acute Lung Injury

TRALI is a serious and potential fatal complication of blood product transfusion. The diagnosis is made by acute lung injury occurring within 6 hours of completed transfusion of blood or blood products, no preexisting lung injury, and no other temporarily associated risk factors for acute lung injury.

A platelet transfusion was suggested by anesthesia and given before induction of anesthesia. The PDR was uneventful, additional transfusions were not necessary, and the procedure was near completion within 3 hours when there was difficulty ventilating and oxygenating the patient. A pneumothorax was ruled out as were other airway issues. After transfer to the ICU, a diagnosis of TRALI was made and a very difficult 6 days to 7 days of ventilatory support and critical care ensued until the episode waned and then resolved. TRALI most often follows platelet transfusion but the incidence is highest after blood transfusion, where the incidence is 1/12,000 transfusions, and is usually self-limiting and resolves without steroids within 48 hours to 96 hours. Pathophysiology involves patient factors, including preexisting inflammatory conditions that cause pulmonary endothelial damage and capillary leak triggered by a transfusion containing HLAs, human neutrophil antibodies, or biologically active lipids. A major abdominal procedure like PDR can lead to an inflammatory state that predisposes patients to TRALI after platelet transfusion.[22] Current risk-reduction approaches include screening against donors who may be alloimmunized followed by antibody testing in selected donors.[23]

UNCOMMON COMPLICATIONS (5%–10% INCIDENCE)
Visceral Artery Pseudoaneurysms

Delayed postpancreatectomy hemorrhage is a complication in 4% to 16% of PDR, with mortality rates as high as 50%.[24–26] Hemorrhage within the first 72 hours after PDR is usually due to venous bleeding from portal-mesenteric tributaries or small arteries and, if not tamponaded by surrounding viscera or clot, may require re-exploration for evacuation and hemostasis. Venous bleeding is low pressure and more apt to stop spontaneously than arterial bleeding.

Late postoperative hemorrhage (1–4 weeks) is initiated by a pancreaticojejunal fistula followed by sepsis from intestinal and biliary bacteria, a pseudoaneurysm, and then hemorrhage.[27] It is the local sepsis that weakens the vessel wall and leads to formation of the pseudoaneurysm.[28] The gastroduodenal artery stump is most often involved, followed by the hepatic, splenic, and intestinal branches of the superior mesenteric artery. An initial transient sentinel gastrointestinal or intraperitoneal bleed(s) heralds subsequent hemorrhage hours to days later.[29] Unanticipated delayed hemorrhage should prompt a computed tomograpy angiogram (CTA) (diagnostic sensitivity >95%).[30] If the amount of contrast used would limit 2 studies and suspicion and experience is high, an angiogram should be done directly. Stenting or embolization of the bleeding pseudoaneurysm is indicated and very successful.[31] Surgical intervention should be infrequently needed because of the great success with angiography and experience that local sepsis persisting after surgery may cause rebleeding and the need for repeat angiography. The reported increased mortality with surgery reflects the critical status of at risk elderly patients with continued bleeding (47% vs 22%, $P = .02$).[32] A multidisciplinary approach, particularly with experienced interventional radiologists, decreases the need for surgery and improves outcomes.[33]

Chylous Ascites

Postoperative chyle leak occurs in 1.3% to 10.8% of patients after pancreatic resection and is due to injury of a major lymphatic channel during an extended lymphadenectomy.[34] Often benign and self-limiting, larger leaks may need occasional oral and intravenous support with medium chain triglycerides, fluids, and electrolytes. Milky drainage fluid with elevated drain triglycerides is diagnostic.[35] Persistent high-volume drainage after PDR may require intravenous fluids and octreotide. Surgical ligation of the cisterna chyli or thoracic duct is infrequently needed. This is a complication best avoided because extended or radical lymphadenectomy adds nothing to survival of pancreatic cancer and is difficult to justify.

Cholangitis

Biliary strictures occur in 3% to 13% of patients after PDR.[36–38] Although attributed to T-tube use or small ducts, the authors' experience is they are rare, are ischemic, and present 8 to 10 or more years after PDR. Stenting and dilatation, either percutaneous or endoscopic, has been succssful treatment. Surgery should rarely be needed.

UNUSUAL COMPLICATIONS (2%–5% INCIDENCE)
Marginal Ulceration

Today gastrojejunal ulceration or marginal ulcers (MUs) after PDR should be unusual. MU after duodenal ulcer surgery was a common complication until H_2-receptor antagonists were introduced. MUs after PDR were uncommon because survival was limited after PDR, and most patients were elderly with hypochlorhydria or achlorhydria, an unlikely population for duodenal ulcers. After distal gastric resection, ulceration can occur on the gastric or jejunal side of the gastrojejunostomy. Ulcerations on the gastric side are due to alkaline reflux and emesis of bile is common. Symptoms are not alleviated by antiulcer therapy. Ulcerations on the jejunal side are peptic in origin and antiulcer therapy relieves symptoms. As indications for PDR were extended to pancreatitis and cystic lesions and younger patients underwent PDR, more MUs were encountered. In 2014, the reported incidence was 2.5% after PDR and 2% after pylorus-preserving PDR. With prophylactic antisecretory medications and compliant patients, rates of ulceration are as low as 1.4%.[39]

Afferent Loop Syndrome

Afferent loop syndrome (ALS) after PDR is due to a partial or complete mechanical obstruction of bile, pancreatic juices, partially digested food, and in a redundant afferent jejunal limb. ALS is usually a late and chronic complication after PDR, and the higher-pressure fluid filled distal limb untwists and rapidly empties often into the stomach and jejunum, which is relieved by emesis. Acute ALS can cause fluid distention in the afferent loop, and dehiscence of a fresh pancreatic or biliary anastamoses or disruption of the limb. Acute ALS has been recognized after gastric resection with a loop gastrojejunostomy, but an acute postoperative presentation is unusual after PDR. Five cases after PDR were cited.[40] All required reoperation with satisfactory outcome. This is best avoided by a nonredundant limb.

Ischemic

The pancreatic head is perfused by the celiac axis and the superior mesenteric artery via the gastroduodenal artery and pancreaticoduodenal arcades. Ischemic complications are exceedingly rare (<2%) given the frequency of PDR and its elderly population. Significant celiac or superior mesenteric artery stenoses is seen in 11% of elderly patients and when diagnosed should be evaluated and stented if necessary preoperatively.[41,42] The consequences of bowel necrosis, anastomotic dehiscence, mesenteric infarction, or hepatic failure and sepsis have a high mortality rate

(83%).[43] This is a situation best avoided by a thorough review of all cross-sectional imaging before surgery is considered.[44–46]

SUMMARY

Complications after PDR occur in at least 30% of patients. Nearly all early complications are a direct result of an intraoperative event, dissection, or anastomoses. By far the most common complications result from a pancreatic enteric leak or fistula. This accounts for the most serious morbidities, sepsis, pseudoaneurysms, and hemorrhage. Rarely, complications are systemic and stem from a compromised or immunosuppresed host or changes in blood flow or pressure during or after surgery. Three rare complications, which were shocking to the authors and were serious or fatal to patients are described: babesiosis, TRALI, and pituitary apoplexy, 2 of which were caused by transfusion of blood and platelets. PDR is a significant operation with serious consequences, and decisions on selection of candidates and safe operations should be thoughtful and always in surgeons' minds.

REFERENCES

1. Ord RL, Lobo CA. Human babesiosis: pathogens, prevalence, diagnosis and treatment. Curr Clin Microbiol Rep 2015;2(4):173–81.
2. Herwaldt BL, Linden JV, Bosserman E, et al. Transfusion-associated babesiosis in the United States: a description of cases. Ann Intern Med 2011;155(8):509–19.
3. White DJ, Talarico J, Chang HG, et al. Human babesiosis in New York State: review of 139 hospitalized cases and analysis of prognostic factors. Arch Intern Med 1998;158(19):2149–54.
4. Vannier EG, Diuk-Wasser MA, Ben Mamoun C, et al. Babesiosis. Infect Dis Clin North Am 2015;29(2):357–70.
5. Krause PJ, Gewurz BE, Hill D, et al. Persistent and relapsing babesiosis in immunocompromised patients. Clin Infect Dis 2008;46(3):370–6.
6. Centers for Disease Control and Prevention (CDC). Babesiosis surveillance - 18 States, 2011. MMWR Morb Mortal Wkly Rep 2012;61(27):505–9.
7. Bish EK, Moritz ED, El-Amine H, et al. Cost-effectiveness of a Babesia microti blood donation intervention based on real-time prospective screening in endemic areas of the United States. Transfusion 2016;56(3):775–7.
8. Goodell AJ, Bloch E, Simon MS, et al. Babesia screening: the importance of reporting and calibration in cost-effectiveness models. Transfusion 2016;56(3):774–5.
9. Simon MS, Leff JA, Pandya A, et al. Cost-effectiveness of blood donor screening for Babesia microti in endemic regions of the United States. Transfusion 2014;54(3 Pt 2):889–99.
10. Liu JK, Nwagwu C, Pikus HJ, et al. Laparoscopic anterior lumbar interbody fusion precipitating pituitary apoplexy. Acta Neurochir (Wien) 2001;143(3):303–6 [discussion: 306–307].
11. Fyrmpas G, Constantinidis J, Foroglou N, et al. Pituitary apoplexy following endoscopic sinus surgery. J Laryngol Otol 2010;124(6):677–9.
12. Mukhida K, Kolyvas G. Pituitary apoplexy following cardiac surgery. Can J Neurol Sci 2007;34(3):390–3.
13. Mura P, Cossu AP, Musu M, et al. Pituitary apoplexy after laparoscopic surgery: a case report. Eur Rev Med Pharmacol Sci 2014;18(22):3524–7.
14. Goel V, Debnath UK, Singh J, et al. Pituitary apoplexy after joint arthroplasty. J Arthroplasty 2009;24(5):826.e7-10.

15. Bailey P. Pathological report of a case of acromegaly with special reference to the lesions in hypophysis cerebri and in the thyroid gland, and a case of hemorrhage into the pituitary. Phila Med J 1898;1:789–92.
16. Randeva HS, Schoebel J, Byrne J, et al. Classical pituitary apoplexy: clinical features, management and outcome. Clin Endocrinol (Oxf) 1999;51(2):181–8.
17. Singh TD, Valizadeh N, Meyer FB, et al. Management and outcomes of pituitary apoplexy. J Neurosurg 2015;122(6):1450–7.
18. Woo HJ, Hwang JH, Hwang SK, et al. Clinical outcome of cranial neuropathy in patients with pituitary apoplexy. J Korean Neurosurg Soc 2010;48(3):213–8.
19. Lubina A, Olchovsky D, Berezin M, et al. Management of pituitary apoplexy: clinical experience with 40 patients. Acta Neurochir (Wien) 2005;147(2):151–7 [discussion: 157].
20. Sibal L, Ball SG, Connolly V, et al. Pituitary apoplexy: a review of clinical presentation, management and outcome in 45 cases. Pituitary 2004;7(3):157–63.
21. Nawar RN, AbdelMannan D, Selman WR, et al. Pituitary tumor apoplexy: a review. J Intensive Care Med 2008;23(2):75–90.
22. Tariket S, Sut C, Hamzeh-Cognasse H, et al. Transfusion-related acute lung injury: transfusion, platelets and biological response modifiers. Expert Rev Hematol 2016;9(5):497–508.
23. Dunbar NM. Current options for transfusion-related acute lung injury risk mitigation in platelet transfusions. Curr Opin Hematol 2015;22(6):554–8.
24. Blanc T, Cortes A, Goere D, et al. Hemorrhage after pancreaticoduodenectomy: when is surgery still indicated? Am J Surg 2007;194(1):3–9.
25. de Castro SM, Busch OR, Gouma DJ. Management of bleeding and leakage after pancreatic surgery. Best Pract Res Clin Gastroenterol 2004;18(5):847–64.
26. Gao F, Li J, Quan S, et al. Risk factors and treatment for hemorrhage after pancreaticoduodenectomy: a case series of 423 patients. Biomed Res Int 2016; 2016:2815693.
27. Feng J, Chen YL, Dong JH, et al. Post-pancreaticoduodenectomy hemorrhage: risk factors, managements and outcomes. Hepatobiliary Pancreat Dis Int 2014; 13(5):513–22.
28. Rumstadt B, Schwab M, Korth P, et al. Hemorrhage after pancreatoduodenectomy. Ann Surg 1998;227(2):236–41.
29. Brodsky JT, Turnbull AD. Arterial hemorrhage after pancreatoduodenectomy. The "sentinel bleed". Arch Surg 1991;126(8):1037–40.
30. Chua AE, Ridley LJ. Diagnostic accuracy of CT angiography in acute gastrointestinal bleeding. J Med Imaging Radiat Oncol 2008;52(4):333–8.
31. Tien YW, Wu YM, Liu KL, et al. Angiography is indicated for every sentinel bleed after pancreaticoduodenectomy. Ann Surg Oncol 2008;15(7):1855–61.
32. Roulin D, Cerantola Y, Demartines N, et al. Systematic review of delayed postoperative hemorrhage after pancreatic resection. J Gastrointest Surg 2011;15(6): 1055–62.
33. Dumitru R, Carbunaru A, Grasu M, et al. Pseudoaneurysm of the splenic artery - an uncommon cause of delayed hemorrhage after pancreaticoduodenectomy. Ann Hepatobiliary Pancreat Surg 2016;20(4):204–10.
34. Assumpcao L, Cameron JL, Wolfgang CL, et al. Incidence and management of chyle leaks following pancreatic resection: a high volume single-center institutional experience. J Gastrointest Surg 2008;12(11):1915–23.
35. Kuboki S, Shimizu H, Yoshidome H, et al. Chylous ascites after hepatopancreatobiliary surgery. Br J Surg 2013;100(4):522–7.

36. Reid-Lombardo KM, Ramos-De la Medina A, Thomsen K, et al. Long-term anastomotic complications after pancreaticoduodenectomy for benign diseases. J Gastrointest Surg 2007;11(12):1704–11.
37. House MG, Cameron JL, Schulick RD, et al. Incidence and outcome of biliary strictures after pancreaticoduodenectomy. Ann Surg 2006;243(5):571–6 [discussion: 576–578].
38. Prawdzik C, Belyaev O, Chromik AM, et al. Surgical revision of hepaticojejunostomy strictures after pancreatectomy. Langenbecks Arch Surg 2015;400(1):67–75.
39. Butler JR, Rogers T, Eckart G, et al. Is antisecretory therapy after pancreatoduodenectomy necessary? Meta-analysis and contemporary practices of pancreatic surgeons. J Gastrointest Surg 2015;19(4):604–12.
40. Nageswaran H, Belgaumkar A, Kumar R, et al. Acute afferent loop syndrome in the early postoperative period following pancreaticoduodenectomy. Ann R Coll Surg Engl 2015;97(5):349–53.
41. Gaujoux S, Sauvanet A, Vullierme MP, et al. Ischemic complications after pancreaticoduodenectomy: incidence, prevention, and management. Ann Surg 2009;249(1):111–7.
42. Park CM, Chung JW, Kim HB, et al. Celiac axis stenosis: incidence and etiologies in asymptomatic individuals. Korean J Radiol 2001;2(1):8–13.
43. Thompson NW, Eckhauser FE, Talpos G, et al. Pancreaticoduodenectomy and celiac occlusive disease. Ann Surg 1981;193(4):399–406.
44. Song SY, Chung JW, Kwon JW, et al. Collateral pathways in patients with celiac axis stenosis: angiographic-spiral CT correlation. Radiographics 2002;22(4):881–93.
45. Blomley MJ, Albrecht T, Williamson RC, et al. Three-dimensional spiral CT angiography in pancreatic surgical planning using non-tailored protocols: comparison with conventional angiography. Br J Radiol 1998;71(843):268–75.
46. Hasegawa K, Imamura H, Akahane M, et al. Endovascular stenting for celiac axis stenosis before pancreaticoduodenectomy. Surgery 2003;133(4):440–2.

Adjuvant or Neoadjuvant Therapy in the Treatment in Pancreatic Malignancies

Where Are We?

Robert A. Wolff, MD

KEYWORDS

- Resectable pancreatic cancer • Borderline resectable pancreatic cancer
- Locally advanced pancreatic cancer • Adjuvant therapy • Neoadjuvant therapy
- Preoperative therapy • Chemotherapy • Resection

KEY POINTS

- Up-front surgery is considered the standard of care for resectable pancreatic cancer despite modest improvements in median overall survival observed over time.
- With few exceptions, surgery first is widely endorsed in the oncology community and this will not change without randomized trials comparing up-front surgery/adjuvant therapy with neoadjuvant therapy/subsequent surgery.
- Until definitive results from these trials are reported, up-front surgery will be used to select patients for adjuvant therapy.
- This strategy places patients at risk for positive surgical margins, poor recovery, and rapid relapse, limiting the delivery of adjuvant therapy.

INTRODUCTION

Ever since A.O. Whipple reported on a 2-stage surgical procedure for removal of ampullary and periampullary neoplasms, variations of the Whipple procedure (pancreatico-duodenectomy) have been widely used for surgical resection of malignant neoplasms of the pancreatic head. By the 1960 to 1970s, it became clear that, despite surgical resection, adenocarcinoma of the pancreas had a propensity to recur locally and metastasize. Early efforts at adjuvant therapy culminated in the report of a randomized trial comparing combined modality therapy with observation after surgery in patients with resected pancreatic cancer. The results, published in 1985, began the era of modern adjuvant therapy for resected pancreatic cancer. In the intervening 30 years, adjuvant

Disclosure: The author has nothing to disclose.
Department of Gastrointestinal Medical Oncology, University of Texas MD Anderson Cancer Center, 1515 Holcombe Boulevard-Unit 421, Houston, TX 77030, USA
E-mail address: rwolff@mdanderson.org

Surg Clin N Am 98 (2018) 95–111
https://doi.org/10.1016/j.suc.2017.09.009
0039-6109/18/© 2017 Elsevier Inc. All rights reserved.

surgical.theclinics.com

therapy has been refined, but improvements in overall survival after surgery have been modest. Moreover, longer survival durations after surgery and adjuvant therapy observed over time are likely partially explained by the availability of newer systemic regimens at the time of relapse. Furthermore, despite improvements in mortality related to pancreatic cancer surgery, it is estimated that only 50% to 60% of patients undergoing surgery with curative intent subsequently receive adjuvant therapy.

In this article, results from modern trials of adjuvant therapy are summarized and followed by a discussion of the flaws in the paradigm of up-front surgery followed by adjuvant therapy. Thereafter, the rationale for preoperative therapy is described with some clinical results. In addition, given the growing appreciation for 3 distinct subsets of localized, nonmetastatic pancreatic cancer (resectable, borderline resectable [BR], and locally advanced [LA] disease), the benefits of a neoadjuvant therapy for these subsets are proposed.

RATIONALE FOR ADJUVANT THERAPY AFTER SURGERY FOR PANCREATIC CANCER

As surgery for carcinoma of the pancreas became widely adopted, postoperative mortality began to decrease and it became increasingly evident that most patients who survived surgical resection ultimately died of disease recurrence. Over time, it became clear that pancreatic cancer had the propensity to recur locally and spread to distant sites. In a review of the experience of the Massachusetts General Hospital (MGH), Tepper and colleagues[1] reported the local failure rate after surgery to be almost 50%, with metastatic disease being observed with less frequency. Hence, early trials of adjuvant therapy were developed using initial chemoradiation, with 5-fluorouracil (5FU) as a radiosensitizer and, in some reports, subsequently delivering 5FU as systemic therapy.

CONFLICTING EARLY EVIDENCE WITH ADJUVANT CHEMORADIATION

In a landmark trial spearheaded by the Mayo Clinic, patients who had undergone complete resection of an adenocarcinoma of the pancreatic head, and who had adequate recovery from surgery, were randomized 1:1 to receive 5FU-based chemoradiation followed by weekly 5FU for up to 2 years, or to undergo observation alone after surgery.[2] Among the 21 patients randomized to chemoradiation, median overall survival was 20 months, whereas the survival for the 22 patients in the observation arm was only 11 months ($P = .03$). The results from this trial could not be confirmed in a subsequent trial performed by the European Organization for Research and Treatment of Cancer (EORTC).[3] Median survival was 17 months for 60 patients with resected pancreatic cancer randomized to receive chemoradiation and 12 months for the 54 patients undergoing observation ($P = .09$). Critics have argued that this was an underpowered positive trial, supporting the role of chemoradiation therapy, whereas others argued against chemoradiation as adjuvant therapy.

The role of chemoradiation in adjuvant therapy was further disputed after the results of the European Study of Pancreatic Cancer showed that the delivery of radiation to adjuvant therapy after surgery led to inferior survival compared with treatment with chemotherapy alone.[4]

Table 1 summarizes the results of several trials in which chemoradiation was a component of therapy.[2–5] Despite efforts spanning more than 20 years, there is no compelling evidence that chemoradiation provides any advantage compared with systemic therapy alone. Of note, the largest ongoing trial of chemotherapy and chemoradiation versus chemotherapy alone has been accruing patients since 2014 and does not expect to reach target accrual of 950 patients until 2020.

Table 1			
Select trials with chemoradiation as a component of adjuvant therapy			
Study/Year	**Number of Patients**	**R1 Resection Rate (%)**	**Adjuvant Chemoradiation Median Survival (mo)**
GITSG 1985	21	0	20
EORTC 1999	60	22	17
ESPAC 2004	280	18	15
RTOG 9704 2008	451	>35	17–20

Abbreviations: EORTC, European Organization for Research and Treatment of Cancer; ESPAC, European Study Group for Pancreatic Cancer; GITSG, Gastrointestinal Tumor Study Group; RTOG, Radiation Therapy Oncology Group.

THE EMERGENCE OF SYSTEMIC THERAPY AS ADJUVANT THERAPY FOR PANCREATIC CANCER

Although progress in adjuvant therapy has been slow, there is now evidence that systemic therapy is superior to observation alone after resection with curative intent, as shown in **Table 2**.[6–10] These results show that (1) chemotherapy improves survival more than observation after surgery, and (2) there is no clear advantage of gemcitabine compared with 5FU when these drugs are given as single agents. However, the combination of gemcitabine with the oral fluoropyrimidine, capecitabine, has recently been reported as superior to gemcitabine alone for resected pancreatic cancer.[9] Thus, the standard of care for patients who undergo up-front surgery with curative intent is gemcitabine and capecitabine given over 24 weeks. This treatment is expected to result in a median overall survival of 28 months with approximately 20% of patients surviving for 5 years.

On first glance at **Table 2**, it seems that adjuvant therapy is improving. Early trials with gemcitabine alone led to overall median survivals of 22 months, whereas the most recent trial shows an improvement in survival to 28 months when gemcitabine and capecitabine are combined. Note that the median survival of patients who receive gemcitabine monotherapy has also steadily increased from 22 months to 25 months. This improvement is possibly explained by better patient selection and improvements

Table 2							
Randomized trials of systemic therapy as adjuvant therapy for resected pancreatic cancer							
Study	**Year**	**Number of Patients**	**R1 Resection Rate (%)**	**Control Arm Median Survival (mo)**	**Experimental Arm Median Survival (mo)**	**P**	**Available Second-Line Therapy**
CONKO 001	2007	368	18	Observation 20.2	Gem 22.1	.06	5FU or gemcitabine
ESPAC 1 and ESPAC 3 (v1)	2009	458	25	Observation 16.8	5FU + Leucovorin 23.2	.003	Gemcitabine
ESPAC 3 v2	2010	1088	35	5FU + Leucovorin 23	Gem 23.6	.39	5FU/oxaliplatin cape/ oxaliplatin
ESPAC 4	2017	730	60	Gem 25.5	Gem + Cape 28	.032	Gem/nab-p or FOLFIRINOX

Abbreviations: cape, capecitabine; gem, gemcitabine; nab-p, nab-paclitaxel.

in perioperative care. However, overall survival may also be influenced by additional anticancer therapy after relapse. In the late 1990s and early 2000s, there was no clear evidence that second-line therapy had any impact on survival for those patients who presented with metastatic disease. With the advent of oxaliplatin, which became available in 2003, investigators have shown some activity of this agent in the second-line setting when combined with 5FU/folinic acid (FOLFOX [folinic acid, 5FU, oxaliplatin] or OFF [oxaliplatin, folinic acid, 5FU]) or capecitabine (XELOX [Xeloda, oxaliplatin]/ CapOx [capecitabine, oxaliplatin]).[11,12] Since that time, 2 newer regimens for advanced pancreatic cancer have been approved. The combination of 5FU, folinic acid, irinotecan, and oxaliplatin (FOLFIRINOX) was accepted as a standard front-line therapy in 2011.[13] In addition, gemcitabine and nab-paclitaxel was subsequently approved in by the US Food and Drug Administration in 2013[14] (both of these regimens showed superiority compared with single-agent gemcitabine in large randomized trials in metastatic pancreatic cancer). Because the options for second-line therapy have expanded over time and were available during the conduct of the recently reported European Study Group for Pancreatic Cancer (ESPAC) 4 trial, some of the incremental prolongation of survival now observed after up-front surgery and adjuvant therapy may therefore be explained by the availability of newer regimens for use at the time of relapse.

In summary, the combination of gemcitabine and capecitabine delivered over 6 months is considered the new standard adjuvant regimen for those patients with adequate recovery from surgery with curative intent. This regimen is expected to result in a median survival of 28 months with a 5-year survival rate of 20%.

THE FLAWED STRATEGY OF UP-FRONT SURGERY AND ADJUVANT THERAPY

Many pancreatic cancer experts continue to endorse the paradigm of up-front surgery followed by adjuvant therapy with continued trials of newer systemic therapies in an effort to make incremental progress. However, data from several sources, including results from the adjuvant trials already reported, suggest that up-front surgery for resectable pancreatic cancer is a flawed strategy and one that hampers more rapid progress for patients. Furthermore, this strategy may limit the number of patients who will benefit from initial surgery.

Ignoring the Denominator

One of the most striking things common to reports of prospective adjuvant therapy trials after initial surgery is the absence of the denominator from which the study population was derived; of the patients taken to the operating room for curative surgery, not all undergo adjuvant therapy. Present estimates from several studies reveal that only 50% to 60% of patients who undergo surgical resection ultimately receive

Table 3
The proportion of patients receiving adjuvant therapy after surgical resection

Data Source	Year	Number of Patients Resection Type	Patients Receiving Adjuvant Therapy (%)
Johns Hopkins	2008	368 R0/R1	53
Mayo Clinic	2008	472 R0 only	60
Medicare/SEER	2011	396 R0/R1	47
NCDB	2014	2047 R0/R1	58

Abbreviations: NCDB, National Cancer Data Base; SEER, Surveillance, Epidemiology and End Results.

adjuvant therapy. **Table 3** summarizes the data in this regard. For example, in a study reported by the group at the Johns Hopkins Hospital (JHH), among 870 patients who underwent an R0 or R1 resection, only 53% underwent adjuvant therapy.[15] The Mayo Clinic also reported their experience for patients who underwent R0 resection; 58% of them received adjuvant therapy.[16] In a more recent analysis derived from the American College of Surgeons (ACS) National Surgical Quality Improvement Program and the National Cancer Data Base (NCDB), among 2047 patients undergoing pancreatic cancer resection, the receipt of subsequent adjuvant therapy was similarly limited to 58%.[17] Other results come from Surveillance, Epidemiology and End Results(SEER)/Medicare data. Among 396 Medicare beneficiaries, adjuvant therapy was given to 47% of resected patients.[18]

Thus, despite the recognition that surgical resection must be linked to the subsequent delivery of adjuvant therapy, a large subset of patients (40%–50%) never receive it. The main factors, discussed in more detail later, are likely related to the complexity of the surgery and resultant complications, potential for early relapse, and postoperative death.

Postoperative Complications Hamper the Delivery of Adjuvant Therapy

Median age of onset for pancreatic cancer is 70 years. Known risk factors for pancreatic cancer include a history of tobacco use, obesity, long-standing diabetes, and metabolic syndrome. Thus, many surgical candidates are of advanced age and often have comorbidities increasing their risk of surgical complications. In the aforementioned analysis from the ACS National Surgical Quality Improvement Program and the NCDB, the rate of serious postoperative complications was 23%; this affected the likelihood of receiving adjuvant therapy. For those patients experiencing at least 1 serious complication, the rate of adjuvant therapy delivery was only 44%. Among those patients with no serious complications, adjuvant therapy was given to 62%. Furthermore, even when adjuvant therapy was ultimately delivered, it was more likely to be delayed by greater than 70 days in patients with serious complications.[17]

Pancreatic Cancer Resections Result in Postoperative Death

Since the early reports of the Whipple procedure, 30-day mortality has steadily declined from around 30% to less than 3% in high-volume centers. However, a recent report shows that this operation remains risky. Among 15,000 patients undergoing resections in centers around the United States, although 30-day mortality was only 3.4%, 90-day mortality was double, increasing to 7.5%.[19]

Pancreatic Cancer Is Locally Invasive

Even before cross-sectional imaging became widely available, it was known that pancreatic cancer has a propensity to recur locally. Similar to the experience at MGH, investigators at the Bethesda Naval Hospital reported a local recurrence rate of 47%, with confirmation based on autopsy or surgical exploration.[20] More recent autopsy data show that local recurrence occurs more frequently than had been estimated through clinical, surgical, or radiographic means. In a rapid autopsy program established at JHH, among 22 patients who died after potentially curative surgery, more than 80% had evidence for local recurrence.[21] Of note, 59% of these patients received chemoradiation as a component of adjuvant therapy.

Furthermore, achieving microscopically negative surgical margins (R0) is increasingly recognized as having more favorable prognosis compared with resections that have microscopically positive margins (R1). Data from several single-institution reports and larger multicenter trials have clearly shown that R1 resections confer worse prognosis compared with R0 resections.[8,9,22] Importantly, evaluation of microscopic margins requires a collaborative approach between the pathologist and the surgeon and methods for rigorous assessment of surgical margins have been developed and published by several groups. This requirement likely explains the increase in the frequency of positive surgical margins reported in adjuvant trials over time, as shown in **Tables 1** and **2**.

Although high-quality dynamic phase cross-sectional imaging has provided the means to characterize tumors as resectable, BR, or LA, even when tumors are radiographically defined as potentially resectable, R1 resections occur frequently.

Verbeke and colleagues[23] suggested that the biology of invading pancreatic cancer cells is distinct from other malignancies in which negative resection margins are also critical for long-term survival. They evaluated the peripheral zone of pancreatic resection specimens, compared them with resected rectal cancers, and found that pancreatic cancer cells were more widely dispersed at the periphery of the tumor compared with resected specimens of rectal cancer. This finding shows one of the insurmountable flaws of up-front surgery, achieving R0 resections based on imaging studies that only provide information at a macroscopic level. It is difficult to imagine that the resolution of future body imaging will become so precise as to allow the visualization of the boundary of the diffusely dispersed and infiltrating border of a pancreatic carcinoma. It is therefore naive to believe that, based on imaging and intraoperative evaluation of the tumor mass, clinicians will observe any meaningful decrease in positive surgical margins with surgery as the first anticancer intervention. Furthermore, if up-front surgery results in an R1 resection, there is no salvage strategy in the postoperative period that offers a significant chance at long-term survival. This flaw in the up-front surgery paradigm is critical, and the "If in doubt, take it out" approach to localized pancreatic cancer is dooming a sizable proportion of patients to inferior survival.

Pancreatic Cancer Is a Systemic Disease

Although many patients present with seemingly localized disease, most harbor microscopic metastases. The rapid autopsy program described earlier found that, among the 22 patients who underwent surgery with curative intent, 88% had metastases at the time of autopsy.[21] However, it is not always appreciated that overt metastatic disease may develop within weeks of presentation with potentially resectable disease. In an analysis of several preoperative trials among patients who were thought to have localized, resectable disease and in whom treatment was initiated with preoperative therapy, 16% developed radiographically evident metastases within 6 to 12 weeks.[22] In another study, the likelihood of encountering unanticipated metastases at the time of surgical exploration increased quickly with every week after preoperative imaging.[24] If only 1 week had passed between the imaging and surgical exploration, 12% of patients had unanticipated metastases, whereas 35% had metastases if the imaging was 6 weeks old.

It is therefore reasonable to expect that, among patients who undergo up-front surgery for resectable disease, at least 15% to 20% will develop clinically evident metastatic disease within the recovery period. No one could argue for up-front surgical intervention as beneficial for this subgroup of patients.

Pancreatic Surgery Is Immunosuppressive

The immunosuppressive nature of major surgical procedures is increasingly recognized and the biological basis of this immunosuppression is currently being elucidated. Recent animal studies show that the stress of major intra-abdominal surgery leads to higher levels of circulating tumor cells compared with levels found in animals undergoing sham procedures.[25] In addition, natural killer cell and antitumor

T-lymphocyte functions are dysregulated after major surgical stress.[26,27] The roles of inflammatory cytokines, coagulation, angiogenic factors, and catecholamines are also thought to play an important role in promoting tumor metastases after resection of the primary tumor.[28] Although surgery after neoadjuvant therapy would also be expected to promote metastases, given the prior delivery of anticancer therapy, the overall microscopic tumor burden may be reduced by preoperative treatment.

In summary, up-front surgery for pancreatic cancer:

- Often leads to incomplete resection of the primary tumor (R1)
- Is sufficiently complex to prevent sufficient recovery to receive adjuvant therapy
- Does not identify patients with aggressive tumor biology who will not benefit from resection
- Can be fatal
- May promote the metastatic compartment by immunosuppressing the patient or through other mechanisms

Thus, up-front surgery is being used to select patients for adjuvant therapy, which is necessary to improve long-term outcomes. Presently, adjuvant therapy is received by only 50% to 60% of patients who undergo surgery as initial therapy, and many of these have undergone an incomplete resection or harbor a higher metastatic tumor burden based on the need to recover for weeks and the immunosuppressive effects of surgery. These circumstances are not optimal for successful delivery of adjuvant therapy.

RATIONALE FOR NEOADJUVANT THERAPY

Taken together, the flaws inherent in up-front surgery as initial cancer therapy argue for the adoption of an alternative approach for the treatment of localized pancreatic cancer.

There are several advantages to the delivery of neoadjuvant therapy rather than up-front surgery.

First, it allows for the delivery of anticancer therapy to patients who have not been physiologically compromised by a major surgical procedure. Second, it provides a period of time to uncover aggressive tumor biology with identification of those patients who have interval development of metastatic disease, contraindicating surgery. This time interval can also reveal underlying patient frailty given the relative rigors of preoperative chemotherapy or chemoradiation. Such patients are likely at higher risk for surgical complications and prove themselves to be unattractive for surgical intervention, something that is not possible with up-front surgery.

From a biological perspective, treatment with chemotherapy or chemoradiation provides early treatment of micrometastatic disease without waiting for recovery from surgery, which is likely to increase the underlying micrometastatic burden. With the primary intact, the tumor mass is also well perfused and the cytotoxic effects of chemotherapy and/or radiation are not compromised by the creation of a more hypoxic, inflammatory, and fibrotic surgical bed. Furthermore, preoperative therapy has the potential to destroy tumor cells, particularly in the periphery of the tumor mass, thereby improving the likelihood of an ultimate R0 resection.

EARLY RESULTS WITH PREOPERATIVE THERAPY

In a series of trials conducted at the University of Texas MD Anderson Cancer Center (UTMDACC), strict radiographic criteria were used to define potentially resectable disease. These criteria, combined with other inclusion and exclusion criteria used consistently over time, have allowed the enrollment of a fairly homogenous patient populations into sequential neoadjuvant trials (**Table 4**). The initial 3 trials were designed

Table 4
Sequential neoadjuvant trials for resectable pancreatic cancer performed at University of Texas MD Anderson Cancer Center 1992 to 2008

Author, Year	Number of Patients	Regimen	Resection Rate (%)	R1 Resection Rate (%)	Median Survival, Resected (mo)
Evans et al,[29] 1992	28	5FU + 50.4 Gy	61	18	Not Stated
Pisters et al,[30] 1998	35	5FU + 30 Gy	57	10	25
Pisters et al,[31] 2002	35	Paclitaxel + 30 Gy	57	32	19
Evans et al,[34] 2008	86	Gemcitabine + 30 Gy	74	11	34
Varadhachary et al,[35] 2008	90	Gem/cis then Gem + 30 Gy	58	4	31

Abbreviation: cis, cisplatin.

using a platform of neoadjuvant chemoradiation with either 5FU or paclitaxel as radiosensitizers.[29–31] The resection rate after preoperative therapy ranged from 57% to 61% with median overall survival for eventually resected patients ranging from 19 to 25 months. These survival durations were similar to those among patients who underwent initial surgery and subsequent adjuvant therapy. However, approximately 40% of enrolled patients were spared the morbidity of surgery based on the discovery of metastatic disease before surgery or intraoperatively. Of note, the results published from UTMDACC were superior to results from a multicenter cooperative group trial conducted through the Eastern Cooperative Oncology Group.[32] The trial enrolled 53 patients and only 45% underwent surgery, with a median survival of 15.7 months.

GEMCITABINE-BASED PREOPERATIVE THERAPY

After gemcitabine showed superiority to weekly bolus 5FU and leucovorin in the treatment of advanced pancreatic cancer, investigators at the University of Michigan reported on the potent radiosensitizing properties of gemcitabine.[33] Our group therefore performed an initial trial of neoadjuvant gemcitabine-based chemoradiation for patients with resectable pancreatic cancer, with a subsequent trial of systemic gemcitabine and cisplatin followed by gemcitabine-based chemoradiation. The results of these trials are also summarized in **Table 4**.[34,35]

Several conclusions can be drawn from these 2 trials. First, gemcitabine-based chemoradiation led to resection rates between 57% and 75%, equivalent to or higher than the rate of delivery of adjuvant therapy after up-front surgery (50%–60%). Second, R0 resection rates were high at approximately 90%. Third, overall median survival for patients undergoing resection was higher than survival durations reported using up-front surgery and adjuvant therapy. These two reports, with a combined enrollment of 176 patients, were published in 2008. Although other groups have reported on their experience using neoadjuvant therapy, smaller numbers of patients have been enrolled in these studies. For example, in a trial of neoadjuvant therapy using gemcitabine and cisplatin without radiation, only 35 patients were enrolled, and 60% were ultimately resected with an 80% R0 resection rate.[36] Median follow-up in this trial was limited but the disease-free and overall survival durations were described as promising.

Nevertheless, results using neoadjuvant therapy in resectable pancreatic cancer remain encouraging. In a prospective analysis of 69 patients treated outside of a clinical trial in the interval from 2004 to 2010 by the group at the Medical College of Wisconsin, the resection rate was 87% and the R0 rate was 97%.[37] The median overall survival for all patients was 31.5 months and the median overall survival for resected patients was 44.9 months.

However, many reports of preoperative therapy have enrolled heterogeneous populations of patients with some having resectable disease, others having BR pancreatic cancer, and others still having LA disease. Under these circumstances, results are more challenging to interpret given the small numbers of patients in each category.

EVIDENCE FOR TREATMENT EFFECT USING NEOADJUVANT THERAPY

Although neoadjuvant therapy followed by surgery has not been shown to be clearly superior to up-front surgery and adjuvant therapy, there is evidence for a treatment effect with the delivery of neoadjuvant therapy.

In reports from several institutions, T stage and N stage are reduced with the delivery of neoadjuvant therapy.[38–40] In addition, overall treatment effect shows that preoperative therapy can result in pathologic complete response or near-complete responses.[41] Such responses are associated with longer survival compared with patients whose resected tumors show lesser degrees of treatment effect.[42] In addition, virtually all reports of preoperative therapy show high rates of R0 resection among the patients who ultimately undergo surgical resection. Moreover, local recurrence after resection may be significantly reduced with the delivery of neoadjuvant therapy.

OTHER LINES OF EVIDENCE SUPPORTING THE DELIVERY OF NEOADJUVANT THERAPY

Using large data sets, several groups have used propensity matching to compare outcomes of patients undergoing neoadjuvant therapy with those of patients undergoing up-front surgery and adjuvant therapy. In at least 3 analyses, neoadjuvant therapy has been shown to be superior to up-front surgery and adjuvant therapy.[43–45] However, in one of these studies among patients with clinical stage I disease, the differences in survival between patients treated with preoperative therapy and surgery and those treated with up-front surgery and adjuvant therapy were not significant.[44] Nevertheless, this same report showed progressive superiority to neoadjuvant therapy for patients with clinical stage II and III pancreatic cancer. Furthermore, neoadjuvant therapy was compared with adjuvant therapy using a Markov decision analysis of 22 studies.[46] Neoadjuvant therapy led to longer life expectancy and longer quality-adjusted life expectancy.

In addition, others have performed cost-analyses comparing neoadjuvant therapy with up-front surgery, showing that the delivery of neoadjuvant therapy is more cost-effective.[47]

In summary, the delivery of preoperative therapy before surgical resection in potentially resectable pancreatic cancer has a sound rationale; has led to high rates of R0 resections; has shown treatment effect that includes complete pathologic responses; and has shown survival durations for resected patients to be at least equivalent, if not superior, to those reported in studies investigating up-front surgery and adjuvant therapy. Furthermore, it provides a selection mechanism to spare patients with unfavorable tumor biology the morbidity of pancreatic cancer surgery.

THE ROLE OF NEOADJUVANT THERAPY IN BORDERLINE RESECTABLE PANCREATIC CANCER

As our group at UTMDACC was conducting studies of preoperative therapy in those patients strictly defined as having potentially resectable disease, we also encountered patients who did not meet our radiographic criteria for resectability based on encasement of the common hepatic artery, significant involvement of the superior mesenteric vein or superior mesenteric-portal venous confluence, or tumor abutment along the superior mesenteric artery or celiac trunk. Nonetheless, we found that, after delivery of multimodality preoperative therapy, a subset of these patients had some evidence of response to treatment without interval development of metastatic disease. Some of these patients were able to undergo R0 or R1 resections, with encouraging survival durations. Based on this experience, we proposed a definition for BR disease and presented 4 cases of patients who were initially considered to have BR tumors and ultimately underwent surgical resection after a period of multimodal therapy.[48]

Importantly, the concept of BR disease was not unique to our group. During this time frame, an appreciation for the distinction between tumors that would now be considered borderline or marginally resectable was emerging.[49] For example, one of the earliest reports using preoperative therapy to downstage what is now known as BR disease was conducted at Stanford University and reported by Mehta and colleagues.[50] The investigators reported on 15 patients they described as having marginally resectable adenocarcinoma of the pancreas, defined as tumors having portal vein, superior mesenteric vein, or artery involvement. These patients were treated with infusional 5-FU and external beam radiation therapy (EBRT) to doses ranging from 50.4 to 56 Gy. Nine patients (60%) underwent surgical resection with negative surgical margins and 2 of 9 (22%) had a complete pathologic response to preoperative treatment. Furthermore, there was a striking difference in overall survival between those patients who did undergo surgical resection and those who did not (30 vs 8 months, respectively).

Thereafter, the authors reported on a series of 160 patients we defined as having BR disease seen at UTMDACC from 1999 to 2006.[51] Of these, 125 (78%) completed preoperative therapy and restaging, and 66 (41%) underwent pancreatectomy with an R0 resection rate of 94%. Median survival was 40 months for the 66 patients who completed all therapy and 13 months for the 94 patients who did not undergo pancreatectomy ($P<.001$).

Other groups are now reporting their single-institutional experiences with BR disease and, depending on the series, resection rates after preoperative therapy range from about 40% to 60%, with most resections classified as R0.[52,53]

Recently, the Alliance for Clinical Trials in Oncology reported on a prospective multicenter pilot trial of induction FOLFIRINOX followed by capecitabine-based chemoradiation in 23 patients deemed to have BR pancreatic cancer.[54] The overall resection rate was 68%, and R0 resections were achieved for 93%. The median overall survival for the population was 21.7 months, and 21.7 months for the resected patients.

The next Alliance trial is being designed as a randomized trial to investigate whether radiation therapy is a necessary component of neoadjuvant therapy for BR disease. Eligible patients with BR tumors will be randomized to receive 8 doses of FOLFIRINOX or 7 doses of FOLFIRINOX followed by radiation therapy.

In the United States, although many centers do not endorse preoperative therapy for potentially resectable disease, there is a growing consensus about the use of neoadjuvant therapy for patients defined as having BR disease. In the National Comprehensive Cancer Network Pancreatic Cancer Subcommittee, there was lack of consensus in this regard in 2006. However, by 2013, most participating centers endorsed neoadjuvant therapy for patients with BR disease.[55] This position is not shared by an expert group of pancreatic cancer specialists in Europe who recommend a neoadjuvant approach to BR disease only in the context of a clinical trial.[56]

NEOADJUVANT THERAPY FOR LOCALLY ADVANCED DISEASE

Although reports have been limited, there have been efforts to downstage LA disease using neoadjuvant therapy. One of the earliest trials reported modest success using infusional 5FU with EBRT in 16 patients with LA disease.[57] Although only 2 (12.5%) were able to undergo surgery with curative intent, the survival of these 2 patients was comparable with that of patients with resectable pancreatic cancer treated with up-front surgery and adjuvant therapy. In a larger trial, the group at Duke University reported on 111 patients treated with preoperative chemoradiation from 1995 to 2000 and included patients with resectable (n = 53) or LA (n = 58) disease.[58] The overall resection rate was superior for patients defined as having resectable disease (53%) compared with the rate for patients with LA disease (19%), with an overall R0 resection rate of 70%.

These and other reports have suggested that, for a subset of patients with pancreatic cancer not initially considered resectable, neoadjuvant therapy could provide sufficient tumor destruction or downstaging to proceed with surgical resection (**Fig. 1**). However, the resection rates reported after neoadjuvant therapy have varied widely from as low as 1% to 60%, with most studies reporting resection rates ranging between 20% and 40%.[51,52,59,60] Patients reported in these studies likely represented a heterogeneous population composed of some having tumor with complete vascular encasement and others having some degree of tumor-vessel contact without encasement.

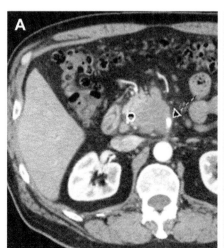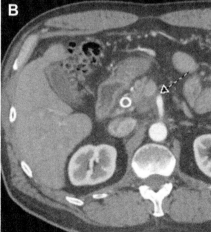

Fig. 1. (*A*) Pretreatment computed tomography (CT) imaging of a locally advanced pancreatic cancer with tumor along the right side of the superior mesenteric artery and extending to the contralateral side. (*B*) Posttreatment CT image of the tumor mass after FOLFIRINOX for 6 doses and capecitabine-based chemoradiation. The residual tumor was resected with skeletonization of the superior mesenteric artery. Histopathology showed a complete pathologic response to neoadjuvant therapy. Arrow in (*A*) and (*B*) depicts the direct contact of tumor with the superior mesenteric artery.

NEOADJUVANT THERAPY AT MD ANDERSON OVER 25 YEARS

Members of our multidisciplinary pancreatic cancer team at UTMDACC have been avid supporters of neoadjuvant therapy for years. Over the past 25 years, we have made an effort to conduct clinical trials in localized pancreatic carcinoma that have used surgical resection as a later step in our patients' anticancer therapy. Using a prospectively collected database, we have tracked patients who have undergone surgery after neoadjuvant therapy either as part of a clinical trial or off protocol. Earlier this year, we published our 25-year experience with surgical resection after neoadjuvant therapy.[61] During the period 1999 to 2014, surgical resections for BR and LA tumors increased. The use of induction systemic chemotherapy and the delivery of postoperative chemotherapy also increased. In addition, R0 resection rates and vascular resection rates increased overall. Despite the increase in resections for patients initially considered to have BR or LA tumors, locoregional recurrence rates remained similar over time, and overall survival improved significantly from a median of 24.1 months in the early 2000s to 43.4 months by 2014 ($P<.0001$). Although the results reported by our group should not be construed as typical, they do represent what is possible using a multidisciplinary approach, and interest in pursuing a neoadjuvant platform in localized pancreatic cancer is growing.

In general, UTMDACC patients defined as having potentially resectable pancreatic cancer are treated on prospective clinical trials whenever available. For those who do not wish to participate, or do not meet eligibility criteria, neoadjuvant therapy with chemoradiation is often advised. For those with BR disease, our approach has been to deliver systemic therapy for 2 to 3 months and if, on restaging, there is no evidence of metastatic disease, we usually recommend a course of chemoradiation. Decisions about patients' surgical candidacy are then made after restaging and formal review in a multidisciplinary pancreatic cancer conference.

THE FUTURE OF ADJUVANT AND NEOADJUVANT THERAPY

There is no definitive evidence supporting the use of postoperative radiation as a component of adjuvant therapy after up-front surgery. Thus, efforts to improve adjuvant therapy have focused on the investigation of combination systemic therapy. At present, there are 2 ongoing randomized trials in this area. The first is comparing gemcitabine with gemcitabine and nab-paclitaxel in the adjuvant setting.[62] In addition, modified FOLFIRINOX is being compared with gemcitabine as systemic adjuvant therapy.[63] Given the survival benefit shown by adding capecitabine to gemcitabine, these 2 trials are likely to be amended to allow gemcitabine/capecitabine as the control arm for both. In neoadjuvant therapy, in which gemcitabine/nab-paclitaxel and FOLFIRINOX are already being used, more novel approaches designed to affect the tumor microenvironment or enhance the patient's immune response are now being investigated.[64,65]

In addition, our group has reported on imaging characteristics of pancreatic adenocarcinoma and has classified primary tumors in the pancreatic parenchyma as either stromal rich or stromal poor.[66] This characterization seems to provide prognostic information, with stromal-poor tumors conferring a worse prognosis for patients after conventional neoadjuvant therapy. In the future, without the need for ample biopsies for molecular interrogation, the ability to tailor neoadjuvant therapy based on imaging characteristics may be feasible.[67]

In summary, neoadjuvant therapy:

- Allows early delivery of cytotoxic therapy before patients are compromised by the stress of a major surgical procedure

- Provides an interval of time to identify aggressive tumor biology and frail patients
- Delivers treatment to tumors that are intact and not altered by surgery with resultant local hypoxia, inflammation, and fibrosis
- Has potential to decrease or even eliminate microscopic metastatic tumor burden
- Can generate treatment effect that increases R0 resection rates and has prognostic significance
- Can expand the population of patients who may ultimately benefit from resection

SUMMARY

Up-front surgery is considered the standard of care for resectable pancreatic cancer despite modest improvements in median overall survival observed over time (20 months in 1985, 28 months in 2017). Nevertheless, with few exceptions, surgery first is widely endorsed in the oncology community and will not change without randomized trials comparing up-front surgery/adjuvant therapy with neoadjuvant therapy/subsequent surgery. Randomized trials of neoadjuvant versus adjuvant therapy are currently enrolling patients.[68] Until definitive results from these trials are reported, up-front surgery will be used to select patients for adjuvant therapy. This strategy places patients at risk for positive surgical margins, poor recovery, and rapid relapse, limiting the delivery of adjuvant therapy.

In contrast, our 25-year experience has shown that neoadjuvant therapy can lead to greater incremental improvements in survival compared with up-front surgery and adjuvant therapy over the same time period. Although there has been a general lack of interest in neoadjuvant therapy for resectable disease, there is growing enthusiasm for neoadjuvant therapy in patients with BR tumors and, in some centers, LA disease. As systemic therapies, radiation techniques, and other locally ablative techniques evolve, resection rates and survival for patients with BR and LA pancreatic cancer are expected to improve.

In addition, for patients undergoing up-front surgery resulting in positive surgical margins, median survival is less than 2 years.[9] Given the demonstrated treatment effect of neoadjuvant therapy, newer drug regimens, and an expanding array of locally ablative and radiation techniques, growing numbers of patients with BR or LA pancreatic cancer are more likely to become surgical candidates with curative potential after application of preoperative therapy.

REFERENCES

1. Tepper J, Nardi G, Sutt H. Carcinoma of the pancreas: review of MGH experience from 1963 to 1973. Analysis of surgical failure and implications for radiation therapy. Cancer 1976;37:1519–24.
2. Kalser MH, Ellenberg SS. Pancreatic cancer. Adjuvant combined radiation and chemotherapy following curative resection. Arch Surg 1985;120:899–903.
3. Klinkenbijl JH, Jeekel J, Sahmoud T, et al. Adjuvant radiotherapy and 5-fluorouracil after curative resection of cancer of the pancreas and periampullary region: phase III trial of the EORTC gastrointestinal tract cancer cooperative group. Ann Surg 1999;230:776–82.
4. Neoptolemos JP, Dunn JA, Stocken DD, et al. Adjuvant chemoradiotherapy and chemotherapy in resectable pancreatic cancer: a randomised controlled trial. Lancet 2001;358:1576–85.
5. Regine WF, Winter KA, Abrams RA, et al. Fluorouracil vs gemcitabine chemotherapy before and after fluorouracil-based chemoradiation following resection

of pancreatic adenocarcinoma: a randomized controlled trial. JAMA 2008;299: 1019–26.

6. Oettle H, Post S, Neuhaus P, et al. Adjuvant chemotherapy with gemcitabine vs observation in patients undergoing curative-intent resection of pancreatic cancer: a randomized controlled trial. JAMA 2007;297:267–77.

7. Neoptolemos JP, Stocken DD, Tudur Smith C, et al. Adjuvant 5-fluorouracil and folinic acid vs observation for pancreatic cancer: composite data from the ESPAC-1 and -3(v1) trials. Br J Cancer 2009;100:246–50.

8. Neoptolemos JP, Stocken DD, Bassi C, et al. Adjuvant chemotherapy with fluorouracil plus folinic acid vs gemcitabine following pancreatic cancer resection: a randomized controlled trial. JAMA 2010;304:1073–81.

9. Neoptolemos JP, Palmer DH, Ghaneh P, et al. Comparison of adjuvant gemcitabine and capecitabine with gemcitabine monotherapy in patients with resected pancreatic cancer (ESPAC-4): a multicentre, open-label, randomised, phase 3 trial. Lancet 2017;389:1011–24.

10. Oettle H, Neuhaus P, Hochhaus A, et al. Adjuvant chemotherapy with gemcitabine and long-term outcomes among patients with resected pancreatic cancer: the CONKO-001 randomized trial. JAMA 2013;310:1473–81.

11. Pelzer U, Schwaner I, Stieler J, et al. Best supportive care (BSC) versus oxaliplatin, folinic acid and 5-fluorouracil (OFF) plus BSC in patients for second-line advanced pancreatic cancer: a phase III-study from the German CONKO-study group. Eur J Cancer 2011;47:1676–81.

12. Xiong HQ, Varadhachary GR, Blais JC, et al. Phase 2 trial of oxaliplatin plus capecitabine (XELOX) as second-line therapy for patients with advanced pancreatic cancer. Cancer 2008;113:2046–52.

13. Conroy T, Desseigne F, Ychou M, et al. FOLFIRINOX versus gemcitabine for metastatic pancreatic cancer. N Engl J Med 2011;364:1817–25.

14. Von Hoff DD, Ervin T, Arena FP, et al. Increased survival in pancreatic cancer with nab-paclitaxel plus gemcitabine. N Engl J Med 2013;369:1691–703.

15. Herman JM, Swartz MJ, Hsu CC, et al. Analysis of fluorouracil-based adjuvant chemotherapy and radiation after pancreaticoduodenectomy for ductal adenocarcinoma of the pancreas: results of a large, prospectively collected database at the Johns Hopkins Hospital. J Clin Oncol 2008;26:3503–10.

16. Corsini MM, Miller RC, Haddock MG, et al. Adjuvant radiotherapy and chemotherapy for pancreatic carcinoma: the Mayo Clinic experience (1975-2005). J Clin Oncol 2008;26:3511–6.

17. Merkow RP, Bilimoria KY, Tomlinson JS, et al. Postoperative complications reduce adjuvant chemotherapy use in resectable pancreatic cancer. Ann Surg 2014;260: 372–7.

18. Lim JE, Chien MW, Earle CC. Prognostic factors following curative resection for pancreatic adenocarcinoma: a population-based, linked database analysis of 396 patients. Ann Surg 2003;237:74–85.

19. Swanson RS, Pezzi CM, Mallin K, et al. The 90-day mortality after pancreatectomy for cancer is double the 30-day mortality: more than 20,000 resections from the national cancer data base. Ann Surg Oncol 2014;21:4059–67.

20. Johnstone PA, Sindelar WF. Patterns of disease recurrence following definitive therapy of adenocarcinoma of the pancreas using surgery and adjuvant radiotherapy: correlations of a clinical trial. Int J Radiat Oncol Biol Phys 1993;27:831–4.

21. Iacobuzio-Donahue CA, Fu B, Yachida S, et al. DPC4 gene status of the primary carcinoma correlates with patterns of failure in patients with pancreatic cancer. J Clin Oncol 2009;27:1806–13.

22. Wolff RA, Varadhachary GR, Evans DB. Adjuvant therapy for adenocarcinoma of the pancreas: analysis of reported trials and recommendations for future progress. Ann Surg Oncol 2008;15:2773–86.
23. Verbeke CS, Knapp J, Gladhaug IP. Tumour growth is more dispersed in pancreatic head cancers than in rectal cancer: implications for resection margin assessment. Histopathology 2011;59:1111–21.
24. Glant JA, Waters JA, House MG, et al. Does the interval from imaging to operation affect the rate of unanticipated metastasis encountered during operation for pancreatic adenocarcinoma? Surgery 2011;150:607–16.
25. Menges P, Klocker C, Diedrich S, et al. Surgical trauma leads to a shorter survival in a murine orthotopic pancreatic cancer model. Eur Surg Res 2015;54:87–94.
26. Tai LH, Zhang J, Auer RC. Preventing surgery-induced NK cell dysfunction and cancer metastases with influenza vaccination. Oncoimmunology 2013;2:e26618.
27. Ananth AA, Tai LH, Lansdell C, et al. Surgical stress abrogates pre-existing protective T cell mediated anti-tumor immunity leading to postoperative cancer recurrence. PLoS One 2016;11:e0155947.
28. Neeman E, Ben-Eliyahu S. Surgery and stress promote cancer metastasis: new outlooks on perioperative mediating mechanisms and immune involvement. Brain Behav Immun 2013;30(Suppl):S32–40.
29. Evans DB, Rich TA, Byrd DR, et al. Preoperative chemoradiation and pancreaticoduodenectomy for adenocarcinoma of the pancreas. Arch Surg 1992;127: 1335–9.
30. Pisters PW, Abbruzzese JL, Janjan NA, et al. Rapid-fractionation preoperative chemoradiation, pancreaticoduodenectomy, and intraoperative radiation therapy for resectable pancreatic adenocarcinoma. J Clin Oncol 1998;16:3843–50.
31. Pisters PW, Wolff RA, Janjan NA, et al. Preoperative paclitaxel and concurrent rapid-fractionation radiation for resectable pancreatic adenocarcinoma: toxicities, histologic response rates, and event-free outcome. J Clin Oncol 2002;20: 2537–44.
32. Hoffman JP, Lipsitz S, Pisansky T, et al. Phase II trial of preoperative radiation therapy and chemotherapy for patients with localized, resectable adenocarcinoma of the pancreas: an Eastern Cooperative Oncology Group Study. J Clin Oncol 1998;16:317–23.
33. Shewach DS, Lawrence TS. Radiosensitization of human solid tumor cell lines with gemcitabine. Semin Oncol 1996;23(5 Suppl 10):65–71.
34. Evans DB, Varadhachary GR, Crane CH, et al. Preoperative gemcitabine-based chemoradiation for patients with resectable adenocarcinoma of the pancreatic head. J Clin Oncol 2008;26:3496–502.
35. Varadhachary GR, Wolff RA, Crane CH, et al. Preoperative gemcitabine and cisplatin followed by gemcitabine-based chemoradiation for resectable adenocarcinoma of the pancreatic head. J Clin Oncol 2008;26:3487–95.
36. Heinrich S, Pestalozzi BC, Schafer M, et al. Prospective phase II trial of neoadjuvant chemotherapy with gemcitabine and cisplatin for resectable adenocarcinoma of the pancreatic head. J Clin Oncol 2008;26:2526–31.
37. Christians KK, Heimler JW, George B, et al. Survival of patients with resectable pancreatic cancer who received neoadjuvant therapy. Surgery 2016;159: 893–900.
38. Roland CL, Yang AD, Katz MH, et al. Neoadjuvant therapy is associated with a reduced lymph node ratio in patients with potentially resectable pancreatic cancer. Ann Surg Oncol 2015;22:1168–75.

39. Townend P, de Reuver PR, Chua TC, et al. Histopathological tumour viability after neoadjuvant chemotherapy influences survival in resected pancreatic cancer: analysis of early outcome data. ANZ J Surg 2017. [Epub ahead of print].

40. Schorn S, Demir IE, Reyes CM, et al. The impact of neoadjuvant therapy on the histopathological features of pancreatic ductal adenocarcinoma - A systematic review and meta-analysis. Cancer Treat Rev 2017;55:96–106.

41. Zhao Q, Rashid A, Gong Y, et al. Pathologic complete response to neoadjuvant therapy in patients with pancreatic ductal adenocarcinoma is associated with a better prognosis. Ann Diagn Pathol 2012;16:29–37.

42. Lee SM, Katz MH, Liu L, et al. Validation of a proposed tumor regression grading scheme for pancreatic ductal adenocarcinoma after neoadjuvant therapy as a prognostic indicator for survival. Am J Surg Pathol 2016;40:1653–60.

43. Mokdad AA, Minter RM, Zhu H, et al. Neoadjuvant therapy followed by resection versus upfront resection for resectable pancreatic cancer: a propensity score matched analysis. J Clin Oncol 2017;35:515–22.

44. Mirkin KA, Hollenbeak CS, Wong J. Survival impact of neoadjuvant therapy in resected pancreatic cancer: a prospective cohort study involving 18,332 patients from the National Cancer Data Base. Int J Surg 2016;34:96–102.

45. Sharma G, Whang EE, Ruan DT, et al. Efficacy of neoadjuvant versus adjuvant therapy for resectable pancreatic adenocarcinoma: a decision analysis. Ann Surg Oncol 2015;22(Suppl 3):S1229–37.

46. de Geus SW, Evans DB, Bliss LA, et al. Neoadjuvant therapy versus upfront surgical strategies in resectable pancreatic cancer: a Markov decision analysis. Eur J Surg Oncol 2016;42:1552–60.

47. Abbott DE, Tzeng CW, Merkow RP, et al. The cost-effectiveness of neoadjuvant chemoradiation is superior to a surgery-first approach in the treatment of pancreatic head adenocarcinoma. Ann Surg Oncol 2013;20(Suppl 3):S500–8.

48. Varadhachary GR, Tamm EP, Abbruzzese JL, et al. Borderline resectable pancreatic cancer: definitions, management, and role of preoperative therapy. Ann Surg Oncol 2006;13:1035–46.

49. Wolff RA. Neoadjuvant chemoradiation for localized adenocarcinoma of the pancreas: great logic, grim reality. Ann Surg Oncol 2001;8:747–8.

50. Mehta VK, Fisher G, Ford JA, et al. Preoperative chemoradiation for marginally resectable adenocarcinoma of the pancreas. J Gastrointest Surg 2001;5:27–35.

51. Katz MH, Pisters PW, Evans DB, et al. Borderline resectable pancreatic cancer: the importance of this emerging stage of disease. J Am Coll Surg 2008;206:833–46.

52. Christians KK, Tsai S, Mahmoud A, et al. Neoadjuvant FOLFIRINOX for borderline resectable pancreas cancer: a new treatment paradigm? Oncologist 2014;19:266–74.

53. Takahashi H, Ohigashi H, Gotoh K, et al. Preoperative gemcitabine-based chemoradiation therapy for resectable and borderline resectable pancreatic cancer. Ann Surg 2013;258:1040–50.

54. Katz MH, Shi Q, Ahmad SA, et al. Preoperative modified FOLFIRINOX treatment followed by capecitabine-based chemoradiation for borderline resectable pancreatic cancer: alliance for clinical trials in oncology trial A021101. JAMA Surg 2016;151:e161137.

55. Tempero MA, Malafa MP, Behrman SW, et al. Pancreatic adenocarcinoma, version 2.2014: featured updates to the NCCN guidelines. J Natl Compr Canc Netw 2014;12:1083–93.

56. Bockhorn M, Uzunoglu FG, Adham M, et al. Borderline resectable pancreatic cancer: a consensus statement by the International Study Group of Pancreatic Surgery (ISGPS). Surgery 2014;155:977–88.
57. Jessup JM, Steele G Jr, Mayer RJ, et al. Neoadjuvant therapy for unresectable pancreatic adenocarcinoma. Arch Surg 1993;128:559–64.
58. White RR, Hurwitz HI, Morse MA, et al. Neoadjuvant chemoradiation for localized adenocarcinoma of the pancreas. Ann Surg Oncol 2001;8:758–65.
59. Kim HJ, Czischke K, Brennan MF, et al. Does neoadjuvant chemoradiation downstage locally advanced pancreatic cancer? J Gastrointest Surg 2002;6:763–9.
60. Gillen S, Schuster T, Meyer Zum Buschenfelde C, et al. Preoperative/neoadjuvant therapy in pancreatic cancer: a systematic review and meta-analysis of response and resection percentages. PLoS Med 2010;7:e1000267.
61. Cloyd JM, Katz MH, Prakash L, et al. Preoperative therapy and pancreatoduodenectomy for pancreatic ductal adenocarcinoma: a 25-year single-institution experience. J Gastrointest Surg 2017;21(1):164–74.
62. Available at: https://clinicaltrials.gov/ct2/show/NCT01964430.
63. Available at: https://clinicaltrials.gov/ct2/show/results/NCT01526135.
64. Sherman MH, Yu RT, Engle DD, et al. Vitamin D receptor-mediated stromal reprogramming suppresses pancreatitis and enhances pancreatic cancer therapy. Cell 2014;159:80–93.
65. Azad A, Yin Lim S, D'Costa Z, et al. PD-L1 blockade enhances response of pancreatic ductal adenocarcinoma to radiotherapy. EMBO Mol Med 2017;9: 167–80.
66. Koay EJ, Truty MJ, Cristini V, et al. Transport properties of pancreatic cancer describe gemcitabine delivery and response. J Clin Invest 2014;124:1525–36.
67. Koay EJ, Amer AM, Baio FE, et al. Toward stratification of patients with pancreatic cancer: past lessons from traditional approaches and future applications with physical biomarkers. Cancer Lett 2016;381(1):237–43.
68. Versteijne E, van Eijck CH, Punt CJ, et al. Preoperative radiochemotherapy versus immediate surgery for resectable and borderline resectable pancreatic cancer (PREOPANC trial): study protocol for a multicentre randomized controlled trial. Trials 2016;17:127.

The Evolving Role of Radiation in Pancreatic Cancer

Evan Landau, MD[a],*, Shalom Kalnicki, MD, FACRO[b]

KEYWORDS

- Pancreatic cancer • Radiation • Chemoradiation therapy • SBRT • SABR • IMRT

KEY POINTS

- The role of radiation in pancreatic cancer is still evolving.
- The data supporting this modality are mixed and likely reflect the systemic nature of this disease.
- Using the correct patient selection, in combination with the newer radiation technology, a role for radiation likely still exists.

Pancreatic cancer is an aggressive malignancy with a poor long-term survival and only mild improvement in outcomes over the past 30 years. Local failure remains a problem and radiation can help improve control. The role of radiation therapy in pancreatic cancer has been controversial and is still evolving. This article reviews the trials of pancreatic cancer and radiation in adjuvant, neoadjuvant, and unresectable lesions. The article reviews the impact and outcomes of evolving radiation technology.

ADJUVANT CHEMORADIATION

The benefit of chemoradiation therapy (CRT) following a pancreatic resection is unclear. There have been 3 randomized trials with conflicting outcomes. The first randomized trial performed by Gastrointestinal Tumor Study Group (GITSG) showed a survival benefit with split-course radiation and 5-fluorouracil (5FU) chemotherapy.[1] A confirmatory trial showed no survival benefit for CRT compared with observation.[2] The most recent data are from a phase 3 randomized trial performed by the European Study Group for Pancreatic Cancer (ESPAC) using a complex 2 by 2 factorial design trial that randomized postresection subjects to 4 arms: observation, 5FU, 5FU plus

The authors have nothing to disclose.
[a] 21st Century Oncology, Broward Health, 1625 Southeast 3rd Avenue, Fort Lauderdale, FL 33316, USA; [b] Radiation Oncology, Montefiore Medical Park, 1625 Poplar Street, Bronx, NY 10461, USA
* Corresponding author.
E-mail address: evan.landau@21co.com

split-course radiation, and 5FU plus split-course radiation therapy followed by 5FU. The trial found that chemotherapy improved projected 5-year survival to 21% versus 8% in the non-chemotherapy arm ($P = .009$). The CRT arm was inferior to the non-CRT arm with a 5-year survival of 10% versus 20% ($P = .05$), respectively.[3] Attempts to combine radiation with gemcitabine using modern radiation techniques have not shown a survival benefit for radiation.[4] Only a single randomized trial from the 1980s showed a survival benefit to CRT, with recent data showing either no benefit or a detriment.

These trials have been criticized for multiple reasons. All 5FU trials used a now anti-quated split-course of radiation with a planned 2 week hiatus, which may be inferior in to the current sequential treatment. In addition, the ESPAC trial, had a complex 2 by 2 factorial design, no quality assurance of radiation therapy planning, and field size and technique were not standardized, which may explain the poor CRT outcomes. A subsequent (Radiation Therapy Oncology Group [RTOG] 97–04) report confirmed that the radiation quality affects survival.[5] Finally, current treatment differ vastly from the randomized trials designed in the 1980–1990. All of these phase 3 trials utilized two dimensional x-ray based targeting with limited motion management, poor image guidance and antiquated radiation planning, and as such raises questions of applicability to modern treatment.

As multiple critiques have been raised, some have pointed to retrospectives series as support for adjuvant CRT. A John Hopkins series of 908 subjects status postpancreatectomy showed a nearly 7-month median survival benefit in CRT (21.2 vs 14.4 months, $P=<.001$).[6] In addition, similar findings were shown in a cohort of 472 subjects, with a 25.5-month versus 19.2-month median survival benefit ($P = .001$).[7] These conflicting data have influenced current guidelines. The National Comprehensive Cancer Network favors chemotherapy alone or induction chemotherapy followed by CRT. The European Society for Radiotherapy and Oncology guidelines do not recommend adjuvant CRT.[8] The RTOG 08-48 is currently accruing subjects for a trial testing 6 months of adjuvant induction chemotherapy and randomization to CRT versus observation in stable subjects. This trial uses modern techniques and has a computed tomography (CT)-based atlas to ensure appropriate target delineation (available at https://www.rtog.org/ClinicalTrials/ProtocolTable/StudyDetails.aspx?study=0848).

Unresectable Pancreatic Cancer

Thirty percent of patients have locally unresectable pancreatic cancer at diagnosis[9] and overall mean survival is limited to 13.6 months.[10] The best management is controversial.

Concurrent chemotherapy and radiation

The benefit of concurrent CRT is controversial because of conflicting trial outcomes. Two initial trails compared antiquated concurrent chemotherapy and radiation versus chemotherapy alone. The GITSG trial of 43 subjects with locally advanced pancreatic cancer (LAPC) showed the combination 5FU and 54 Gy of radiation showed an improved 10-week survival but toxicity in the CRT was "severe" in 50% of patients.[11] In 1985, a study of LAPC patients of 5FU versus 5FU and 40 Gy radiation, and showed no benefit of CRT with nearly identical median survival.[12]

After the acceptance of gemcitabine as standard chemotherapy, 2 CRT versus chemotherapy trials were published, again with different outcomes. The Federation Francophone de Cancerologie Digestive (FFCD) group randomized LAPC subjects to a high dose of radiation of 60 Gy with infusional 5FU and intermittent cisplatin versus gemcitabine alone. This trial showed a statistically significant decrease in median survival with CRT of 8.6 months versus gemcitabine alone of 13 months (P = .03). This trial has been criticized for the high dose of radiation and combination regime which was not previously tested, poor compliance with treatment, and high CRT toxicity of 78% grade 3 or 4.[13] Eastern Cooperative Oncology Group (ECOG) randomized LAPC subjects to full-dose gemcitabine alone versus CRT with 3D CT and dose-reduced gemcitabine (600 mg/m^2). The trial was closed early secondary to poor accrual but was still powered to show a survival benefit in the CRT arm of 11.1 to 9.2 months (P = .017). However, toxicity was high in CRT arm with 41% at grade 4 or 5.[14]

Which chemotherapy with radiation: concurrent capecitabine–5-fluorouracil or gemcitabine?

The initial CRT trials used 5FU-based chemotherapy as the radiation sensitizing agent. However, gemcitabine has become a standard due to significant systemic efficacy and improved survival.[15,16] In addition, it is a potent radiation sensitizer,[17] although initial experience noted significant toxicity when combined with radiation.[18] Even in the phase III setting, the combined approach has yielded many side effects. Multiple studies have consistently demonstrated success with both acceptable toxicity and encouraging overall survival with gemcitabine as a radiation sensitizer, with some trials using a full-dose regime.[19]

The SCALOP trial addressed the question of which concurrent agent is better. The investigators successfully treated 114 subjects with LAPC to induction chemotherapy, then randomized the subjects to combination gemcitabine and radiation or capecitabine and radiation. There was no statistical improvement in the capecitabine arm, with overall survival of 17.6 months versus 14.6 months in the gemcitabine arm (P = .185); however, the per treatment and multivariate analysis found a benefit to capecitabine and radiation.[20] In addition the hematologic side effects rate was higher in the gemcitabine arm and, in both arms, only 68% to 74% of subjects completed the total radiation dosing.[21]

LAP07 (Chemoradiation vs Chemotherapy Trial)

The findings from a Groupe Coopérateur Multidisciplinaire en Oncologie or GERCOR induction chemotherapy study led to most recent and influential CRT versus chemotherapy trial, the LAP07.[22] This 2 by 2 French trial randomized subjects to 2 induction options: gemcitabine (1000 mg/m^2) versus gemcitabine (1000 mg/m^2) plus 100 mg/d of erlotinib. Of the subjects, 442 were randomized to chemotherapy and 269 subjects did not progress after the 4 months induction period and were randomized to same-dose chemotherapy versus 54 Gy plus capecitabine. The radiation was 3D CT-based without prophylactic lymph node irradiation but with a sizable margin of 3 cm superior to inferior. In the final analysis, no survival benefit was found with the addition of radiation. A 14% local control benefit was noted and the CRT had a similar toxicity to chemotherapy except for more nausea.[10] This trial has had a significant impact on the national guidelines. The American Society of Clinical Oncology guidelines consider chemotherapy as the standard with CRT if no progression is noted.[23]

Who should get radiation based off the trial outcomes?

Based on the mixed and equivocal data of radiation therapy in the adjuvant and LAPC setting, the benefit and role of radiation in pancreatic cancer is uncertain. The authors hold that radiation therapy has a role in pancreatic cancer for several reasons. First, patient selection strongly influences outcome; second, the anatomic complexity and motion of the pancreas during treatment may explain some of the mixed data; third, new technology may offer better therapy and improved outcomes; and, finally, using this new technology for neoadjuvant chemoradiation may be the preferred treatment application.

Patient selection

Distant failure is all too common in pancreatic cancer, and local treatment should only be offered to patients with local disease or a local failure pattern. Upfront chemotherapy may help stratify risk and has become the recommended standard of care in LAPC.[23] The rationale for this standard is compelling. First, pancreatic cancer has a high metastatic rate and nearly a quarter of LAPCs will have rapid distant progression during the initial course of treatment.[10] Therefore, systemic therapy should be offered early in the course of management. Second, CRT has toxicity and should only be offered to patients who have been shown to have local disease. Finally, chemotherapy is effective[15] and it may make the target more receptive and amenable to radiation. Clinical data support this approach. The MD Anderson group looked at a retrospective analysis of their patients who underwent induction chemotherapy followed by CRT, versus CRT alone. They found a 3-month survival improvement in the induction group.[24] In a subgroup analysis of multiple prospective phase II and III GERCOR group studies, a comparison of CCR induction chemotherapy followed by CRT versus chemotherapy alone also yielded a survival benefit in the induction group.[22]

Predicting local failure: SMAD4 Gene and CA19-9 Tumor Marker

Local failure remains a significant problem in pancreatic cancer. In 3 cited studies using chemotherapy alone, it ranged from 34% to 46%. Ideally, radiation should be offered to patients when preventing local failure might affect survival. SMAD4 (dpc4) is a histologic marker that has been shown to correlate with failure pattern. In a rapid autopsy series dpc4 was highly correlated with metastatic disease.[25] In a phase 2 trial examining the benefits of Erbitux, with induction chemotherapy and then with concurrent chemoradiation, a secondary analysis on SMAD4 mutation showed that an intact SMAD4 was associated with an increased risk of local progression, whereas loss of SMAD4 was associated a distant dominant progression.[26] However, the predictive failure pattern of SMAD4 in post-Whipple cases is uncertain.[27,28]

Questions remain about the application and predictability of SMAD4 because the local patterns of recurrence may not correlate with the usual radiation field. An additional difficulty may exist because needle biopsy may provide insufficient sampling for SMAD4. One study of preoperative cytology, via Endoscopic Ultrasound Guided Fine Needle Aspiration, incorrectly classified the SMAD4 in 29% of the sample compared with the final pathologic results.[29]

Ca19-9 a marker used to predict survival in pancreatic cancer[30] has been suggested as a risk stratifier following induction chemotherapy. In the SCALOP trial, a Ca19-9 following induction chemotherapy and before chemoradiation of less than 46 U/mL was associated with improved survival at 12 months; therefore, patients with a Ca19-9 below may be better candidates for subsequent chemoradiation.[20]

Anatomic complexity and motion

Pancreatic cancer offers multiple complexities in the successful administration of radiation treatment and the initial radiation technology was limited in meeting these challenges. First, the pancreas is anatomically adjacent to multiple organs sensitive to radiation, including the kidneys, liver, stomach, and small bowel, as well as, in particular, the duodenum. Therefore, for radiation therapy to be successful the dose must be sculpted to the cancer and excess radiation to the normal adjacent organs avoided. This was not available in older trials, which used 2D targeting and limited organ sparing. Second, the pancreas is a moving target and during 1 respiratory cycle moves 1.5 to 3.5 cm.[31–33] Therefore, to cover the target during the respiratory cycles, early series added a motion margin of 2 cm to 3 cm.[10,13] Increasing the margin may allow better coverage of the target but with increased treatment morbidity. This may partially explain the high toxicity rate in early papers on ablative radiation in which a larger margin was used and the late grade 2 morbidity was 94%.[34]

New technology
Radiation has benefited from multiple technological innovations during the past 15 years, which may combat some of these issues. Significant progress has been made in reducing the target size. Modern external radiation treatment benefits from real-time image guidance, which includes daily conebeam and kilovoltage (kV) imaging. This technology allows for accurate daily matching and decreases in target margin. In addition, better preradiation 3D-imaging technology provides more accurate tumor delineation.

Smaller Targets: Avoiding Elective Nodal Irradiation

The radiation target in pancreatic cancer has also changed. Typically, nodal groups and the primary tumor were included in the radiation field because regional nodes are involved in at least 30% of pancreatic cancer.[35] However, as radiation doses escalated, nodal irradiation was deemed too morbid. Most new series of radiation of pancreatic cancer avoid elective lymph node irradiation and only target tumors.[19,36] In addition, patterns of failure series have helped better define the peripancreatic area as the site of greatest risk.[37] Finally, and somewhat provocatively, without elective nodal irradiation tumor control is consistently better, or as good as, when electively nodes were included in radiation treatment. This brings up the question of whether there is any benefit to elective nodal treatment at all.

Dose Sculpting

Intensity-modulated radiation therapy
Intensity-modulated radiation therapy (IMRT) is a technology that divides radiation into small beamlets and shapes them around the target to improve sparing of adjacent organs. In addition, complex planning algorithms are used to maximize therapy. Efforts have been made to utilize this technology as a means of increasing the dose of radiation and avoiding toxicity.[38]

Gemcitabine is a potent radiation sensitizer[17] but early combinations with radiation led to high toxicity. A dose escalation trial in unresectable subjects that used IMRT concurrent with gemcitabine (1000 mg/m^2) delivered 55 Gy in 25 fractions showed an encouraging 24% resectability rate and a 14.8-month overall survival.[19] A confirmatory retrospective series indicated a mean overall survival of 22.9 months and a resection rate of 29%.[39] In addition, IMRT has lessened the toxicity versus 2D or 3D technology.[32]

An MD Anderson group published a provocative concept of treating LAPC with induction chemotherapy and hypofractionated IMRT. IMRT was used to create hotspots of dosage in the tumor and spare the adjacent organs by respiratory motion management.[40] They compared it to the standard dose and found a better 3-year survival of 31% versus 9%.[41] This concept was adopted for a prospective phase II RTOG trial that was terminated because of slow accrual (available at https://www.rtog.org/LinkClick.aspx?fileticket=HQpVTl4rE58%3D&tabid=290).

Stereotactic Body Radiation Therapy or Stereotactic Ablative Radiation

Stereotactic body radiation therapy (SBRT) has shown much promise in pancreatic cancer and is rapidly setting a new standard. SBRT technology uses high doses of radiation per fraction (>6 Gy) and fewer fractions (1–5) in a conformal radiation field.[42] The pancreas as a target for ablative radiations offers several challenges. The lesions are adjacent to radiation sensitive organs, particularly the duodenum, and the pancreas is a moving target because of respiratory motion.[33] Technology has been developed to combat this issue. Motion management via either robotic hybrid tracking technology with fiducial markers or with linear accelerator-based abdominal compression, gating, and image guidance have been effective, and have reduced the set up margin from 2 to 3 cm to 2 to 3 mm.[43]

Stereotactic body radiation therapy prospective data

The SBRT literature is limited, without phase III studies, and has only a few prospective or phase II studies. Early publications showed excellent local control (>90%)[44] but concerns about late grade 3 toxicity greater than 33%.[34] Toxicity has been lowered by adopting a 5 to 6 fraction course. A recent publication showed a 2-year local recurrence rate of 90% and no grade 3 toxicity.[45] These treatments can be completed in a week and all full-dose systemic therapy can be continued. Finally, SBRT has shown progress in borderline resectable subjects. One retrospective study of 101 subjects treated with gemcitabine, docetaxel, capecitabine, and SBRT showed that 54.5% underwent resection, 96.4% had complete resection (R)-0, and there was a 33-month survival for resectable subjects (**Table 1**).[46]

Stereotactic body radiation therapy versus intensity-modulated radiation therapy

There are no comparative studies between IMRT using 25 to 28 treatments versus the SBRT 1 to 5 fractions. The prolonged treatment with IMRT allows for the integration of systemic chemotherapy as a sensitizer but may delay full-dose chemotherapy. SBRT allows for a short course but it is not sensitized by chemotherapy and, because it uses an ablative dose in its therapy, it may be limited by the risk of adjacent small bowel damage. SBRT may allow for a smaller target volumes as in one series the SBRT target was 1/3 the size of the standard CRT treatment.[47] Wild and colleagues[48] suggested that the larger radiation field and additional fractions of IMRT may have an associated morbidity because significantly increased amounts of circulating blood lymphocytes are irradiated. These lymphocytes may be active in tumor kill, and lymphopenia was found to be a prognostic finding in CRT pancreatic subjects (**Tables 2 and 3**).

Future developments: stereotactic body radiation therapy and immunotherapy

SBRT may offer tumor-related immunogenic modulation that may not be found in CRT cases. SBRT has been associated with a host of changes in the tumor

| Table 1 | | | | | |
| Stereotactic body radiation therapy for unresectable cancer | | | | | |
Trial	N	Dose	FFLP	Overall Survival	Toxicity (Late)
Rashid et al,[46] 2016	49	6.6 Gy/5 fx	78% at 1 y	13.9 mo	10.6% > grade 2
Chang et al,[36] 2009	77	25 Gy/1 fx	84% at 1 y	11.9 mo	25% > grade 2 9% > grade 3
Comito et al,[45] 2017	45	45 Gy/6 fx	90% at 2 y	19 mo	4% > grade 2 0% > grade 3

Abbreviation: fx, fractions of radiation treatment.

Table 2
Induction chemotherapy: 3-Dimensional Chemoradiation Therapy versus Intensity-Modulated Radiation Therapy versus Stereotactic Body Radiation therapy for Unresectable Pancreatic Cancer

Trial	Induction	Concurrent Chemotherapy and Radiation Technique	N	Overall Survival Median	Toxicity grade 3	FFLP	Surgery Rate
LAPC07[10]	Gemcitabine	Capecitabine 3D Radiation	109	15.2	24%	—	4%
Ben Josef et al,[19] 2012	Gemcitabine	Gemcitabine IMRT	50	14.8	24%	59% at 2 y	20%
Herman et al,[6] 2015	Gemcitabine	SBRT	49	13.9	6%	78% at 1yr	8%

Abbreviations: FFLP, freedom from local progression; SBRT, Stereotactic body radiation therapy.

microenvironment that can be presented to the immune system, including release of tumor debris, inflammatory cytokines, and tumor associated antigens. This response has been shown in vivo models to be dose-dependent and ablative dosing of SBRT may lead these tumor cells to function as an antitumor vaccine.[49] This combination approach is currently being tested in multiple prospective trials.[50]

Dose escalation
In general, curable dosing of gross disease is normally in excess of 70 Gy but most past series have limited dosing to 40 to 50 Gy. Early efforts in dose escalation have met significant toxicities[34,51] and no outcome improvement.[13,52] These initial failures may reflect toxicities from poor technique. However, in recent literature there are suggestions that increases in dosing may lead to better local control. The IMRT escalation studies have shown encouraging improvement in outcome and local control with some morbidity.[19] Two retrospective comparison studies showed survival benefit with dose escalation.[41,53] Ablative dosing with SBRT, in both single fraction and multiple fraction, has excellent local control.[45] In addition, intraoperative radiation allows for organ-sparing dose escalation and has demonstrated encouraging results.[54]

Neoadjuvant Chemoradiation

The best option for cure for a patient with pancreatic cancer is a surgical excision. However, only a small subset of all patients present with resectable disease;

Table 3
Intensity-modulated radiation therapy versus stereotactic body radiation therapy linear accelerator or robotic radiosurgery

	IMRT	SBRT Liniac/Robotic Radiosurgery
Number of treatments, length	25–28, 5–6 wk	1-5, 1 wk
Dosing	45–50 Gy	25–33 Gy
Chemotherapy	Concurrent	Sequential
Image guidance	Conebeam	Conebeam or KV-hybrid tracking
Respiratory management	Abdominal compression gating	Abdominal compression gating fiducial tracking
Target size	300–500 mL	100 mL
Elective nodal treatment	Can allow	Very limited

therefore, this cure option is not available to most patients. In addition, even among patients with resectable cancer at presentation, the cure rate is limited and the rate of positive margins at surgery is common with a R1 resection rate of 17% to 42%. Finally, surgery can be associated with significant morbidity and a significant percentage of patients develop metastatic disease rapidly after surgical excision. The benefit of adjuvant therapy has been primarily flat during the past 25 years. This has led many investigators to pursue a neoadjuvant approach of chemotherapy and radiation.

This approach may offer multiple theoretic advantages. First, nonsurgically manipulated tissue may allow for a better vascular supply to the tumor and possibly a higher response rate to induction chemotherapy and radiation. Second, this approach may shrink the size of the tumor and improve resectability, R0 resection, and lymph node sterilization. Third, this technique allows investigators and clinicians to assess the response to the tumor. Fourth, a delay in systemic therapy may lead to rapid progression of distant metastatic disease. However, questions remain.

Does neoadjuvant therapy in fact improve the resectability and is it better than upfront resection?

Prospective phase II trials have shown encouraging outcomes with neoadjuvant approach. The resectability rate was improved in a heterogeneous metaanalysis of 111 subjects, by 73% for resectable cancers and 33% for LAPC or borderline cases.[55] In addition, the R0 resection rate has been reported to be high following neoadjuvant therapy. A metaanalysis of subjects with neoadjuvant gemcitabine-based therapy showed an improvement of 89% in resectable and 60% in unresectable patients.[56] In resectable patients a phase II trial of 86 patient who underwent a Gemcitabine (400mg/m^2) CRT showed that 13 patients progressed, and 73 underwent surgery, the overall population had an encouraging 22.7 months median survival.[57] In a large phase II trial of 188 resectable subjects treated with neoadjuvant gemcitabine (1000 mg/m^2) with fractionated 50 Gy in 25 fractions yielded a resection rate of 87%, an R0 of 99%, and a very encouraging 5-year survival of 57%.[58] Similar findings were reported in a smaller US multi-institutional series.[12,59]

The question of whether neoadjuvant or adjuvant therapy is the better approach can only be answered in a randomized trial. One randomized trial was attempted and failed to accrue subjects. Some retrospective data suggest a benefit to neoadjuvant treatment. In a single retrospective comparison of borderline or LAPC subjects undergoing FOLFIRNOX (fluorouracil [5-FU], leucovorin, irinotecan and oxaliplatin) plus or minus radiation, the 50% who had surgery versus an upfront surgical series showed an improved outcome with the neoadjuvant approach, a decrease in margin positivity, lower lymph node positivity, and lower operative morbidity.[60] A second retrospective comparison series between resectable subjects undergoing upfront surgery versus neoadjuvant chemotherapy and SBRT showed a decrease in positive margins, similar morbidity and improved survival of 33.5 vs 23.1 months, ($P = .057$).[61] In addition, a population-based study of operable pancreatic cancer found an improvement in survival for neoadjuvant versus adjuvant treatment.[62] However, theses data may reflect a selection bias in favor of the neoadjuvant patients because the patients who progressed during neoadjuvant were not included.

Does neoadjuvant therapy allow for the clinician to assess response?

Neoadjuvant therapy likely offers a histologic response; however, radiographic changes may be limited. In a large metaanalysis of 111 studies, the investigators reported that combined radiographic and histologic response rate was 33%.[55] In addition, histologic responses on surgical pathologic reports have been shown to be high at 50% in a series.[63] However, recent data cast doubt on the benefit of neoadjuvant treatment to yield a radiographic change. A single institution experience of subjects with borderline resectable cases treated with neoadjuvant CRT only yielded a radiographic change in less than 1% of subjects.[12,64] A similar study of 40 subjects undergoing neoadjuvant treatment showed that radiographic findings may show a decrease in tumor size but radiographic downstaging was unreliable.[60] In the SBRT literature, the response rate can be high but significant radiographic regression may not be noted.[43] These finding may reflect CTs inability to differentiate tumor from fibrosis; in 1 surgical series a 56% fibrosis rate was noted following neoadjuvant therapy.[65]

SUMMARY

The role of radiation in pancreatic cancer is still evolving. The data supporting this modality are mixed and likely reflect the systemic nature of this disease. Using correct patient selection in combination with the newer radiation technology, a role for radiation likely still exists.

REFERENCES

1. Kalser MH, Ellenberg SS. Pancreatic cancer. Adjuvant combined radiation and chemotherapy following curative resection. Arch Surg 1985;120(8):899–903.
2. Klinkenbijl JH, Jeekel J, Sahmoud T, et al. Adjuvant radiotherapy and 5-fluorouracil after curative resection of cancer of the pancreas and periampullary region: phase III trial of the EORTC gastrointestinal tract cancer cooperative group. Ann Surg 1999;230(6):776–82 [discussion: 782–4].
3. Neoptolemos JP, Stocken DD, Friess H, et al, European Study Group for Pancreatic, C. A randomized trial of chemoradiotherapy and chemotherapy after resection of pancreatic cancer. N Engl J Med 2004;350(12):1200–10.
4. Van Laethem JL, Hammel P, Mornex F, et al. Adjuvant gemcitabine alone versus gemcitabine-based chemoradiotherapy after curative resection for pancreatic cancer: a randomized EORTC-40013-22012/FFCD- 9203/GERCOR phase II study. J Clin Oncol 2010;28(29):4450–6.
5. Abrams RA, Winter KA, Regine WF, et al. Failure to adhere to protocol specified radiation therapy guidelines was associated with decreased survival in RTOG 9704–a phase III trial of adjuvant chemotherapy and chemoradiotherapy for patients with resected adenocarcinoma of the pancreas. Int J Radiat Oncol Biol Phys 2012;82(2):809–16.
6. Herman JM, Swartz MJ, Hsu CC, et al. Analysis of fluorouracil-based adjuvant chemotherapy and radiation after pancreaticoduodenectomy for ductal adenocarcinoma of the pancreas: results of a large, prospectively collected database at the Johns Hopkins Hospital. J Clin Oncol 2008;26(21):3503–10.
7. Corsini MM, Miller RC, Haddock MG, et al. Adjuvant radiotherapy and chemotherapy for pancreatic carcinoma: the Mayo Clinic experience (1975-2005). J Clin Oncol 2008;26(21):3511–6.
8. Ducreux M, Cuhna AS, Caramella C, et al. Cancer of the pancreas: ESMO Clinical Practice Guidelines for diagnosis, treatment and follow-up. Ann Oncol 2015; 26(Suppl 5):v56–68.
9. Hidalgo M. Pancreatic cancer. N Engl J Med 2010;362(17):1605–17.
10. Hammel P, Huguet F, van Laethem JL, et al. Effect of chemoradiotherapy vs chemotherapy on survival in patients with locally advanced pancreatic cancer

controlled after 4 months of gemcitabine with or without Erlotinib: the LAP07 randomized clinical trial. JAMA 2016;315(17):1844–53.

11. Treatment of locally unresectable carcinoma of the pancreas: comparison of combined-modality therapy (chemotherapy plus radiotherapy) to chemotherapy alone. Gastrointestinal Tumor Study Group. J Natl Cancer Inst 1988;80(10): 751–5.

12. Klaassen DJ, MacIntyre JM, Catton GE, et al. Treatment of locally unresectable cancer of the stomach and pancreas: a randomized comparison of 5- fluorouracil alone with radiation plus concurrent and maintenance 5-fluorouracil–an Eastern Cooperative Oncology Group study. J Clin Oncol 1985;3(3):373–8.

13. Chauffert B, Mornex F, Bonnetain F, et al. Phase III trial comparing intensive induction chemoradiotherapy (60 Gy, infusional 5-FU and intermittent cisplatin) followed by maintenance gemcitabine with gemcitabine alone for locally advanced unresectable pancreatic cancer. Definitive results of the 2000-01 FFCD/SFRO study. Ann Oncol 2008;19(9):1592–9.

14. Loehrer PJ Sr, Feng Y, Cardenes H, et al. Gemcitabine alone versus gemcitabine plus radiotherapy in patients with locally advanced pancreatic cancer: an Eastern Cooperative Oncology Group trial. J Clin Oncol 2011;29(31):4105–12.

15. Oettle H, Neuhaus P, Hochhaus A, et al. Adjuvant chemotherapy with gemcitabine and long-term outcomes among patients with resected pancreatic cancer: the CONKO-001 randomized trial. JAMA 2013;310(14):1473–81.

16. Oettle H, Post S, Neuhaus P, et al. Adjuvant chemotherapy with gemcitabine vs observation in patients undergoing curative-intent resection of pancreatic cancer: a randomized controlled trial. JAMA 2007;297(3):267–77.

17. Lawrence TS, Chang EY, Hahn TM, et al. Radiosensitization of pancreatic cancer cells by 2',2'-difluoro-2'-deoxycytidine. Int J Radiat Oncol Biol Phys 1996;34(4): 867–72.

18. Wolff RA, Evans DB, Gravel DM, et al. Phase I trial of gemcitabine combined with radiation for the treatment of locally advanced pancreatic adenocarcinoma. Clin Cancer Res 2001;7(8):2246–53.

19. Ben-Josef E, Schipper M, Francis IR, et al. A phase I/II trial of intensity modulated radiation (IMRT) dose escalation with concurrent fixed-dose rate gemcitabine (FDR-G) in patients with unresectable pancreatic cancer. Int J Radiat Oncol Biol Phys 2012;84(5):1166–71.

20. Hurt CN, Falk S, Crosby T, et al. Long-term results and recurrence patterns from SCALOP: a phase II randomised trial of gemcitabine- or capecitabine-based chemoradiation for locally advanced pancreatic cancer. Br J Cancer 2017; 116(10):1264–70.

21. Mukherjee S, Hurt CN, Bridgewater J, et al. Gemcitabine-based or capecitabine-based chemoradiotherapy for locally advanced pancreatic cancer (SCALOP): a multicentre, randomised, phase 2 trial. Lancet Oncol 2013;14(4):317–26.

22. Balaban EP, Mangu PB, Khorana AA, et al. Locally advanced, unresectable pancreatic cancer: American Society of Clinical Oncology clinical practice guideline. J Clin Oncol 2016;34(22):2654–68.

23. Krishnan S, Rana V, Janjan NA, et al. Induction chemotherapy selects patients with locally advanced, unresectable pancreatic cancer for optimal benefit from consolidative chemoradiation therapy. Cancer 2007;110(1):47–55.

24. Huguet F, Andre T, Hammel P, et al. Impact of chemoradiotherapy after disease control with chemotherapy in locally advanced pancreatic adenocarcinoma in GERCOR phase II and III studies. J Clin Oncol 2007;25(3):326–31.

25. Iacobuzio-Donahue CA, Fu B, Yachida S, et al. DPC4 gene status of the primary carcinoma correlates with patterns of failure in patients with pancreatic cancer. J Clin Oncol 2009;27(11):1806–13.

26. Crane CH, Varadhachary GR, Yordy JS, et al. Phase II trial of cetuximab, gemcitabine, and oxaliplatin followed by chemoradiation with cetuximab for locally advanced (T4) pancreatic adenocarcinoma: correlation of Smad4(Dpc4) immunostaining with pattern of disease progression. J Clin Oncol 2011;29(22): 3037–43.

27. Shin SH, Kim HJ, Hwang DW, et al. The DPC4/SMAD4 genetic status determines recurrence patterns and treatment outcomes in resected pancreatic ductal adenocarcinoma: a prospective cohort study. Oncotarget 2017;8(11):17945–59.

28. Winter JM, Tang LH, Klimstra DS, et al. Failure patterns in resected pancreas adenocarcinoma: lack of predicted benefit to SMAD4 expression. Ann Surg 2013;258(2):331–5.

29. Kharofa JR, Barnes C, Mackinnon A, et al. Correlation of SMAD4 expression in pretreatment cytologic specimens and postneoadjuvant treatment surgical specimens in patients with pancreatic cancer. Int J Radiat Oncol Biol Phys 2016;96(2):S141.

30. Berger AC, Garcia M Jr, Hoffman JP, et al. Postresection CA 19-9 predicts overall survival in patients with pancreatic cancer treated with adjuvant chemoradiation: a prospective validation by RTOG 9704. J Clin Oncol 2008;26(36):5918–22.

31. Bryan PJ, Custar S, Haaga JR, et al. Respiratory movement of the pancreas: an ultrasonic study. J Ultrasound Med 1984;3(7):317–20.

32. Cardenes HR, Moore AM, Johnson CS, et al. A phase II study of gemcitabine in combination with radiation therapy in patients with localized, unresectable, pancreatic cancer: a Hoosier Oncology Group study. Am J Clin Oncol 2011; 34(5):460–5.

33. Mori S, Hara R, Yanagi T, et al. Four-dimensional measurement of intrafractional respiratory motion of pancreatic tumors using a 256 multi-slice CT scanner. Radiother Oncol 2009;92(2):231–7.

34. Hoyer M, Roed H, Sengelov L, et al. Phase-II study on stereotactic radiotherapy of locally advanced pancreatic carcinoma. Radiother Oncol 2005;76(1):48–53.

35. Sun W, Leong CN, Zhang Z, et al. Proposing the lymphatic target volume for elective radiation therapy for pancreatic cancer: a pooled analysis of clinical evidence. Radiat Oncol 2010;5:28.

36. Chang DT, Schellenberg D, Shen J, et al. Stereotactic radiotherapy for unresectable adenocarcinoma of the pancreas. Cancer 2009;115(3):665–72.

37. Dholakia AS, Kumar R, Raman SP, et al. Mapping patterns of local recurrence after pancreaticoduodenectomy for pancreatic adenocarcinoma: a new approach to adjuvant radiation field design. Int J Radiat Oncol Biol Phys 2013;87(5): 1007–15.

38. Spalding AC, Jee KW, Vineberg K, et al. Potential for dose-escalation and reduction of risk in pancreatic cancer using IMRT optimization with lexicographic ordering and gEUD-based cost functions. Med Phys 2007;34(2):521–9.

39. Badiyan SN, Olsen JR, Lee AY, et al. Induction chemotherapy followed by concurrent full-dose gemcitabine and intensity-modulated radiation therapy for borderline resectable and locally advanced pancreatic adenocarcinoma. Am J Clin Oncol 2016;39(1):1–7.

40. Crane CH. Hypofractionated ablative radiotherapy for locally advanced pancreatic cancer. J Radiat Res 2016;57(Suppl 1):i53–7.

41. Krishnan S, Chadha AS, Suh Y, et al. Focal radiation therapy dose escalation improves overall survival in locally advanced pancreatic cancer patients receiving induction chemotherapy and consolidative chemoradiation. Int J Radiat Oncol Biol Phys 2016;94(4):755–65.

42. Solberg TD, Balter JM, Benedict SH, et al. Quality and safety considerations in stereotactic radiosurgery and stereotactic body radiation therapy: executive summary. Pract Radiat Oncol 2012;2(1):2–9.

43. Schellenberg D, Kim J, Christman-Skieller C, et al. Single-fraction stereotactic body radiation therapy and sequential gemcitabine for the treatment of locally advanced pancreatic cancer. Int J Radiat Oncol Biol Phys 2011;81(1):181–8.

44. Koong AC, Christofferson E, Le QT, et al. Phase II study to assess the efficacy of conventionally fractionated radiotherapy followed by a stereotactic radiosurgery boost in patients with locally advanced pancreatic cancer. Int J Radiat Oncol Biol Phys 2005;63(2):320–3.

45. Comito T, Cozzi L, Clerici E, et al. Can stereotactic body radiation therapy be a viable and efficient therapeutic option for unresectable locally advanced pancreatic adenocarcinoma? Results of a phase 2 study. Technol Cancer Res Treat 2017;16(3):295–301.

46. Rashid OM, Pimiento JM, Gamenthaler AW, et al. Outcomes of a clinical pathway for borderline tesectable pancreatic cancer. Ann Surg Oncol 2016;23(4):1371–9.

47. Wild AT, Herman JM, Dholakia AS, et al. Lymphocyte-sparing effect of stereotactic body radiation therapy in patients with unresectable pancreatic cancer. Int J Radiat Oncol Biol Phys 2016;94(3):571–9.

48. Wild AT, Ye X, Ellsworth SG, et al. The association between chemoradiation-related lymphopenia and clinical outcomes in patients with locally advanced pancreatic adenocarcinoma. Am J Clin Oncol 2015;38(3):259–65.

49. Bernstein MB, Krishnan S, Hodge JW, et al. Immunotherapy and stereotactic ablative radiotherapy (ISABR): a curative approach? Nat Rev Clin Oncol 2016; 13(8):516–24.

50. Kang J, Demaria S, Formenti S. Current clinical trials testing the combination of immunotherapy with radiotherapy. J Immunother Cancer 2016;4:51.

51. Schellenberg D, Goodman KA, Lee F, et al. Gemcitabine chemotherapy and single-fraction stereotactic body radiotherapy for locally advanced pancreatic cancer. Int J Radiat Oncol Biol Phys 2008;72(3):678–86.

52. Moertel CG, Frytak S, Hahn RG, et al. Therapy of locally unresectable pancreatic carcinoma: a randomized comparison of high dose (6000 rads) radiation alone, moderate dose radiation (4000 rads + 5-fluorouracil), and high dose radiation + 5-fluorouracil: the Gastrointestinal Tumor Study Group. Cancer 1981;48(8): 1705–10.

53. Chung SY, Chang JS, Lee BM, et al. Dose escalation in locally advanced pancreatic cancer patients receiving chemoradiotherapy. Radiother Oncol 2017;123(3): 438–45.

54. Krempien R, Roeder F. Intraoperative radiation therapy (IORT) in pancreatic cancer. Radiat Oncol 2017;12(1):8.

55. Gillen S, Schuster T, Meyer Zum Buschenfelde C, et al. Preoperative/neoadjuvant therapy in pancreatic cancer: a systematic review and meta-analysis of response and resection percentages. PLoS Med 2010;7(4):e1000267.

56. Andriulli A, Festa V, Botteri E, et al. Neoadjuvant/preoperative gemcitabine for patients with localized pancreatic cancer: a meta-analysis of prospective studies. Ann Surg Oncol 2012;19(5):1644–62.

57. Evans DB, Varadhachary GR, Crane CH, et al. Preoperative gemcitabine-based chemoradiation for patients with resectable adenocarcinoma of the pancreatic head. J Clin Oncol 2008;26(21):3496–502.
58. Takahashi H, Ohigashi H, Gotoh K, et al. Preoperative gemcitabine-based chemoradiation therapy for resectable and borderline resectable pancreatic cancer. Ann Surg 2013;258(6):1040–50.
59. Talamonti MS, Small W Jr, Mulcahy MF, et al. A multi-institutional phase II trial of preoperative full-dose gemcitabine and concurrent radiation for patients with potentially resectable pancreatic carcinoma. Ann Surg Oncol 2006;13(2):150–8.
60. Ferrone CR, Marchegiani G, Hong TS, et al. Radiological and surgical implications of neoadjuvant treatment with FOLFIRINOX for locally advanced and borderline resectable pancreatic cancer. Ann Surg 2015;261(1):12–7.
61. Mellon EA, Strom TJ, Hoffe SE, et al. Favorable perioperative outcomes after resection of borderline resectable pancreatic cancer treated with neoadjuvant stereotactic radiation and chemotherapy compared with upfront pancreatectomy for resectable cancer. J Gastrointest Oncol 2016;7(4):547–55.
62. Artinyan A, Anaya DA, McKenzie S, et al. Neoadjuvant therapy is associated with improved survival in resectable pancreatic adenocarcinoma. Cancer 2011; 117(10):2044–9.
63. Le Scodan R, Mornex F, Girard N, et al. Preoperative chemoradiation in potentially resectable pancreatic adenocarcinoma: feasibility, treatment effect evaluation and prognostic factors, analysis of the SFRO-FFCD 9704 trial and literature review. Ann Oncol 2009;20(8):1387–96.
64. Katz MH, Fleming JB, Bhosale P, et al. Response of borderline resectable pancreatic cancer to neoadjuvant therapy is not reflected by radiographic indicators. Cancer 2012;118(23):5749–56.
65. Sasson AR, Wetherington RW, Hoffman JP, et al. Neoadjuvant chemoradiotherapy for adenocarcinoma of the pancreas: analysis of histopathology and outcome. Int J Gastrointest Cancer 2003;34(2–3):121–8.

Nonoperative Ablation of Pancreatic Neoplasms

Cristina Marrocchio, MD*,1, Susan Dababou, MD1, Carlo Catalano, MD,
Alessandro Napoli, MD, PhD

KEYWORDS

- Pancreatic cancer • Minimally invasive therapies • High-intensity focused ultrasound
- Radiofrequency ablation • Cryotherapy • Irreversible electroporation
- Microwave ablation

KEY POINTS

- The prognosis of pancreatic cancer remains dismal. Although surgical resection is the only curative treatment, almost 80% of patients are diagnosed in advanced unresectable stages.
- The noninvasiveness, high-safety, and multimodal approach suggest high-intensity focused ultrasound as a possible treatment in management of unresectable advanced pancreatic cancer, with promising results in terms of pain palliation and tumor control.
- Radiofrequency ablation, microwave ablation, irreversible electroporation, and cryoablation have been used for the management of unresectable locally advanced pancreatic cancer. There is some experience with their intraoperative use; however, in the future, an important role may be fulfilled by percutaneous approaches to reduce risks and morbidity.
- Minimally invasive therapies are promising for unresectable pancreatic cancers to achieve symptoms palliation and local tumor control.

The prognosis of pancreatic cancer remains dismal.[1] Although surgical resection is thought by many to be the only curative treatment, due to the aggressive nature of the cancer and the nonspecificity of symptoms, almost 80% of patients are diagnosed in advanced unresectable stages.[2]

For this reason, in the past few years, a strong effort has been made to investigate the application of minimally invasive ablative techniques for unresectable, locally advanced pancreatic cancer. These procedures, associated with lower morbidity and mortality, have demonstrated positive results on local tumor control and palliation

Disclosure Statement: The authors have nothing to disclose.
Department of Radiological Sciences, Sapienza University of Rome, V.le Regina Elena 324, Rome 00180, Italy
1 These authors contributed equally to this work.
* Corresponding author.
E-mail address: cristinamarrocchio@gmail.com

of symptoms. The main limitations and challenges of the treatments are the organ location and the risk to develop pancreatitis or to damage the contiguous neurovascular structures. Studies have described the use of high-intensity focused ultrasound (HIFU), radiofrequency ablation (RFA), microwave ablation (MWA), cryotherapy, and irreversible electroporation (IRE). Some experience has accumulated with the intraoperative use of these techniques; however, in the future, an important step may be fulfilled by percutaneous approaches to reduce morbidity and mortality. Although the clinical applications of minimally invasive therapies for pancreatic cancers are still in their infancy, the results are promising.

HIGH-INTENSITY FOCUSED ULTRASOUND

HIFU is a new totally noninvasive technique approved by the US Food and Drug Administration for the treatment of painful bone metastases, uterine fibroids, and essential tremor. Recently, new applications in oncology, including the management of unresectable pancreatic cancer, are undergoing study and are showing promising results.[3] HIFU, either ultrasound (US)-guided focused US (FUS) (USgFUS) or MRI-guided FUS (MRgFUS), generates and focuses a beam of high-energy US to a precisely defined region of few millimeters, called the sonication spot. In few seconds the energy accumulates, inducing a steep increase in temperature that causes coagulative necrosis in the targeted tissue. HIFU has considerable advantages over other minimally invasive techniques in that it is totally noninvasive, does not use ionizing radiations, and, if MRI-guided, monitors in real-time the temperature reached in the tissue, ensuring a safe and effective ablation.

PREOPERATIVE PLANNING AND PATIENT PREPARATION

Although some variation may be present among the studies, some steps are universally performed before treatment. The patient should be fasting and procedures to displace the bowel from the US beam, such as drinking degassed water or intestinal cleaning, may be used to decrease the chance of adverse events. The patient is positioned prone on the treatment bed with the region to be treated cleaned, examined to exclude the presence of scars, and aligned with the US transducer. A coupling gel or immersion of the area to be treated in degassed water increases the contact with the transducer eliminating any interposed air. The main precaution to reduce any risk of adverse outcomes is to ensure the patient has neither air nor scars interposed in the beam trajectory because they may reflect or absorb heat, causing collateral damage and decreasing the effective dose delivered. MRgFUS and USgFUS require general anesthesia, whereas in pulsed USgFUS local anesthesia is sufficient and sometimes no anesthesia is necessary. Vital signs are monitored during the procedure. If the patient is conscious, a stop button is provided to interrupt the treatment in case of unpleasant sensations.

TREATMENT
Planning

Before the treatment starts, the patient position is checked and the acoustic window is optimized using the diagnostic probe incorporated in the transducer in USgFUS or acquiring T1-weighted and T2-weighted MRI sequences, with and without fat saturation, at the inspiration phase in MRgFUS.

The treatment plan is assessed in 4 phases:

1. Calibration: The orientation and position of the transducer in relation to the target lesion is assessed.

2. Segmentation: On acquired 2-dimensional cross-slice images, the operator manually outlines the region of treatment to be ablated, the skin border, and the limited energy density regions that may be damaged by the US beam (nerves, bowel, and bones). Anatomic fiducials are placed to detect any movement of the patient.
3. Planning: The software automatically calculates the optimal ablation coverage of the region of treatment, planning the number and position of sonications, and ensures a safe margin between the beam and neighboring viscera. Manual adjustments of the US beam orientation and the number and location of the sonications ensure a safe complete ablation of the target.
4. Verification: A series of sonications below the ablative threshold are performed to confirm the correct targeting.

Procedure

After the planning, treatment is started by increasing the power and energy of the sonications to reach ablative temperatures between 60°C and 80°C. For pancreatic cancer, the authors use a threshold of 65°C to define successful ablation. The treatment includes a specific number of sonications separated by a cooling time to allow heat dissipation and avoid damage in the near-fields or far-fields. For each sonication, the operator can change sonication parameters: duration, location, size of the spot, power, energy, angulation of the US beam, and cooling time (**Fig. 1**). USgFUS relies on the detection of a hyperechogenic change in the targeted region to assess the ablation status. MRgFUS provides more accurate monitoring using MRI thermometry sequences that detect temperature changes based on heat-induced changes in the hydrogen bonds of water contained within the tissue. It displays a thermal map where

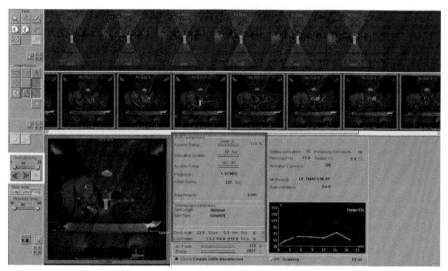

Fig. 1. MRgFUS (ExAblate 2100 type 1.1, InSightec, Haifa, Israel) coupled with a 3T-MRI system (General Electric Health Care, Milwaukee, WI, USA) treatment of pancreatic cancer. This treatment screen illustrates the intraprocedural MRI and parameters of sonication number 15 (*yellow outline*). On the right, a panel (*red outline*) displays the sonication parameters with the possibility of manual adjustments of the settings by the operator. The actually delivered energy and power are reported below (*orange outline*). The temperature reached in the spot can be monitored on the temperature curves at the bottom right. Note in the top row the MRI thermometry sequences.

regions that achieved a sufficient temperature for ablation are colored and easily visualized. The temperature in the surrounding tissues is also monitored (**Fig. 2**). At the end of the MRgFUS procedure, hypointense regions on gadolinium-enhanced T1-weighted images are considered ablated.

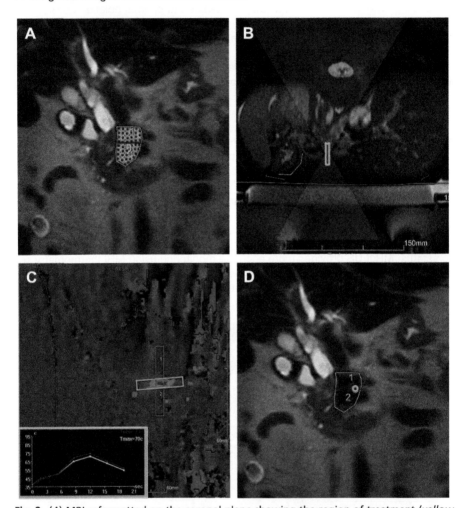

Fig. 2. (*A*) MRI reformatted on the coronal plane showing the region of treatment (*yellow line*) delineated during the segmentation phase of the procedure. The green circles are the sonication spots computed by the software; the operator is free to change and adjust them based on tumor features. (*B*) MRI reformatted on the axial plane displaying the sonication spot (*blue rectangular box*) with the acoustic window highlighted as a blue cone. It is important to exclude air and scar tissue from the acoustic window because they can interact with the US beam, causing adverse events. (*C*) MRI thermometry sequence that allows visualization in real-time of the deposition of energy and the increase in tissue temperature during the treatment. The sonicated area is indicated by the blue rectangular box; inside, the region that reached the ablative temperature threshold is colored. A cursor allows monitoring of the temperature in the surrounding tissue. The temperature graph below provides quantitative information of tissue heating. (*D*) MRI reformatted on the coronal plane shows the ablated area (*blue*) inside the region of treatment (*yellow*) and the next sonication spot (*light blue circle*) that is going to be targeted.

Postanesthesia, the vital signs and pancreatic function are monitored, and the skin is monitored for burns. Analgesics or antiemetics are administered as needed. We hospitalize all patients for 24 hours and all receive intravenous steroids (40 mg methylprednisolone) to avoid vascular compression from edema of the lesion or surrounding tissue.

REVIEW OF THE LITERATURE

The 2 main imaging guidance methods for HIFU are US or MRI. For pancreatic cancer most use USgFUS, whereas MRI guidance has been used only in the authors' center. USgFUS is less expensive, more accessible and allows easier control of respiratory displacement of the target and easy visualization of interfering interphase in the US beam.[4] Two different devices have been used. The first involves the application of continuous high-intensity US, which requires general anesthesia and hospitalization, but potentially treats the entire lesion in a single session. The second uses pulsed lower energy sonications, which permits treatment with conscious sedation or, at times, without anesthesia and hospitalization but requires multiple sessions per patient.[5] Both result in reasonably successful treatments.[6] The largest clinical trials published are from China and are not available in English language. In Western countries, the application of HIFU to pancreatic cancer is quite recent and the publications are mostly retrospective. Prospective randomized clinical trials are expected in the future.

In the literature, the inclusion criteria vary. The most selective treat only body and tail lesions of the pancreas and exclude pancreatic head lesions to avoid posttreatment edema. Most patients had stage III or IV pancreatic adenocarcinoma.

Partial tumor responses range from 14% to 100%.[6] Debate exists on assessing effective ablation in USgFUS because the hyperechogenic change of lesions may differ with the postablation computed tomography (CT) scan. CT or contrast-enhanced MRI are preferred postablation. Recently, PET-CT is being evaluated to determine the metabolic tumor changes.[6]

Importantly, some investigators have reported downstaging of unresectable lesions to resectable ones after HIFU therapy.[7,8] HIFU has been used to treat liver and other metastases, to gain better tumor control.[9,10] HIFU treatment of the liver can be challenging but was successful in all reported cases.

A greater tumor response and longer survival has been obtained when HIFU is combined with concurrent chemotherapy or radiotherapy.[11] Because the overall survival has not been rigorously addressed and randomized controlled studies are lacking, it is not possible to compare survival with HIFU and other therapies. Vidal-Jove and colleagues[12] evaluated retrospectively 48 pancreatic cancers after HIFU with chemotherapy. The overall median survival was 16 months, with 14 patients alive at the time of the report. The study identified patients with stage III cancers and minimal vascular invasion who were not candidates for surgical resection as a subpopulation that could benefit from HIFU for a long-term disease-free survival. In a retrospective analysis on 689 patients with unresectable pancreatic cancer, 436 were treated with HIFU alone or HIFU combined with other therapies. A stratified analysis found a survival benefit after HIFU combined with other therapies compared with only HIFU, and for repeated HIFU for tumor recurrence compared with single HIFU. The major survival advantage was found in stage IV pancreatic cancers.[13]

HIFU has a high safety profile. No deaths were reported in the published reports. Mild complications occurred, mostly skin burns of first and second degree, skin redness, edema and pain in the treated region, induration of subcutaneous tissue, transient edema, and low-grade fever.[14] A pancreatic pseudocyst has been observed.[7,15] These events can be minimized by adopting the necessary precautions in the treatment preparation. Jaundice has also been reported secondary to HIFU ablation.[16] The transient amylase and lipase increase detected in some patients is usually asymptomatic and clinical pancreatitis is rarely encountered.[16] This may be explained by the mechanism of cell death induced by HIFU: when the cell's temperature reaches the ablative threshold, there is a degradation of pancreatic enzymes followed by cell death (thermal fixation).[17] The feared complication is bowel perforation due to the interposition of intestinal loops along the US beam. The literature reports a few cases of pancreaticoduodenal fistula.[9] One case of portal vein thrombosis requiring hospitalization occurred. The pancreatic cancer was compressing the vessel and the edema after the procedure may have increased the impingement.[18]

Other Pancreatic Lesions

Although most of the studies use HIFU for pancreatic adenocarcinoma, there are case reports of HIFU and other pancreatic lesions.

Currently, there is no standard management for patients with unresectable pancreatic neuroendocrine tumors.[19] In these cases, HIFU may palliate symptoms and ameliorate survival and quality of life. In a case report by Chen and colleagues,[19] an 80-year-old patient diagnosed with a very large lesion (10.1–9.4 cm) on CT scan was experiencing significant clinical symptoms. Because other treatment modalities were not feasible because of comorbidities or refusal, HIFU was used to palliate the pain and achieve local tumor control. After 3 cycles of pulsed FUS, pain decreased from a baseline numeric rating scale (NRS) of 8 out of 10 to a posttreatment NRS of 1 out of 10. The patient was still alive at article writing, with stable disease according to World Health Organization Criteria for Response.

Orgera and colleagues[20] described the palliative treatment of 3 patients with unresectable insulinomas with lung and liver metastases. These patients were suffering severe episodes of nocturnal hypoglycemia, uncontrolled by medical therapy. After undergoing a combined regiment of HIFU, chemotherapy, and radiotherapy, the tumors were successfully ablated with no occurrence of side effects and resolution of the episodes of nocturnal hypoglycemia.

Orsi and colleagues[18] described HIFU combined with radiotherapy and chemotherapy for 1 unresectable neuroendocrine pancreatic tumor. A complete response was observed on posttreatment images with no side effects. The same group treated a metastatic anaplastic pancreatic carcinoma infiltrating the splenic artery and superior mesenteric vein. After 5 cycles of systemic chemotherapy, the patient underwent HIFU and other 5 more cycles of chemotherapy. After HIFU, a large necrosis was present in the center of the tumor with a reduction in the mass and paraaortic lymph nodes size. Dyspepsia and dorsal pain were resolved.[21]

Orgera and colleagues[22] described the treatment of a pancreatic metastatic lesion from a renal cell carcinoma. After resection of the primary renal cell carcinoma, staged as T3bN0M0 according to the TNM classification of Malignant Tumours, a nodule was detected in the pancreatic head by CT scan at a 3-month follow-up. The patient was not considered a suitable candidate for surgery due to the short disease-free interval. During follow-up, further progression was seen and the patient underwent HIFU. After the treatment, there was a complete lack of enhancement without any injury to the surrounding organs. At 9-month follow-up after HIFU, the decreased size of the mass and lack of enhancement were confirmed, without evidences of recurrence.

These preliminary reports support the efficacy of HIFU in the treatment of numerous types of pancreatic lesions. Further clinical trials are needed to evaluate the efficacy, safety, and long-term results.

THE AUTHORS EXPERIENCE WITH MRI-GUIDED FOCUSED US

At the authors' center, the HIFU clinic was established in 2010 with the acquisition of a MRgFUS machine (ExAblate, Insightec, Haifa, Israel) mounted on a 3T-MRI guiding device. The first applications were limited to uterine fibroids and bone metastases, but expansion of the program included pancreas, liver, prostate, breast, and osteoid osteoma.[3,23–28]

The authors' interest in the HIFU therapy arose from its noninvasive features, safety, and low morbidity, with multiple applications to palliate patients with cancer. The high degree of safety and precise targeting are particularly useful for pancreatic cancer, a lesion surrounding or involving major vessels and contiguous organs. HIFU is unique among minimally invasive procedures because it avoids insertion of needles or probes, and allows uniform heating. An additional benefit in recurrent tumors is that it can easily be repeated because ionizing radiations are not used and there is no concern with chemotherapy use.

The effect of HIFU on the disease includes a thermally induced ablation of the tumor mass, plus additional therapeutic benefits to improve quality of life. Pancreatic cancer-associated pain can be debilitating and difficult to control. As many as 81% of patients experience pain relief after HIFU, with sustained response reported even 17 months after therapy.[29] Other cancer-related symptoms also improve, such as fatigue and loss of appetite, with an improvement in the Karnofsky Performance Scale.[30]

HIFU, similar to other minimally invasive techniques, such as cryoablation and RFA, seems to increase the tumor-specific immunity, which contributes to the control of micrometastases and helps maintain a disease-free survival.[31] The level of CD4+ and the CD4+ to CD8+ ratio increases after HIFU. The probable underlying mechanism is the localized inflammation and lysis of tumor cells that leads to the exposure of previously sequestered cancer antigens. Immune components, such as dendritic cells and macrophages, also increase.[32]

A third effect of HIFU therapy is potentiation of concomitant treatments. HIFU increases the radiosensitivity of cancer cells, and increases the sensitivity and permeability of the tumor to chemotherapy.[11] The relative lack of perfusion and the anatomic composition of pancreatic cancer generally limits the entry of chemotherapy particles. HIFU favors the entrance of drugs by a transient increase in permeability of blood vessels and cellular membranes (sonoporation), a result of the mechanical effect of US energy on the tissue.[33,34]

MRI guidance favors a better contrast resolution, with detailed morphologic depiction of the complicated neurovascular anatomy, and a monitoring of the temperature reached within the lesion.[4]

For all these reasons, we began to treat patients with unresectable pancreatic cancer with MRgFUS. A preliminary study on 2 patients with unresectable adenocarcinoma of the pancreatic neck showed that 80% and 85% of the tumor volumes were nonperfused, indicating successful ablation. Pain palliation was achieved with reduction in the visual analog scale (VAS) score from a mean of 7 out of 10 to 3 out of 10. No complications occurred.[27] We confirmed these results in 6 patients with unresectable pancreatic adenocarcinoma in the body or neck.[35] Although successful USgFUS treatments for lesions in the head of the pancreas have been reported without complications, some fear an increased risk of posttreatment duodenal or vascular obstruction, and we have excluded these lesions.

The main difficulty in treating abdominal organs with HIFU is targeting the lesion while taking into account the organs' displacement secondary to respiratory or peristaltic movements. Although promising automatic respiratory gating devices are being developed, they are not available for clinical practice.[36] This limit is even more relevant in MRgFUS because it relies on scanner images acquired before or during treatment, without the continuous US probe assessment of the organs possible in USgFUS. In our experience, all patients were treated under general anesthesia with controlled respiration and images were acquired at the inspiration phase with a fixed amount of inhaled airflow and duration of apnea, to confirm an identical organ shift and lesion positioning. A recovery period of 2 minutes between apneas was established for blood oxygen saturation.

Our preliminary results are encouraging. All 6 patients who underwent MRgFUS experienced pain palliation with a mean VAS score decrease from 7 out of 10 to 3 out of 10 in the week after treatment. Pain medications were stopped after 2 days, except 1 patient who continued paracetamol as needed for 1 month and 2 patients who continued paracetamol as needed for the entire follow-up. The results were long-lasting with continued palliation at 6 months. All patients had a technically successful treatment, with a mean devascularization of 80% (SD of 5%) of the tumor volume without regrowth in 5 patients at 6-month follow-up. One patient had a cluster of solid enhancing tissues at the periphery of the ablated area at 6 months, but it was negligible and did not extend beyond the outer borders of the originally ablated lesion. Except for 1 patient who had a significant shrinkage of the mass, the volume of the tumor remained essentially stable over time. This is a common finding after HIFU, with the volume of the mass sometimes increasing because of edema. Indeed, the reduction of mass size is not considered reliable in evaluating treatment success. All treatments were successful, even in case of vascular encasement by the tumor (**Fig. 3**). We addressed the areas close to large vessels with a mildly increased amount of energy to avoid any heat dissipation from the circulating blood. The noninvasiveness and accurate planning ensured safety without bowel perforation or skin burns in our patients.

MINIMALLY INVASIVE ABLATIVE THERAPIES

The image-guided minimally invasive procedures can be roughly divided into 2 groups: thermal ablative techniques (RFA, MWA, cryoablation) and nonthermal ablative techniques (IRE).[14] The main challenges with these therapeutic approaches are the anatomic and histologic features of the pancreas that entail a significant risk to the close sensitive structures with thermal energy and to pancreatitis. Improvements in imaging and energy monitoring would improve the efficacy and safety of the procedures.

Radiofrequency Ablation

RFA uses high-frequency alternating current, conveyed by 1 or more needle electrodes inserted in the neoplastic tissue. The local increase in temperature leads to coagulative necrosis and protein denaturation inside the neoplastic tissue.[31] The treatment is performed under US or CT guidance and the ablation is achieved by increasing the local tissue temperature for a short time interval. Several studies suggest reaching 90°C to ensure ablation without complications.[37] The tissue echogenicity change is the main parameter for the assessment of the efficacy; the tissue impedance can also be used because it increases when necrosis occurs. The temperature reached within the tissue can be directly detected by the electrode tip, which can be multiple or single, depending on the needle used.[37]

The dimension of the mass does not represent an absolute limit for this technique because it is applicable for tumor masses of 5 cm or more.[31] RFA can be performed at laparotomy, percutaneously, or during laparoscopy. The approach most commonly

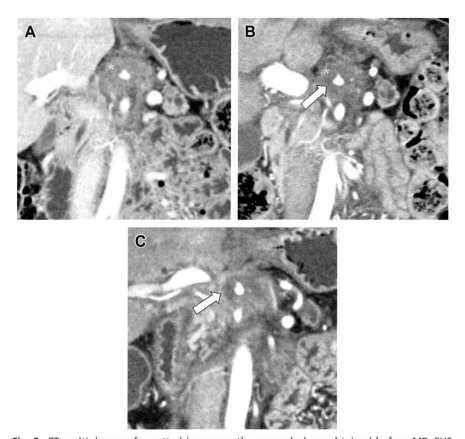

Fig. 3. CT multiplanar reformatted image on the coronal plane obtained before MRgFUS treatment (*A*), immediately posttreatment (*B*), and at 1-year follow-up (*C*). (*A*) The tumor (*yellow asterisk*) with encasement of both the celiac axis and the superior mesenteric artery. Immediately posttreatment (*B*) there is devascularization and necrosis (*arrow*) of the ablated area associated with clinical reduction in pain. At 1-year follow-up (*C*), the tumor still presents devascularized area with no symptoms recurrence.

described is to use RFA via laparotomy with US-guidance. Nevertheless, its use in locally advanced pancreatic cancer has been questioned for the invasiveness of the procedure and an often incomplete ablation. The ring of neoplastic tissue that is not ablated to ensure safety of close structures is often targeted with chemotherapy or radiotherapy because the tissue becomes more vulnerable and sensitive after RFA.[31]

A few studies have described percutaneous RFA and most are case reports of various pancreatic tumors (functional and nonfunctional neuroendocrine tumors, metastases, and ductal adenocarcinomas).[14] D'Onofrio and colleagues[38] treated 18 patients who had locally advanced adenocarcinoma in the pancreatic body and tail with vascular encasement unsuitable for surgery after chemotherapy. The verification of the needle path and its insertion into the center of the mass was carefully monitored through US and the efficacy assessed with hyperechoic changes in the ablated tissue. Technical success, defined as the ablation of 50% or more of the targeted mass, was obtained in 93% of the patients without complications.

The capacity of RFA to successfully ablate a pancreatic tumor, in addition to the difficult location, is limited by the increased impedance linked to the necrotic tissue change, which self-limits the ablation.[37,39] Moreover, although new needle technology is improving heat deposition, this is still heterogeneous due to the intrinsic tissue features and it cannot currently be monitored in real-time during the procedure. Safety is nevertheless ensured because the heat conduction occurs mainly inside the neoplastic mass due to the specific tissue conductibility (thermal diffusivity effect).[37]

The main adverse events reported with percutaneous RFA are abdominal pain, the self-limiting form of pancreatitis, minimal peripancreatic inflammatory reaction with little fluid collection, and slight and transient increase in serum amylase and lipase.[14]

Microwave Ablation

MWA uses microwave radiations to locally increase the temperature by agitating the water molecules contained in the tissue, causing cellular death via coagulation necrosis. The procedure can be done openly, endoscopically, or percutaneously. US or CT image guidance is used to verify the correct and safe position of the probe (antenna).[37]

Even if further studies are needed to assess its efficacy, this technique has some advantages compared with RFA. It can treat larger areas and reach local higher temperatures, measured with a thermocouple probe. The effect of microwaves does not depend on tissue type, is not limited by tissue impedance, and pancreatic regions close to vascular structures can be treated with no heat-sink effect experienced.[40] The procedure is faster and more than 1 applicator can be used, avoiding multiple procedures. The pain experienced is less than with RFA and generally occurs after percutaneous and endoscopic MWA, during which the patient is under conscious sedation.[14,41] On the other hand, the ablation area is very sensitive to the type of antenna, its position and frequency. A study reporting percutaneous MWA for the treatment of 5 subjects with pancreatic ductal adenocarcinoma concluded that this procedure may increase the patients' quality of life and seems to be a feasible palliative treatment of pancreatic head tumors.[42]

Cryoablation

Cryoablation is a thermal technique that uses low temperature to induce tumor ablation. The cold local environment causes tissue necrosis and apoptosis through both intracellular and extracellular ice formation. The technique consists in the insertion of a cryoprobe into the tumor, with multiple probes often necessary for the ablation of lesions larger than 3 cm.[37] It can be performed percutaneously or surgically, under CT or US guidance. Cryoablation is based on a freezing-thawing cycle, usually repeated twice, although more cycles are necessary for larger lesions. First, the temperature decreases to $-160°C$ with the formation of an ice ball, which is predictive of the ablated area and can be easily visualized with US.[43] Then, the temperature slowly thaws to zero and another cycle is repeated. As for RFA, the maintenance of a safety margin to close sensitive structures is advised, with 5 mm distance ensuring safe ablation.[37]

Results with percutaneous cryoablation for pancreatic cancer and neuroendocrine pancreatic tumor are promising in terms of pain palliation, increased overall survival, and improved performance status.[44] The largest retrospective study of 67 subjects observed an increase in the overall survival of metastatic pancreatic cancer following US-guided and CT-guided percutaneous or open cryoablation.[45] The median overall survival of the cryotherapy group was 7 months compared with 3,5 months in the chemotherapy group. Multiple sessions of cryoablation associated with immunotherapy are linked to better results, with a median overall survival of 13 months. Combinations of cryotherapy and iodine seed implantation has also been studied in 38 subjects by Xu and colleagues.[46] Of the subjects, 23.6% had a total response,

42.1% had partial response, 26.3% had stable disease, and 7.9% experienced disease progression with a median overall survival of 12 months.

Cryotherapy is a feasible and potentially safe therapeutic option for locally advanced and unresectable pancreatic cancer even in the presence of metastases.[47] Also, neuroendocrine tumors in multiple endocrine neoplasia type 1 have been treated achieving good symptoms control.[44]

The rate of complications following cryoablation is not high, with the main adverse events being mild abdominal pain and delayed gastric emptying. Major adverse events reported include bleeding, pancreatic and biliary leak, acute pancreatitis, and cryoprobe needle metastasis.[37,42,48] Also, cryoshock may occur following the rapid release of cellular debris in the systemic circulation after the reperfusion of the ablated area. This phenomenon is rare with heat-based ablation.[37]

Irreversible Electroporation

IRE is a nonthermal technique delivering short high-voltage electric current pulses that trigger apoptotic pathways through disruption of the cellular homeostasis with induction of irreversible permeabilization of lipid membranes. The innovation of this ablative technique is the preservation of the supporting connective extracellular structures, which allows a fast recovery; and of the close surrounding structures, such as vital tissues, nerves, and vessels, which allows the treatment of tumors encasing major peripancreatic vessels.[31]

Electrodes, from 2 to 6 needles, are introduced into the pancreatic tumor mass through a percutaneous or surgical approach.[49] US or CT can be used for image guidance and the treatment protocol is computed based on tissue conductivity and needle position. As a general rule, it is preferred to treat lesion sizes of 3 to 3.5 cm.[31] The patient is under general anesthesia with complete muscular paralysis and the electric pulses are electrocardiogram-synchronized to avoid triggering arrhythmias. Indeed, the electric fields applied can cause cardiac muscle contraction.[37] Therefore, IRE is not indicated for patients with history of cardiac arrhythmia, congestive heart failure, or symptomatic coronary artery disease. Biliary metallic stents must be removed for concern of thermal injuries.[31] These limitations of IRE may decrease the number of patients who could benefit from the treatment. Immediately after the procedure, treatment efficacy is assessed with hyperechogenic changes and is confirmed after an hour as a hypodense lesion on CT.[49]

A recent prospective study investigated the safety of percutaneous IRE and evaluated the quality of life, pain perception, and efficacy in terms of local tumor progression and survival. The median size of the tumors treated was 4 cm. The pain control was moderate, with recurrence of a pain difficult to control with analgesics 6 months after the procedure. The patients experienced a decrease in general functioning at 3-month and 6-month follow-up on quality of life scores. The median overall survival after IRE was 11 months.[50] Minor adverse events reported were nausea, vomiting, diarrhea, delayed gastric emptying, abdominal pain, and loss of appetite. Edematous pancreatitis, massive hematemesis caused by duodenal wall ulcer, and new onset biliary obstruction were observed among the major adverse events.[50]

IRE is a relatively new technique that is still performed only in few centers and more studies are needed to assess its efficacy. The main factors limiting its wider application are the need of general anesthesia with muscular block and the exclusion of patients with cardiac problems and/or biliary stents. For now, IRE is limited to stage III and IV pancreatic cancer with centimetric liver metastases, and is often offered as a bridge therapy before radical surgical resection.[49]

SUMMARY

Minimally invasive techniques are promising for local tumor control and palliation of symptoms from unresectable pancreatic cancer to improve the quality of life and to reduce the tumor burden. Further studies are needed to standardize the clinical indications and the technical parameters to maximize the results minimizing morbidity and mortality. Considering all the advantages of HIFU and the future expected technological improvements, this technique has the potential to have a dominant role in the management of unresectable locally advanced pancreatic cancer.

REFERENCES

1. Siegel R, Naishadham D, Jemal A. Cancer statistics, 2013. CA Cancer J Clin 2013;63(1):11–30.
2. Zuckerman DS, Ryan DP. Adjuvant therapy for pancreatic cancer. Cancer 2008; 112(2):243–9.
3. Napoli A, Anzidei M, Ciolina F, et al. MR-guided high-intensity focused ultrasound: current status of an emerging technology. Cardiovasc Intervent Radiol 2013;36(5):1190–203.
4. Wu F. Extracorporeal high intensity focused ultrasound in the treatment of patients with solid malignancy. Minim Invasive Ther Allied Technol 2006;15(1):26–35.
5. Wu F. High intensity focused ultrasound: a noninvasive therapy for locally advanced pancreatic cancer. World J Gastroenterol 2014;20(44):16480.
6. Khokhlova TD, Hwang JH. HIFU for Palliative Treatment of Pancreatic Cancer. In: Escoffre JM, Bouakaz A, editors. Therapeutic Ultrasound. Advances in Experimental Medicine and Biology, vol 880. Springer: Cham (Switzerland); 2016.
7. Sofuni A, Moriyasu F, Sano T, et al. Safety trial of high-intensity focused ultrasound therapy for pancreatic cancer. World J Gastroenterol 2014;20(28):9570.
8. Zhao H, Yang G, Wang D, et al. Concurrent gemcitabine and high-intensity focused ultrasound therapy in patients with locally advanced pancreatic cancer. Anticancer Drugs 2010;21(4):447–52.
9. Sung HY, Jung SE, Cho SH, et al. Long-term outcome of high-intensity focused ultrasound in advanced pancreatic cancer. Pancreas 2011;40(7):1080–6.
10. Wu F, Wang ZB, Zhu H, et al. Feasibility of US-guided high-intensity focused ultrasound treatment in patients with advanced pancreatic cancer: initial experience. Radiology 2005;236(3):1034–40.
11. Li CC, Wang YQ, Li YP, et al. High-intensity focused ultrasound for treatment of pancreatic cancer: a systematic review. J Evid Based Med 2014;7(4):270–81.
12. Vidal-Jove J, Perich E, del Castillo MA. Ultrasound guided high intensity focused ultrasound for malignant tumors: the Spanish experience of survival advantage in stage III and IV pancreatic cancer. Ultrason Sonochem 2015;27:703–6.
13. Ning ZY, Cheng CS, Xie J, et al. A retrospective analysis of survival factors of high intensity focused ultrasound (HIFU) treatment for unresectable pancreatic cancer. Discov Med 2016;21(118):435–45.
14. Ierardi AM, Lucchina N, Bacuzzi A, et al. Percutaneous ablation therapies of inoperable pancreatic cancer: a systematic review. Ann Gastroenterol 2015;28(4): 431.
15. Xiong LL, Hwang JH, Huang XB, et al. Early clinical experience using high intensity focused ultrasound for palliation of inoperable pancreatic cancer. JOP 2009; 10(2):123–9.
16. Wang K, Zhu H, Meng Z, et al. Safety evaluation of high-intensity focused ultrasound in patients with pancreatic cancer. Oncol Res Treat 2013;36(3):88–92.

17. Jang HJ, Lee JY, Lee DH, et al. Current and future clinical applications of high-intensity focused ultrasound (HIFU) for pancreatic cancer. Gut Liver 2010; 4(Suppl.1):S57–61.
18. Orsi F, Zhang L, Arnone P, et al. High-intensity focused ultrasound ablation: effective and safe therapy for solid tumors in difficult locations. AJR Am J Roentgenol 2010;195(3):W245–52.
19. Chen Q, Zhu X, Chen Q, et al. Unresectable giant pancreatic neuroendocrine tumor effectively treated by high-intensity focused ultrasound: a case report and review of the literature. Pancreatology 2013;13(6):634–8.
20. Orgera G, Monfardini L, Della Vigna P, et al. High-intensity focused ultrasound (HIFU) in patients with solid malignancies: evaluation of feasibility, local tumour response and clinical results. Radiol Med 2011;116(5):734–48.
21. Ungaro A, Orsi F, Casadio C, et al. Successful palliative approach with high-intensity focused ultrasound in a patient with metastatic anaplastic pancreatic carcinoma: a case report. Ecancermedicalscience 2016;10:635.
22. Orgera G, Krokidis M, Monfardini L, et al. Ultrasound-guided high-intensity focused ultrasound(USgHIFU) ablation in pancreatic metastasis from renal cell carcinoma. Cardiovasc Intervent Radiol 2012;35(5):1258–61.
23. Cavallo Marincola B, Pediconi F, Anzidei M, et al. High-intensity focused ultrasound in breast pathology: non-invasive treatment of benign and malignant lesions. Expert Rev Med Devices 2015;12(2):191–9.
24. Marigliano C, Panzironi G, Molisso L, et al. First experience of real-time elastography with transvaginal approach in assessing response to MRgFUS treatment of uterine fibroids. Radiol Med 2016;121(12):926–34.
25. Napoli A, Anzidei M, De Nunzio C, et al. Real-time magnetic resonance–guided high-intensity focused ultrasound focal therapy for localised prostate cancer: preliminary experience. Eur Urol 2013;63(2):395–8.
26. Napoli A, Anzidei M, Marincola BC, et al. MR imaging–guided focused ultrasound for treatment of bone metastasis. Radiographics 2013;33(6):1555–68.
27. Anzidei M, Napoli A, Sandolo F, et al. Magnetic resonance-guided focused ultrasound ablation in abdominal moving organs: a feasibility study in selected cases of pancreatic and liver cancer. Cardiovasc Intervent Radiol 2014;37(6):1611–7.
28. Napoli A, Mastantuono M, Cavallo Marincola B, et al. Osteoid osteoma: MR-guided focused ultrasound for entirely noninvasive treatment. Radiology 2013; 267(2):514–21.
29. Dababou S, Marrocchio C, Rosenberg J, et al. A meta-analysis of palliative treatment of pancreatic cancer with high intensity focused ultrasound. J Ther Ultrasound 2017;5(1):9.
30. Zhou Y. High-intensity focused ultrasound treatment for advanced pancreatic cancer. Gastroenterol Res Pract 2014;2014:205325.
31. Paiella S, Salvia R, Ramera M, et al. Local ablative strategies for ductal pancreatic cancer (radiofrequency ablation, irreversible electroporation): a review. Gastroenterol Res Pract 2016;2016:4508376.
32. Wu F, Wang ZB, Lu P, et al. Activated anti-tumor immunity in cancer patients after high intensity focused ultrasound ablation. Ultrasound Med Biol 2004;30(9): 1217–22.
33. Yuh EL, Shulman SG, Mehta SA, et al. Delivery of systemic chemotherapeutic agent to tumors by using focused ultrasound: study in a Murine model. Radiology 2005;234(2):431–7.
34. Liang HD, Tang J, Halliwell M. Sonoporation, drug delivery, and gene therapy. Proc Inst Mech Eng H 2010;224(2):343–61.

35. Anzidei M, Marincola BC, Bezzi M, et al. Magnetic resonance–guided high-intensity focused ultrasound treatment of locally advanced pancreatic adenocarcinoma: preliminary experience for pain palliation and local tumor control. Invest Radiol 2014;49(12):759–65.

36. Ries M, De Senneville BD, Roujol S, et al. Real-time 3D target tracking in MRI guided focused ultrasound ablations in moving tissues. Magn Reson Med 2010;64(6):1704–12.

37. D'Onofrio M, Ciaravino V, De Robertis R, et al. Percutaneous ablation of pancreatic cancer. World J Gastroenterol 2016;22(44):9661.

38. D'Onofrio M, Barbi E, Girelli R, et al. Radiofrequency ablation of locally advanced pancreatic adenocarcinoma: an overview. World J Gastroenterol 2010;16(28): 3478–83.

39. Iida H, Aihara T, Ikuta S, et al. Effectiveness of impedance monitoring during radiofrequency ablation for predicting popping. World J Gastroenterol 2012;18(41): 5870–8.

40. Carrafiello G, Laganà D, Mangini M, et al. Microwave tumors ablation: principles, clinical applications and review of preliminary experiences. Int J Surg 2008;6: S65–9.

41. Wright AS, Lee FT, Mahvi DM. Hepatic microwave ablation with multiple antennae results in synergistically larger zones of coagulation necrosis. Ann Surg Oncol 2003;10(3):275–83.

42. Carrafiello G, Ierardi AM, Fontana F, et al. Microwave ablation of pancreatic head cancer: safety and efficacy. J Vasc Interv Radiol 2013;24(10):1513–20.

43. Keane MG, Bramis K, Pereira SP, et al. Systematic review of novel ablative methods in locally advanced pancreatic cancer. World J Gastroenterol 2014; 20(9):2267–78.

44. Li J, Zhang C, Chen J, et al. Two case reports of pilot percutaneous cryosurgery in familial multiple endocrine neoplasia type 1. Pancreas 2013;42(2):353–7.

45. Niu L, Chen J, He L, et al. Combination treatment with comprehensive cryoablation and immunotherapy in metastatic pancreatic cancer. Pancreas 2013;42(7): 1143–9.

46. Xu K-C, Niu L-Z, Hu Y-Z, et al. A pilot study on combination of cryosurgery and ^{125}iodine seed implantation for treatment of locally advanced pancreatic cancer. World J Gastroenterol 2008;14(10):1603–11.

47. Luo XM, Niu LZ, Chen JB, et al. Advances in cryoablation for pancreatic cancer. World J Gastroenterol 2016;22(2):790.

48. Petrou A, Moris D, Tabet PP, et al. Ablation of the locally advanced pancreatic cancer: an introduction and brief summary of techniques. J BUON 2016;21(3): 650–8.

49. Tasu JP, Vesselle G, Herpe G, et al. Irreversible electroporation for locally advanced pancreatic cancer: where do we stand in 2017? Pancreas 2017; 46(3):283–7.

50. Scheffer HJ, Vroomen LG, de Jong MC, et al. Ablation of locally advanced pancreatic cancer with percutaneous irreversible electroporation: results of the phase I/II PANFIRE study. Radiology 2017;282(2):585–97.

Incidental Intraductal Papillary Mucinous Neoplasm, Cystic or Premalignant Lesions of the Pancreas

The Case for Aggressive Management

Alexander T. El Gammal, MD, Jakob R. Izbicki, MD*

KEYWORDS

- Intraductal papillary mucinous neoplasm • Cystic intrapancreatic lesion
- Cystic pancreatic tumor differentiation

KEY POINTS

- Because main-duct and mixed type intraductal papillary mucinous neoplasms are highly associated with malignant transformation, they both should be treated with surgical-oncologic intent.
- Serous cystadenoma (SC) is the only lesion that may appear microcystic; computed tomography often reveals a sponge or honeycomb-like lesion with countless small cysts separated by slender septa.
- SCs are benign cystic tumors that derive from pancreatic centroacinar cells.

INTRODUCTION

Incidental cystic intrapancreatic lesions are daily findings in abdominal radiology. In fact, previously undetected cystic intrapancreatic lesions are found in 1.2% to 2.6% of abdominal multidetector computed tomography (CT) examinations and in 13.5% to 19.9% of abdominal MRI studies.[1–5] Although there have been major efforts to systematically define a standard of care for these lesions,[6–8] there is currently no consensus how these lesions should be managed.[5] Postmortem

The authors have nothing to disclose.
Department of General, Visceral and Thoracic Surgery, University Medical Center Hamburg-Eppendorf, Martinistrasse 5220246, Hamburg, Germany
* Corresponding author.
E-mail address: izbicki@uke.de

autopsies revealed intrapancreatic cystic lesions in up to 25% of autopsies.[9] Therefore, it is not surprising that the discovery of incidental pancreatic lesions is increasingly common with technologic diagnostic advancements. Clinical recommendations for the treatment of incidental pancreatic lesions are urgently needed. This article provides a perspective and guideline on the clinical management of incidental intraductal papillary mucinous neoplasms (IPMNs) and cystic or premalignant lesions of the pancreas.

Generally, 4 major types of cystic intrapancreatic incidentalomas are distinguished based on location, main pancreatic duct communication, and occurrence of septae, loculations, or calcifications: (1) unilocular or oligolocular (pseudocyst, IPMN, serous cystadenoma [SC], mucinous cystic neoplasm [MCN]), or multilocular (oligocystic SCs, branch-duct IPMN [BD-IPMN], MCN); (2) microcystic SC; (3) macrocystic (MCN, SC, or IPMN); and (4) cysts with a solid component (IPMN, MCN).[5,10]

Unilocular or Oligolocular Cysts

Unilocular cysts associated with a history of pancreatitis are pseudocysts in most cases.[5] If diagnosed in elderly women, however, unilocular cysts located in the pancreatic head featuring a lobulated contour but lacking wall enhancement or mural nodules may be specific for SC.[5] Calcification in the tumor periphery can be a characteristic for MCN.[5,10–12]

Multilocular Cystic Lesions

Multilocular intrapancreatic cystic lesions can be pleomorphic, lobulated, or feature a smooth shape with septations.[5,10,12,13] Oligocystic SCs usually feature a lobulated shape with either internal septations or no septation at all.[5,10,12,13] A pleomorphic shape is typical for BD-IPMNs. A smooth shape with septation is specific for MCNs.[5,10,12,13]

Differentiation of cystic tumors may be difficult because of their overlapping morphology.[14] However, oligocystic SC appears as multicystic or cystic-lobulated with septations, whereas MCN features a smooth shape, with or without septations. SCs typically show central calcification within the fibrous stroma. MCN may feature peripheral eggshell calcification.[5,10,15,16]

Microcystic Lesions

SC is the only lesion that may appear microcystic. CT often reveals a sponge or honeycomb-like lesion with countless small cysts separated by slender septa. In about 20% of SCs, the septa may merge into a central stellate scar, which may calcify. Because microcystic lesions (**Fig. 1**) may easily be mistaken for solid structures in CT scans, a T2-weighted MRI and endoscopic ultrasonography (EUS) should be performed.[5,10,17,18]

Cysts with or Without a Solid Component

Cysts with solid components should be considered highly suspicious for malignancy. Solid tumors with cystic components may be solid pseudopapillary tumors, malignant adenocarcinoma, cystic pancreatic endocrine tumor, and metastasis. Cystic tumors with a solid component may be MCNs and IPMNs that transformed to malignant tumors or cystic degeneration.[5,10] Either way, incidentalomas with this appearance are highly suspicious for malignancy.

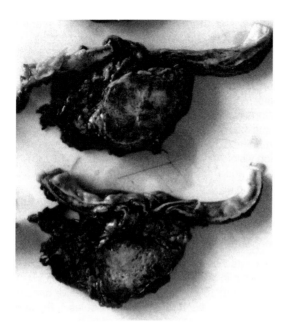

Fig. 1. Macroscopic pathologic examination of a microcystic cystadenoma.

Cystic Lesions with or Without Pancreatic Duct Communication

In radiologic practice, communication of the cystic lesion to the pancreatic main and branch duct may indicate an IPMN. Rarely, this can be observed in MCNs.[19]

TYPES OF CYSTIC INCIDENTALOMAS

The classification of cystic pancreatic neoplasms is based on the type of epithelium and a mucinous or nonmucinous content.[20–22] MCNs and IPMNs account for most mucinous neoplasms.[22–24] The following nonmucinous cystic lesions may occur in the pancreas: cystic pancreatic ductal adenocarcinomas (PDAs), serous cystic neoplasms (SCNs), cystic pancreatic neuroendocrine tumors (PNETs), pseudocysts, solid pseudopapillary neoplasms (SPNs), and other rare lesions.[22] PDA, PNET, MCN, IPMN, and SPN are considered neoplastic or have high-risk potential for malignancy, whereas pseudocysts (**Fig. 2**), serous cysts, and simple cysts are nonneoplastic or have low-risk potential for malignancy.[22,25,26]

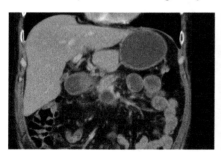
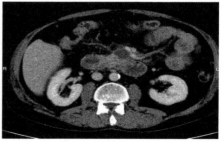

Fig. 2. Incidental occurrence of a pancreatic pseudocyst. CT scan of a pancreatic pseudocyst. Incidental occurrence of a pancreatic pseudocyst. CT scan of a pancreatic pseudocyst. Coronal ct scan of the abdomen (*left*). Transversal ct scan of the abdomen (*right*).

Previous studies have shown that SC, MCN, and IPMN account for most of the pancreatic cysts found in asymptomatic individuals.[16]

Serous Cystadenomas

SCs are benign cystic tumors that derive from pancreatic centroacinar cells (**Fig. 3**). SCs usually manifest as numerous fluid-filled cysts and occur in any part of the pancreas.[26] Occasionally, SC appear as an oligocystic lesion, which can be challenging to differentiate from MCN if found in the pancreatic tail or body.[26–29] On radiologic imaging, SC manifests as a focal, well-demarcated lesion with a central scar or sunburst calcification visible in 20% of SCs.[26] EUS, on the other hand, often reveals a honeycomb-like appearance.[21,26] When acquired, cytologic analysis exhibits cuboidal glycogen-staining cells in 50% of cases.[26,30–32] Therefore, cytologic diagnosis can be difficult. SCs are considered benign and should only be resected if symptomatic or if malignancy cannot be fully excluded.[26]

Mucinous Cystic Neoplasm

MCNs are mucinous cysts that contain ovarian-like stroma (**Figs. 4** and **5**). They occur almost exclusively in women and usually present as unilocular cysts in the body and/or tail of the pancreas.[33] About 15% of MCNs contain invasive cancer.[33,34] Risk factors for malignancy include size greater than 6 cm and nodules.[34] Previous studies demonstrated that the risk of high-grade dysplasia or invasive cancer decreases dramatically to less than 0.4% when MCNs are smaller than 3 cm and without nodules.[35]

Intraductal Papillary Mucinous Neoplasms

IPMNs (**Fig. 6**) were first described by Ohhashi and colleagues[36] in 1982 and are considered a specific tumor-entity. By definition they can be distinguished from PDAs and MCNs.[36] Histopathologically, IPMNs feature dysplastic changes of the epithelium, with grade of dysplasia ranging from low or intermediate to high (IPMN

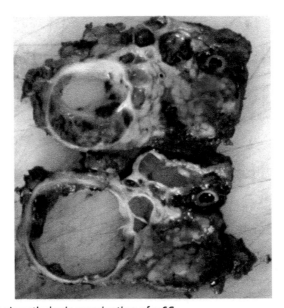

Fig. 3. Macroscopic pathologic examination of a SC.

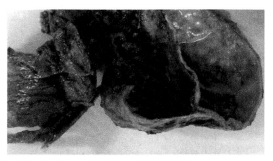

Fig. 4. Macroscopic pathologic examination of an MCN.

with carcinoma in situ), which are considered to be noninvasive up to IPMNs with invasive carcinoma (invasive IPMN).[37–39] Currently, IPMNs are the most frequently resected cystic lesion.[40] The World Health Organization defines IPMNs as follows: An intraductal papillary mucin-producing neoplasm, arises in the main pancreatic duct or its major branches. The papillary epithelium component, and the degree of mucin secretion, cystic duct dilatation, and invasiveness are variable. Intraductal papillary-mucin neoplasms are divided into benign, borderline, and malignant noninvasive or invasive lesions.[41]

Most IPMNs are in the head of the pancreas and derived from the main pancreatic duct and its branches.[41–44] Usually, IPMN lesions involve either a single cystic mass or a segmental duct; however, diffuse involvement has also been described.[41,45–47]

In general, IPMNs are subdivided into different types depending on the involvement of pancreatic ductal system microscopically and macroscopically[24,39,41]: main-duct

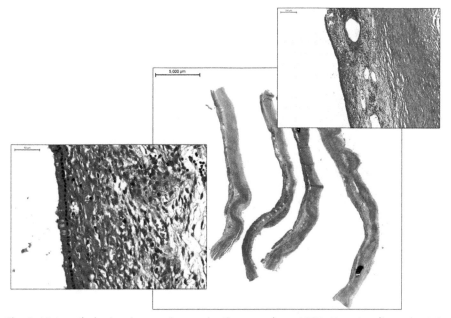

Fig. 5. Histopathologic microscopic examination reveals an MCN. Hematoxylin-eosin stain (H&E stain).

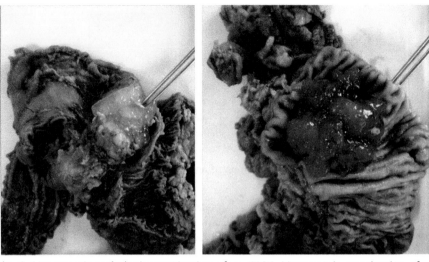

Fig. 6. Macroscopic pathologic examination of an IPMN. Macroscopic examination of an IPMN. In macroscopic examination the cystic formation might feature different shapes and colors (*left, right*).

IPMN (MD-IPMN) (**Figs. 7** and **8**), BD-IPMN (**Figs. 9** and **10**), and mixed-duct IPMN (XD-IPMN). For further details see **Table 1**. Generally speaking, risk factors for malignant IPMNs include solid components, main pancreatic duct dilation, cyst size greater than 3 cm, and nodules.[33,34]

Diagnostics of Incidentalomas of the Pancreas

When approaching incidental pancreatic cysts, the following aspects should be addressed:

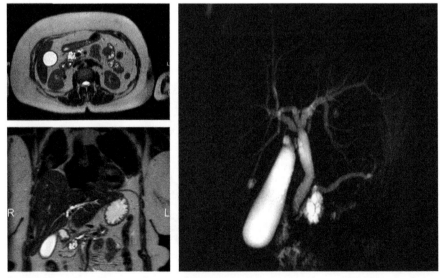

Fig. 7. MRI and MRCP scan of an incidental main-duct IPMN with a multilocular configuration. MRI and MRCP scan of an incidental main-duct IPMN with a multilocular configuration. Transversal MRI scan (*upper left*). Coronal MRI scan (*downer left*). MRCP scan (*right*).

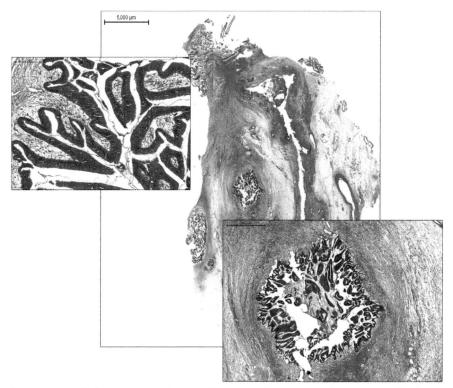

Fig. 8. Histopathologic examination reveals a main-duct IPMN with an intestinal subtype. H&E stain.

1. Type of cyst
   a. Mucinous or nonmucinous? Mucinous cysts show a much higher potential for malignancy than nonmucinous cysts; therefore, it is crucial to distinguish mucinous from nonmucinous cysts.
      i. Multidetector CT is able to identify mucinous cysts with an accuracy of 71% to 84%.[52–55] However, accuracy for diagnosing the specific type of cyst is lower (40%–70%).[52–55] SCs usually have a higher attenuation than pseudocysts, MCNs, and IPMNs; lower attenuation than insulinomas; and comparable attenuation to pancreatic adenocarcinomas.[56]

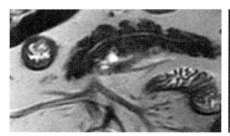
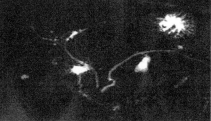

Fig. 9. Incidental cystic pancreatic lesions. MRCP scan indicates a BD-IPMN. Incidental cystic pancreatic lesions in MRI scan (*left*). MRCP scan indicates a BD-IPMN (*right*).

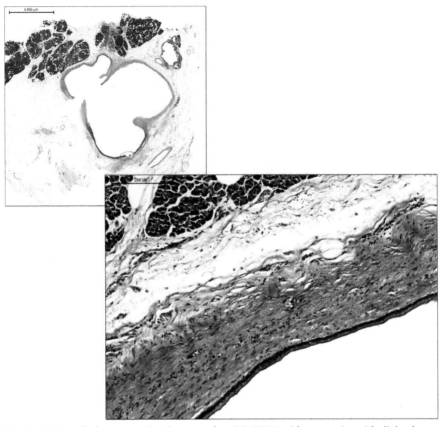

Fig. 10. Histopathologic examination reveals a BD-IPMN with a gastric epithelial subtype. H&E stain.

Table 1 Types of intraductal papillary mucinous neoplasm		
MD-IPMN	**BD-IPMN**	**XD-IPMN**
• Cystic tumor that involves only the main pancreatic duct which features diffuse or segmental dilatation to >5 mm[24,33] • *Histologic characteristics: mostly intestinal epithelial subtype*[48] • *High frequency of malignancy (>60%)*[24,33,49,50]	• Tumor involves only branch-ducts, no dilatation of main pancreatic duct[7] • *Histologic characteristics: mostly gastric epithelial subtype*[48] • Lower frequency of malignancy (26%)[24] • 20% to 30% of BD-IPMN ultimately turn out to be mixed type IPMN on histopathologic examination after surgical pathologic assessment[33,51]	• Tumor involves both the main pancreatic duct and its side branches[24] • *Histologic characteristics: both gastric and intestinal epithelial subtype, depending on ratio MD-IPMN to BD-IPMN*[48] • XD-IPMN has a comparable malignant potential to MD-IPMN[33,48]

ii. Compared with multidetector CT, MRI is superior in identifying mucinous cysts with an accuracy of 79% to 82%; however, for diagnosing specific types of cysts it is comparable to multidetector CT.[52,55] Therefore, MRI or magnetic resonance cholangiopancreatography (MRCP) is the preferred imaging technique because it better detects septa, nodules, and duct communication.[6,20,52]

iii. High-resolution imaging of pancreatic cystic lesions can be provided by EUS[21,22] and allows cytologic and biochemical fluid analysis of the cystic fluid when combined with EUS-guided fine-needle aspiration.[22,57] However, EUS imaging alone is insufficient for mucinous cysts with only 56% sensitivity, 45% specificity, and 51% accuracy.[52,57]

2. Is the cyst currently malignant?

a. Unfortunately, diagnostic differentiation between benign and premalignant lesions can be tricky.[26,58,59] In addition, cystic fluid analysis studies currently fail to clearly distinguish among the different pancreatic cyst types or to predict the behavior of these lesions.[14,58,59] Overall accuracy of preoperative diagnosis of pancreatic cysts is currently only 68% compared with surgical histopathologic assesment.[59,60] One study suggested a preoperative diagnostic accuracy of only 47%.[59,61] Malignant pancreatic lesions are lethal in most cases. Therefore, the following principle should be obeyed: if in doubt take it out! Especially considering that a tailored surgical approach, for example, segmental resection. Duodenum-preserving pancreatic head resection, also done by laparoscopy, can be offered to the patient.

3. If not, what is the malignant potential of the cyst?[52,59] If it is high or if there is doubt about it being benign, it should be treated with oncological intent.

4. Important considerations include a patient's biological age, comorbidities, fitness, tumor localization, and the planned surgical approach; what is the benefit-risk ratio? Young, surgically fit patients with long life expectancies will most likely benefit from a surgical approach, whereas biologically old patients with serious life-limiting comorbidities will most likely not benefit.

Treatment of Intraductal Papillary Mucinous Neoplasms

Surgical decisions for IPNM must be based on the type of IPMN diagnosed.[49] The risk of malignancy in MD-IPMN and XD-IPMN is 60% to 90%, therefore these 2 entities represent major indications for oncological surgical treatment that includes a formal pancreatic resection and lymphadenectomy.[24,49,50] However, for BD-IPMN, indications for surgery should be more balanced because malignancy occurs in approximately 20% to 25% (**Figs. 11** and **12**).[7,49,62,63]

Surgical Treatment of Main-Duct and Mixed-Duct Intraductal Papillary Mucinous Neoplasm Lesions

Because MD-IPMN and XD-IPMN are highly associated with malignant transformation, they both should be treated with surgical-oncologic intent. The type of surgical procedure will vary and depends on the localization of the lesions. The surgical standard procedures include partial, distal, and total pancreatectomy.[39,49,64]

Treatment of Branch-Duct Intraductal Papillary Mucinous Neoplasm

Currently, the guidelines recommend resection of BD-IPMN with a diameter of more than 3 cm. Smaller BD-IPMN should only be resected when high-risk stigmata, including mural nodules, positive cytology, symptoms, or a synchronously dilated main duct, are evident.[49] Recent studies, however, show that the incidence of

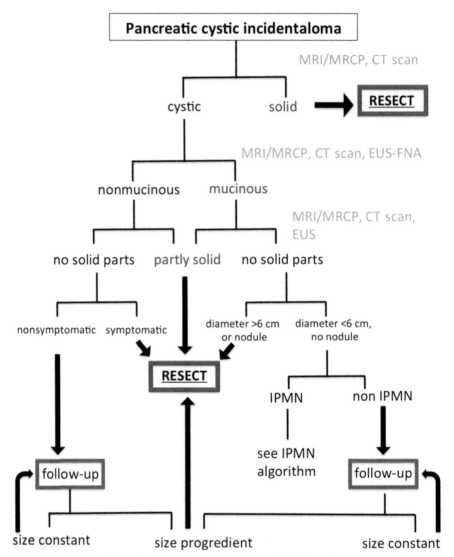

Fig. 11. Decision-making algorithm for pancreatic cystic incidentalomas. FNA, fine-needle aspiration.

malignancy is approximately 25% in BD-IPMN less than 3 cm[49,62,65–67] and neither the existence of mural nodules nor clinical symptoms correlated with malignancy.[49,67]

According to the Sendai guidelines,[24,68] BD-IPMNs have been treated according to risk stratification. However, several large series have implied that even small and asymptomatic side-branch IPMNs without suspicious radiologic features contain a risk of invasive carcinoma that may be as high as 20%.[51,65,66,69] Also, cyst size may be inaccurate for predicting malignant risk.[69] In fact, so-called Sendai-negative IPMNs have a malignant findings in 14% to 25.5% of final histologic examination of the resected pancreatic specimen.[24,51,60,62]

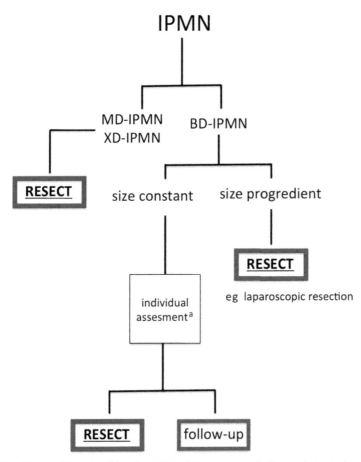

Fig. 12. Decision-making algorithm for IPMNs. [a] Assessment of all morphological and clinical factors, including imaging, tumor markers, symptoms, progression, and prior patient history.

Currently, diagnostic and prognostic markers fail to be sufficiently reliable to distinguish between cysts at risk of malignant transformation and those with no risk. Therefore, surgery for BD-IPMNs should be considered in all fit patients.[51,62] Preferably, the surgery should be performed in specialized high-volume centers with high operative and clinical experience in pancreatic surgery.

Suspected malignant BD-IPMN should be treated similarly to the location-based approach of MD-IPMN. Depending on the location of the lesion, either a partial pancreaticoduodenectomy or distal pancreatectomy should be performed.[49] Because the surgical treatment of BD-IPMN is also focused on prevention of malignancy, less extensive surgical approaches may be considered, for example, laparoscopic enucleations or central pancreatectomies.[49,70–75]

REFERENCES

1. Laffan TA, Horton KM, Klein AP, et al. Prevalence of unsuspected pancreatic cysts on MDCT. AJR Am J Roentgenol 2008;191(3):802–7.
2. Lee KS, Sekhar A, Rofsky NM, et al. Prevalence of incidental pancreatic cysts in the adult population on MR imaging. Am J Gastroenterol 2010;105(9):2079–84.

3. Spinelli KS, Fromwiller TE, Daniel RA, et al. Cystic pancreatic neoplasms: observe or operate. Ann Surg 2004;239(5):651–7 [discussion: 657–9].

4. Zhang XM, Mitchell DG, Dohke M, et al. Pancreatic cysts: depiction on single-shot fast spin-echo MR images. Radiology 2002;223(2):547–53.

5. Gore RM, Wenzke DR, Thakrar KH, et al. The incidental cystic pancreas mass: a practical approach. Cancer Imaging 2012;12:414–21.

6. Berland LL, Silverman SG, Gore RM, et al. Managing incidental findings on abdominal CT: white paper of the ACR incidental findings committee. J Am Coll Radiol 2010;7(10):754–73.

7. Tanaka M. Controversies in the management of pancreatic IPMN. Nat Rev Gastroenterol Hepatol 2011;8(1):56–60.

8. Sahani DV, Lin DJ, Venkatesan AM, et al. Multidisciplinary approach to diagnosis and management of intraductal papillary mucinous neoplasms of the pancreas. Clin Gastroenterol Hepatol 2009;7(3):259–69.

9. Hruban RH, PM, Klimstra DS. Atlas of tumor pathology: tumors of the pancreas. 4th edition. American Registry of Pathology and Armed Forces Institute of Pathology; 2007. Available at: https://www.ncbi.nlm.nih.gov/nlmcatalog/101478799. Accessed October 27, 2017.

10. Cho HW, Choi JY, Kim MJ, et al. Pancreatic tumors: emphasis on CT findings and pathologic classification. Korean J Radiol 2011;12(6):731–9.

11. Werner JB, Bartosch-Harlid A, Andersson R. Cystic pancreatic lesions: current evidence for diagnosis and treatment. Scand J Gastroenterol 2011;46(7–8): 773–88.

12. Sakorafas GH, Smyrniotis V, Reid-Lombardo KM, et al. Primary pancreatic cystic neoplasms revisited: part II. Mucinous cystic neoplasms. Surg Oncol 2011;20(2): e93–101.

13. Testini M, Gurrado A, Lissidini G, et al. Management of mucinous cystic neoplasms of the pancreas. World J Gastroenterol 2010;16(45):5682–92.

14. Megibow AJ, Baker ME, Gore RM, et al. The incidental pancreatic cyst. Radiol Clin North Am 2011;49(2):349–59.

15. Adsay NV. Cystic neoplasia of the pancreas: pathology and biology. J Gastrointest Surg 2008;12(3):401–4.

16. Parra-Herran CE, Garcia MT, Herrera L, et al. Cystic lesions of the pancreas: clinical and pathologic review of cases in a five year period. JOP 2010;11(4):358–64.

17. Wargo JA, Fernandez-del-Castillo C, Warshaw AL. Management of pancreatic serous cystadenomas. Adv Surg 2009;43:23–34.

18. Sahara S, Kawai N, Sato M, et al. Differentiation of pancreatic serous cystadenoma from endocrine tumor and intraductal papillary mucinous neoplasm based on washout pattern on multiphase CT. J Comput Assist Tomogr 2012;36(2):231–6.

19. Morel A, Marteau V, Chambon E, et al. Pancreatic mucinous cystadenoma communicating with the main pancreatic duct on MRI. Br J Radiol 2009; 82(984):e243–5.

20. Waters JA, Schmidt CM, Pinchot JW, et al. CT vs MRCP: optimal classification of IPMN type and extent. J Gastrointest Surg 2008;12(1):101–9.

21. Brugge WR, Lauwers GY, Sahani D, et al. Cystic neoplasms of the pancreas. N Engl J Med 2004;351(12):1218–26.

22. Khashab MA, Kim K, Lennon AM, et al. Should we do EUS/FNA on patients with pancreatic cysts? The incremental diagnostic yield of EUS over CT/MRI for prediction of cystic neoplasms. Pancreas 2013;42(4):717–21.

23. Singh M, Maitra A. Precursor lesions of pancreatic cancer: molecular pathology and clinical implications. Pancreatology 2007;7(1):9–19.

24. Tanaka M, Fernandez-del Castillo C, Adsay V, et al. International consensus guidelines 2012 for the management of IPMN and MCN of the pancreas. Pancreatology 2012;12(3):183–97.
25. Khashab MA, Shin EJ, Amateau S, et al. Tumor size and location correlate with behavior of pancreatic serous cystic neoplasms. Am J Gastroenterol 2011; 106(8):1521–6.
26. Khalid A, Brugge W. ACG practice guidelines for the diagnosis and management of neoplastic pancreatic cysts. Am J Gastroenterol 2007;102(10):2339–49.
27. Compagno J, Oertel JE. Microcystic adenomas of the pancreas (glycogen-rich cystadenomas): a clinicopathologic study of 34 cases. Am J Clin Pathol 1978; 69(3):289–98.
28. Pyke CM, van Heerden JA, Colby TV, et al. The spectrum of serous cystadenoma of the pancreas. Clinical, pathologic, and surgical aspects. Ann Surg 1992; 215(2):132–9.
29. Lundstedt C, Dawiskiba S. Serous and mucinous cystadenoma/cystadenocarcinoma of the pancreas. Abdom Imaging 2000;25(2):201–6.
30. Frossard JL, Amouyal P, Amouyal G, et al. Performance of endosonography-guided fine needle aspiration and biopsy in the diagnosis of pancreatic cystic lesions. Am J Gastroenterol 2003;98(7):1516–24.
31. Jones EC, Suen KC, Grant DR, et al. Fine-needle aspiration cytology of neoplastic cysts of the pancreas. Diagn Cytopathol 1987;3(3):238–43.
32. Centeno BA, Lewandrowski KB, Warshaw AL, et al. Cyst fluid cytologic analysis in the differential diagnosis of pancreatic cystic lesions. Am J Clin Pathol 1994; 101(4):483–7.
33. Chiang AL, Lee LS. Clinical approach to incidental pancreatic cysts. World J Gastroenterol 2016;22(3):1236–45.
34. Scheiman JM, Hwang JH, Moayyedi P. American gastroenterological association technical review on the diagnosis and management of asymptomatic neoplastic pancreatic cysts. Gastroenterology 2015;148(4):824–48.e22.
35. Nguyen D, Dawson DW, Hines OJ, et al. Mucinous cystic neoplasms of the pancreas: are we overestimating malignant potential? Am Surg 2014;80(10): 915–9.
36. Ohashi K, Murakami Y, Maruyama M, et al. Four cases of mucus-secreting pancreatic cancer. Prog Digest Endosc 1982;20:348–51.
37. Hruban RH, Takaori K, Klimstra DS, et al. An illustrated consensus on the classification of pancreatic intraepithelial neoplasia and intraductal papillary mucinous neoplasms. Am J Surg Pathol 2004;28(8):977–87.
38. Bosman FT, Hruban RH, Carneiro F, et al. 4th edition. WHO classification of tumors of the digestive system, vol. Lyon (France): IARC Press; 2010.
39. Paini M, Crippa S, Scopelliti F, et al. Extent of surgery and implications of transection margin status after resection of IPMNs. Gastroenterol Res Pract 2014;2014: 269803.
40. Fernandez-del Castillo C, Adsay NV. Intraductal papillary mucinous neoplasms of the pancreas. Gastroenterology 2010;139(3):708–13, 713.e1–2.
41. Longnecker DS, Adler G, Hruban RH, et al. Intraductal papillary-mucinous neoplasms of the pancreas. In: Hamilton SR, AL, editors. World Health Organization classification of tumors. Lyon (France): IARC Press; 2000. p. 237–40. Available at: https://www.iarc.fr/en/publications/pdfs-online/pat-gen/bb2/BB2.pdf. Accessed October 27, 2017.

42. Solcia E, Capella C, Kloppel G. Tumors of the pancreas. In: Armed Forces Institute of Pathology, editor. Atlas of tumor pathology, vol. fascicle 20. Washington, DC: Armed Forces Institute of Pathology; 1997.

43. Conley CR, Scheithauer BW, van Heerden JA, et al. Diffuse intraductal papillary adenocarcinoma of the pancreas. Ann Surg 1987;205(3):246–9.

44. Austin DF. Etiological clues from descriptive epidemiology: squamous carcinoma of the rectum or anus. Natl Cancer Inst Monogr 1982;62:89–90.

45. Longnecker DS. Observations on the etiology and pathogenesis of intraductal papillary-mucinous neoplasms of the pancreas. Hepatogastroenterology 1998; 45(24):1973–80.

46. Sho M, Nakajima Y, Kanehiro H, et al. Pattern of recurrence after resection for intraductal papillary mucinous tumors of the pancreas. World J Surg 1998;22(8): 874–8.

47. Traverso LW, Peralta EA, Ryan JA Jr, et al. Intraductal neoplasms of the pancreas. Am J Surg 1998;175(5):426–32.

48. Sahora K, Fernandez-del Castillo C, Dong F, et al. Not all mixed-type intraductal papillary mucinous neoplasms behave like main-duct lesions: implications of minimal involvement of the main pancreatic duct. Surgery 2014;156(3):611–21.

49. Hackert T, Fritz S, Buchler MW. Main- and branch-duct intraductal papillary mucinous neoplasms: extent of surgical resection. Viszeralmedizin 2015;31(1): 38–42.

50. Kappeli RM, Muller SA, Hummel B, et al. IPMN: surgical treatment. Langenbecks Arch Surg 2013;398(8):1029–37.

51. Fritz S, Werner J, Buchler MW. Reply to letter: "liberal resection for (presumed) Sendai negative branch-duct IPMN–also not harmless". Ann Surg 2014;259(3): e46.

52. Lee LS. Diagnostic approach to pancreatic cysts. Curr Opin Gastroenterol 2014; 30(5):511–7.

53. Sainani NI, Saokar A, Deshpande V, et al. Comparative performance of MDCT and MRI with MR cholangiopancreatography in characterizing small pancreatic cysts. AJR Am J Roentgenol 2009;193(3):722–31.

54. Mohamadnejad M, Eloubeidi MA. Cystsic lesions of the pancreas. Arch Iran Med 2013;16(4):233–9.

55. Sahani DV, Kambadakone A, Macari M, et al. Diagnosis and management of cystic pancreatic lesions. AJR Am J Roentgenol 2013;200(2):343–54.

56. Chu LC, Singhi AD, Hruban RH, et al. Characterization of pancreatic serous cystadenoma on dual-phase multidetector computed tomography. J Comput Assist Tomogr 2014;38(2):258–63.

57. Brugge WR, Lewandrowski K, Lee-Lewandrowski E, et al. Diagnosis of pancreatic cystic neoplasms: a report of the cooperative pancreatic cyst study. Gastroenterology 2004;126(5):1330–6.

58. Al-Haddad M, Schmidt MC, Sandrasegaran K, et al. Diagnosis and treatment of cystic pancreatic tumors. Clin Gastroenterol Hepatol 2011;9(8):635–48.

59. Lee LS. Incidental cystic lesions in the pancreas: resect? EUS? Follow? Curr Treat Options Gastroenterol 2014;12(3):333–49.

60. Correa-Gallego C, Ferrone CR, Thayer SP, et al. Incidental pancreatic cysts: do we really know what we are watching? Pancreatology 2010;10(2–3):144–50.

61. Cho CS, Russ AJ, Loeffler AG, et al. Preoperative classification of pancreatic cystic neoplasms: the clinical significance of diagnostic inaccuracy. Ann Surg Oncol 2013;20(9):3112–9.

62. Fritz S, Klauss M, Bergmann F, et al. Small (Sendai negative) branch-duct IPMNs: not harmless. Ann Surg 2012;256(2):313–20.
63. Goh BK, Tan DM, Ho MM, et al. Utility of the Sendai consensus guidelines for branch-duct intraductal papillary mucinous neoplasms: a systematic review. J Gastrointest Surg 2014;18(7):1350–7.
64. Hackert T, Tjaden C, Buchler MW. Developments in pancreatic surgery during the past ten years. Zentralbl Chir 2014;139(3):292–300 [in German].
65. Schmidt CM, White PB, Waters JA, et al. Intraductal papillary mucinous neoplasms: predictors of malignant and invasive pathology. Ann Surg 2007;246(4): 644–51 [discussion: 651–4].
66. Jang JY, Kim SW, Lee SE, et al. Treatment guidelines for branch duct type intraductal papillary mucinous neoplasms of the pancreas: when can we operate or observe? Ann Surg Oncol 2008;15(1):199–205.
67. Kato Y, Takahashi S, Gotohda N, et al. Risk factors for malignancy in branched-type intraductal papillary mucinous neoplasms of the pancreas during the follow-up period. World J Surg 2015;39(1):244–50.
68. Tanaka M, Chari S, Adsay V, et al. International consensus guidelines for management of intraductal papillary mucinous neoplasms and mucinous cystic neoplasms of the pancreas. Pancreatology 2006;6(1–2):17–32.
69. Walsh RM, Vogt DP, Henderson JM, et al. Management of suspected pancreatic cystic neoplasms based on cyst size. Surgery 2008;144(4):677–84 [discussion: 684–5].
70. Hackert T, Hinz U, Fritz S, et al. Enucleation in pancreatic surgery: indications, technique, and outcome compared to standard pancreatic resections. Langenbecks Arch Surg 2011;396(8):1197–203.
71. Crippa S, Bassi C, Salvia R, et al. Enucleation of pancreatic neoplasms. Br J Surg 2007;94(10):1254–9.
72. Sauvanet A, Gaujoux S, Blanc B, et al. Parenchyma-sparing pancreatectomy for presumed noninvasive intraductal papillary mucinous neoplasms of the pancreas. Ann Surg 2014;260(2):364–71.
73. Turrini O, Schmidt CM, Pitt HA, et al. Side-branch intraductal papillary mucinous neoplasms of the pancreatic head/uncinate: resection or enucleation? HPB (Oxford) 2011;13(2):126–31.
74. Goudard Y, Gaujoux S, Dokmak S, et al. Reappraisal of central pancreatectomy a 12-year single-center experience. JAMA Surg 2014;149(4):356–63.
75. Muller MW, Friess H, Kleeff J, et al. Middle segmental pancreatic resection: an option to treat benign pancreatic body lesions. Ann Surg 2006;244(6):909–18 [discussion: 918–20].

Nonfunctioning Incidental Pancreatic Neuroendocrine Tumors: Who, When, and How to Treat?

Marina Gorelik, DO*, Mahmoud Ahmad, MD, MBA,
David Grossman, MD, Martin Grossman, MD,
Avram M. Cooperman, MD

KEYWORDS

- Pancreatic neuroendocrine tumor (PNET)
- Nonfunctioning pancreatic neuroendocrine tumor (NF-PNET) • Surveillance

KEY POINTS

- More than 50% nonfunctioning (NF) pancreatic neuroendocrine tumors (PNETs) are incidental findings on cross-sectional imaging.
- Asymptomatic NF-PNETs are indolent, and surveillance is safe and reasonable.
- Size is a less important determinant of therapy than grade, Ki-67, symptoms, and imaging.
- Surgical options include enucleation, distal and central pancreatectomy, and pancreaticoduodenectomy resection.
- A multidisciplinary approach with colleagues and informed consent with patients and families are essential.

INTRODUCTION

Pancreatic neuroendocrine tumors (PNETs) are an interesting, diverse, rare group of neoplasms with a varied course and prognosis. They account for 1% to 2% of all pancreatic neoplasms and have a low incidence of 0.43 per 100,000.[1] With a prognosis far better than pancreatic adenocarcinoma, they range from benign to low-grade malignant lesions and much less often as high-grade or metastatic lesions.[2–4], More than 50% of NF-PNETs are incidental findings[2–5] on cross-sectional imaging and most of these lesions are asymptomatic and indolent and found in elderly patients with comorbidities.[3,5] Despite consensus management recommendations, which not surprisingly are surgery based or biased, legitimate doubts persist regarding the need to treat and which NF-PNETs may be observed. This article reviews the natural history,

The authors have nothing to disclose.
Department of General Surgery, Aventura Hospital and Medical Center, 20900 Biscayne Blvd, Aventura, FL 33180, USA
* Corresponding author.
E-mail address: mgorelik0610@gmail.com

presentation, and guidelines for therapy for NF-PNET, reflective of the authors' understanding and unintended biases.

CLASSIFICATION

The PNET cell of origin was believed to originate from islet cells, but recent studies suggest that a pluripotent stem cell of the ductal-acinar system may be the precursor cell.[6,7] PNETs demonstrate important genetic differences from pancreatic adenocarcinoma that involve distinct mutations from adenocarcinoma.[6–8]

PNETs are classified as functional (F) or Non functioning (NF). F-PNETs hypersecrete single or multiple hormones, causing a constellation of symptoms and often a dramatic presentation[4]; 60%-90% of all PNETs are NF and do not produce clinical syndromes[9]; 90% of PNETs are sporadic and 10% are associated with genetic syndromes, such as multiple endocrine neoplasia type 1 (MEN1), von Hippel-Lindau disease, neurofibromatosis type 1, and tuberous sclerosis.4,6 The most common pancreatic neoplasms in MEN1 are gastrinomas and insulinomas.[4,6]

CLINICAL PRESENTATION

NF-PNETs are diagnosed most often by imaging or endoscopic studies as incidental findings. Less often patients present with nonspecific symptoms[9] abdominal pain,weight loss, and/or jaundice.[5,9] Symptoms are caused by tumor invasion or encroachment or displacement of contiguous structures, and symptomatic lesions are larger than nonsymptomatic lesions.[5] NF-PNETs may not produce hormones or peptides, produce them at low levels and without symptoms, or secrete peptides that cause no symptoms[4,5]; 60% to 100% of NF-PNETs secrete 1 or more peptides, such as chromogranin A (CgA), neuron-specific enolase, pancreatic polypeptide, ghrelin, neurotensin, motilin, or subunits of human chorionic gonadotrophin, which do not cause symptoms.[10]

F-PNETs have a wide range of clinical presentations, depending on which hormone(s) is/are hypersecreted. The most common F-PNETs include insulinomas, gastrinomas, glucagonomas, VIPomas, and somatostatinomas. Other unusual F-PNETs have been reported. F-PNETs are summarized in **Table 1**.[5,11–15]

DIAGNOSIS

Symptomatic patients require laboratory and imaging studies to identify and localize the hypersecreted hormones. With NF neoplasms, measurement of nonspecific circulating markers, such as CgA, pancreatic polypeptide, neuron-specific enolase, and pancreastatin, help establish a diagnosis.[10,16–18] CgA is the most sensitive marker, with a sensitivity of 60% and specificity of 80%.[17–19] Higher CgA levels correlate with greater tumor burden, metastatic disease and may be used to assess response to therapy.[17,18] Neuron-specific enolase is an insensitive tumor marker (30%–40%), but its specificity is almost 100%.[18,19]

Incidental NF-PNETs, are localized on discovery but further evaluation may include a pancreatic protocol CT scan, MRI, endoscopic ultrasound (EUS), and/or somatostatin receptor studies. PNETs usually hyperenhance with intravenous contrast in the arterial phase of a triple-phase CT scan.[20,21] The benefits of MRI include less radiation and better detection of liver metastasis.[21] PNETs have low signal intensity on T1-weighted images and high signal intensity on T2 images.[21] Although most PNETs are solid, approximately 10% are cystic with smooth margins and enhance peripherally on arterial and portal phases.[21] EUS is quite sensitive for diagnosing and staging most NF-PNETs, by fine-needle aspiration of the lesion and suspicious lymph nodes.[22,23]

Table 1
Functional neuroendocrine tumors

Name	Hormone	Tumor Location	Functional Pancreatic Neuroendocrine Tumor (%)	Malignant (%)	Symptoms
Insulinoma	Insulin	Pancreas	35–40	<10	Hypoglycemia Anxiety, tremors, palpitations Weight loss
Gastrinoma	Gastrin	75% gasrtrinoma triangle 25% duodenum	16–30	60–90	Epigastric pain Diarrhea Refractory or complicated ulcer disease
VIPoma	Vasoactive intestinal peptide	75% pancreas 20% neurogenic 5% duodenum	<10	50–70	Secretory diarrhea Achlorhydria Hypokalemia Dehydration
Glucagonoma	Glucagon	Pancreas	<10	60–80	Necrolytic migratory erythema Glucose intolerance Stomatitis
Somatostatinoma	Somatostatin	66% pancreas 33% duodenal	<5	>70	Diabetes Cholelithiasis Steatorrhea
GRFoma	Growth hormone–releasing hormone	Pancreas 30% Lung 54% Jejunum 7% Other 13%	Unknown	>60	Acromegaly
ACTHoma	ACTH (corticotropin)	Pancreas	Unknown	>95	Cushing syndrome
Others	Carcinoid Parathyroid hormone–, related protein Renin Luteinizing hormone Erythropoietin Cholecystokinin Glucagon-like peptide 1				

Somatostatin scintigraphy uses the overexpression of somatostatin receptors present on many NF-PNETS to allow identification and to predict therapeutic response to labeled somatostatin analogs.[24–26] There are 2 primary types of somatostatin receptor–based images available. The octreoscan, which uses the ligand indium In 111–DPTA-D-Phe-1-octreotide, and the newest somatostatin receptor–based imaging modality, which uses the positron emitter gallium Ga 68 to label somatostatin analogs.[24–29] The most common of these analogs are ^{68}Ga-DOTATATE, ^{68}Ga-DOTATOC, and ^{68}Ga-DOTANOC.[25–30] The PET images are fused with CT to enhance resolution. ^{68}Ga-DOTATATE PET/CT detects 95.1% of lesions, significantly higher than the 45.3% with CT or MRI and the 30.9% with ^{111}In-pentetreotide SPECT/CT, and has the additional benefits[29] of staging and detecting recurrence after treatment.[27–29]

Fludeoxyglucose F 18 (FDG) PET is used to detect many malignancies, but most neuroendocrine tumors (NETs) are metabolically inactive and do not take up the tracer.[30] Higher-grade NETs are more apt to uptake FDG, suggesting a more aggressive lesion.[30] FDG avidity correlates with early tumor progression and increased mortality.[30]

STAGING

Over the past decade, there has been a shift from "benign" or "malignant" to "170 stratification," which identifies factors that predict behavior. The current classification and staging systems were proposed by the World Health Organization (WHO), the European Neuroendocrine Tumor Society (ENETS), and the American Joint Committee on Cancer (AJCC).[5] The WHO system is based on tumor proliferation rates and in 2010 classified PNETs into 3 main groups: NETs (NET-G1 and NET-G2) and neuroendocrine carcinoma G3.[5,31] Ki-67 is a nuclear protein that is expressed only during active but not resting phases of cell cycles.[31] NET-G1 and NET-G2 tumors are considered well-differentiated neoplasms.[31] NET-G1 neoplasms have a mitotic count of less than 2 per 10 high-power fields (HPFs) and a Ki-67% less than or equal to 2%.[31] NET-G2s have mitotic counts of 2 to 20 per 10 HPFs and a Ki-67% of 3% to 20%.[31] while NET-G3 is characterized by mitotic counts greater than 20 per 10 HPFs and a Ki-67 greater than 20.[31]

ENETS and AJCC staging is based on the tumor-nodes-metastasis (TNM) classification. In 2010, the AJCC proposed a specific TNM staging system for PNETs, which includes local disease (stage I), locally advanced/resectable tumors (stage II), locally advanced/unresectable tumors (stage III), and distant metastatic tumors (stage IV).[5] **Tables 2** and **3** present the current WHO, AJCC, and ENETS classification systems.[31] Both the ENETS and the AJCC system have been validated and provide important prognostic information for PNETs.[2,5]

MOLECULAR BIOLOGY

The most frequent genetic alterations in PNETs occur in the *MEN1* gene, death-domain–associated protein (DAXX)/mental retardation syndrome X-linked gene (alpha

Table 2
2010 World Health Organization classification of neuroendocrine tumor

Grade	Mitotic Count (Mitoses per 10% High-power Fields)	Ki-67 Index	Differentiation
G1 (low)	<2	≤2	Well differentiated
G2 (intermediate)	2–20	3–20	Well differentiated
G3 (high)	>20	>20	Poorly differentiated

Table 3	
American Joint Committee on Cancer and European Neuroendocrine Tumor Society staging classification	
American Joint Committee on Cancer	**European Neuroendocrine Tumor Society**
T1—tumor limited to pancreas, <2 cm	T1—tumor limited to pancreas, <2 cm
T2—tumor limited to pancreas, >2 cm	T2—tumor limited to pancreas, 2–4 cm
T3—tumor extension beyond pancreas, but not involving celiac axis or SMA	T3—tumor limited to the pancreas, >4 cm, or tumor invading duodenum or common bile duct
T4—tumor involves celiac axis or SMA	T4—tumor invades adjacent structures
N0—no regional lymph node metastasis	N0—no regional lymph node metastasis
N1—regional lymph node metastasis	N1—regional lymph node metastasis
M0—no distant metastasis	M0—no distant metastasis
M1—distant metastasis	M1—distant metastasis
Stage IA—T1N0M0	Stage I—T1N0M0
Stage IB—T2N0M0	Stage IIA—T2N0M0
Stage IIA—T3N0M0	Stage IIB—T3N0M0
Stage IIB—T1-3N1M0	Stage IIIA—T4N0M0
Stage III—T4N0-1M0	Stage IIIB—any T, N1M0
Stage IV—any T, any N, M1	Stage IV—any T, any N, M1

Data from Edge SB, Byrd DR, Compton CC, et al. AJCC Cancer Staging Manual. 7th Edition. New York: Springer; 2010.

thalassemia/mental retardation syndrome X-linked (ATRX)), and the mammalian target of rapamycin pathway (mTOR).[8,32] WHO grade 3 neoplasms, or neuroendocrine carcinomas, are genetically distinct, with TP53 and RB mutations found frequently.[33]

The protein menin, encoded by the MEN1 gene, regulates gene transcription by coordinating chromatin remodeling.[8,33] This mutation is observed in sporadic and hereditary lesions, and inactivating mutations in MEN1 are detected in 25% to 30% of sporadic PNET cases.[33] There is no current way to clinically target MEN1 mutations.[33]

The mTOR pathway is a key driver of pancreatic NETs.[8,32,33] Exome sequencing has shown that a large number of well-differentiated PNETs have somatic genetic mutations that encode proteins in the mTOR pathway.[33] Several therapeutic agents that target elements of the mTOR pathway have been developed.[32] The mTOR inhibitor, everolimus, markedly extended the progression-free survival in unresectable PNETs in the phase III RADIANT-3 and 4 trials.[32,33]

The proteins encoded by ATRX and DAXX are related to chromatin remodeling at telomeres.[32] Loss of ATRX/DAXX function is associated with the alternative lengthening of telomeres, a telomerase-independent mechanism, important for survival of telomerase-negative cancer cells.[33] Somatic inactivating mutations in ATRX and DAXX were detected in 18% and 25% of PNET's, [32] but as yet there is no way to target and treat DAXX/ATRX mutations.[32]

PNETs highly express many proangiogenic molecules, such as hypoxia-inducible factor 1α and vascular endothelial growth factor (VEGF).[33] Antiangiogenic strategies, including the VEGF inhibitor bevacizumab and the VEGF receptor–targeted tyrosine kinase inhibitor sunitinib, are currently used.[33]

MANAGEMENT

Significant refinements in resolution of CT and MRI have resulted in display of smaller incidental prostate, breast, and pancreatic neuroendocrine lesions (incidentalomas).[34]

Most never become symptomatic, alter lifespan, or require therapy and are overdiagnosed. Overdiagnoses have resulted in costly and unnecessary intervention for lesions that might never manifest clinically. This is the genesis of the "Who, When and How to Treat" controversy of NF-PNETs. Unlike incidental prostate and breast lesions in which overdiagnosis is well documented, it is suggested in NF-PNETs because experience and studies are fewer.

Stanley Hoerr's adage, "It is hard to make asymptomatic patients better,"[35] is appropriate when deciding treatment of indolent asymptomatic NF-PNETs. Absent controlled trials, logic, tumor characteristics, markers, and individual experience are invoked to predict course and outcomes. Some investigators favor resecting all NF-PNETs to avoid growth and progression[36–40]; others are more selective, using size and growth on serial scans to determine therapy[41–54]; whereas others favor biopsy to evaluate the molecular markers that correlate with behavior.[49,51–53]

The concern that all NF-PNET will grow, metastasize, and become fatal has led some to advise resection for all PNETs. Gratian and colleagues reviewed the National Cancer Database of 1854 NF-PNETs less than or equal to 2 cm, identified by *International Classification of Disease for Oncology* (3rd edition) codes; 39% presented with regional lymph node metastases and 10% with distant metastases. The 5-year overall survival for nonoperated patients was 27.6% compared with 83.0% for partial pancreatectomy and 72.3% for pancreaticoduodenectomy. The investigators favor resection because all NF-PNETs are potentially malignant. These outcomes are at marked variance with all current studies. Patients were not separated into F or NF, symptomatic or indolent, or incidentally diagnosed PNETs. Also, preoperative biopsy, grading, and nuclear studies were not mentioned.

Other groups favor surveillance for NF-PNETs. A Mayo Clinic study by Lee and colleagues[41] reviewed patients with NF-PNETs from 2000 to 2011. There were 77 observed and 56 resected patients. The 77 patients had a median tumor size of 1.0 cm (0.3–3.2 cm) and a mean follow-up of 45 months. Tumor size did not change throughout follow-up and disease did not progress, and there was no disease-related mortality. Of the 56 operated patients, the median tumor size was 1.8 cm (0.5–3.6 cm) and the mean follow-up was 52 months. Operated patients also had no mortality or recurrence, but 46% had significant complications, half of which were pancreatic fistulas. This study confirmed that many PNETs are indolent and dormant and can be observed, and there is significant morbidity with pancreatic surgery regardless of surgeon experience and expertise.

Many favor 2 cm as the cutoff size to treat or follow. Bettini and colleagues[49] correlated tumor size and malignant potential and noted higher grade and Ki-67 in larger lesions. In addition to a size greater than 2 cm, symptoms were an independent predictor of malignancy. Gaujoux and colleagues[50] followed 41 patients with asymptomatic sporadic NF-PNETs less than 2 cm. After a median follow-up of 34 months, no patient had distant or nodal metastases on imaging. Other studies have found that larger NF-PNET size up to 3 cm did not correlate with behavior and factors other than size are more important.[45] Jiang and colleagues found a correlation between radiologic tumor diameter of 2.5 cm, high tumor grade, symptoms, and lymph node metastases. Sallinen and colleagues[52] stratified NF-PNETs into 3 groups: less than 2 cm, 2 cm to 4 cm and greater than 4 cm and noted size alone did not predict behavior. Aggressive behavior correlated with symptomatic disease and bile/pancreatic duct obstruction and dilatation even in tumors less than 2 cm. No small asymptomatic tumor developed distant disease or mortality. WHO 2010 grade was highly correlated with overall and disease-free survival. A WHO tumor grade 2 or 3 may be a better indicator of aggressive biology than size and incidental tumors were 4 times less likely to progress than symptomatic patients. These findings suggest that incidental tumors remain indolent and tumor grade and degree of differentiation predict behavior, recurrence, and overall survival. The benefits of observation were reinforced in a matched case-control study by Sadot and colleagues[54], who demonstrated 5-year progression-free survival rates of 95% and 91% ($P = .3$) for observation and resection, respectively. At a median of 7 years, no patient developed cancer. The inclusion cutoff size was 3 cm, again suggesting that size is an inaccurate predictor of malignancy and progression.

A few small NF-PNETs are not dormant and display activity, usually by size increase and less often by symptoms; 19 patients in 3 crossover studies underwent surgery because of increase in tumor size, development of symptoms, or pancreatic duct dilatation.[55] None with malignancy died or had recurrence.[55] This suggests that observation does not compromise outcomes, even if surgery is indicated later, and most NF-PNETs are well behaved citizens.

Risk stratification involves determination of grade, which requires tissue samples acquired by fine-needle aspiration or core biopsy. Calcifications on preoperative CT scans may suggest aggressive behavior.[56,57] Calcifications were present in 321% of PNET's in one series and correlated this finding with higher tumor grade, lymph node, and liver metastasis.[56] Worhunsky and colleagues[57] studied tumor enhancement on CT and correlated it with clinicopathologic factors and overall survival in 118 patients with well-differentiated PNETs. Hypoenhancing PNETs were larger and more often intermediate grade, with higher rates of lymph node and synchronous liver metastases. Hypoenhancing lesions had a poorer prognosis than isoenhancing and hyperenhancing tumors (5-year survival rates, 54% vs 89% vs 93%, respectively).

Surgical treatment, if needed for NF-PNET, depends on tumor size and location within the pancreas. When resection is necessary, 4 operations are favored: enucleation for lesions not contiguous to the pancreatic duct, distal resection of the tail and a segment of the body for distal lesions, central resection for lesions over the superior mesenteric vein not amenable to enucleation, and pancreaticoduodenal resection for some lesions in the head/uncinate of the pancreas.[58–60]

Some technical tips that may be helpful are as follows. Enucleation is associated with a varying rate of pancreatic fistula. For lesions near the pancreatic duct, a preoperative stent placed by ERCP may help identify the duct tumor interface and serve as a stent if the duct is entered. If a stent is not used and intraoperative concern about a fistula is raised, an injection of secretin, which increases pancreatic secretion, resolves the issue. Finally, for central resection, the authors favor closing the distal duct rather than anastomosing it. This has limited fistula rates. The authors drain all resections and enucleations.

SUMMARY

Asymptomatic NF-PNETs are indolent, slow-growing tumors and surveillance is safe and reasonable. Despite consensus, size is less sensitive than grade and Ki-67. Decisions regarding therapy are multifactorial, and a multidisciplinary approach and decision making are a shared process with colleagues, patients, and families. Decisions are balanced by patient morbidities, preferences, and risks. As molecular diagnostics evolves, preoperative acquisition of tissue samples may become even more important in selecting surveillance or resection.

REFERENCES

1. Lawrence B, Gustafsson B, Chan A, et al. The epidemiology of gastroentero-pancreatic neuroendocrine tumors. Endocrinol Metab Clin N Am 2011;40(1):1–18.
2. Cloyd JM, Poultsides GA. Non-functional neuroendocrine tumors of the pancreas: Advances in diagnosis and management. World J Gastroenterol 2015;21(32):9512–25.
3. Vagefi PA, Razo O, Deshpande V, et al. Evolving patterns in the detection and outcomes of pancreatic neuroendocrine neoplasms: the Massachusetts general hospital experience from 1977 to 2005. Arch Surg 2007;142(4):347–54.
4. Ro C, Chai W, Yu VE, et al. Pancreatic neuroendocrine tumors: biology, diagnosis, and treatment. Chin J Cancer 2013;32(6):312–24.
5. Bar-Moshe Y, Mazeh H, Grozinsky-Glasberg S. Non-functioning pancreatic neuroendocrine tumors: Surgery or observation? World J Gastrointest Endosc 2017;9(4):153–61.
6. McKenna LR, Edil BH. Update on pancreatic neuroendocrine tumors. Gland Surg 2014;3(4):258–75.
7. Vortmeyer AO, Huang S, Lubensky I, et al. Nonislet origin of pancreatic islet cell tumors. J Clin Endocrinol Metab 2004;89:1934–8.
8. Jiao Y, Shi C, Edil BH, et al. DAXX/ATRX, MEN1, and mTOR pathway genes are frequently altered in pancreatic neuroendocrine tumors. Science 2011;331:1199–203.
9. Kuo JH, Lee JA, Chabot JA. Nonfunctional pancreatic neuroendocrine tumors. Surg Clin North Am 2014;94:689–708.
10. Oberg K, Modlin IM, De Herder W, et al. Consensus on biomarkers for neuroen-docrine tumour disease. Lancet Oncol 2015;16(9):e435–46.
11. De Herder WW, Niederle B, Scoazec JY, et al. Well-differentiated pancreatic tu-mor/carcinoma: insulinoma. Neuroendocrinology 2006;84:183–8.
12. Jensen RT. Management of the Zollinger-Ellison syndrome in patients with multi-ple endocrine neoplasia type 1. J Intern Med 1998;243:477–88.
13. Van Beek AP, De Haas ER, Van Vloten WA, et al. The glucagonoma syndrome and necrolytic migratory erythema: a clinical review. Eur J Endocrinol 2004;151(5):531–7.
14. Moayedoddin B, Booya F, Wermers RA, et al. Spectrum of malignant somatostatin-producing neuroendocrine tumors. Endocr Pract 2006;12:394–400.
15. Nesi G, Marcucci T, Rubio CA, et al. Somatostatinoma: clinico-pathological fea-tures of three cases and literature reviewed. J Gastroenterol Hepatol 2008;23:521–6.
16. Gut P, Czarnywojtek A, Fischbach J, et al. Chromogranin A – unspecific neuroen-docrine marker. Clinical utility and potential diagnostic pitfalls. Arch Med Sci 2016;12(1):1–9.
17. Modlin IM, Gustafsson BI, Moss SF, et al. Chromogranin A- biological function and clinical utility in neuro-endocrine tumor disease. Ann Surg Oncol 2010;17:2427–43.
18. Dumlu EG, Karakoç D, Özdemir A. Nonfunctional pancreatic neuroendocrine tu-mors: advances in diagnosis, management, and controversies. Int Surg 2015;100(6):1089–97.
19. Jun E, Kim SC, Song KB, et al. Diagnostic value of chromogranin A in pancreatic neuroendocrine tumors depends on tumor size: a prospective observational study from a single institute. Surgery 2017;162(1):120–30.

20. Rockall AG, Reznek RH. Imaging of neuroendocrine tumours (CT/MR/US). Best Pract Res Clin Endocrinol Metab 2007;21:43–68.
21. Maxwell JE, Howe JR. Imaging in neuroendocrine tumors: an update for the clinician. Int J Endocr Oncol 2015;2(2):159–68.
22. Puli SR, Kalva N, Bechtold ML, et al. Diagnostic accuracy of endoscopic ultrasound in pancreatic neuroendocrine tumors: A systematic review and meta analysis. World J Gastroenterol 2013;19(23):3678–84.
23. Khashab MA, Yong E, Lennon AM, et al. EUS is still superior to multidetector computerized tomography for detection of pancreatic neuroendocrine tumors. Gastrointest Endosc 2011;73:691–6.
24. Treglia G, Castaldi P, Rindi G, et al. Diagnostic performance of Gallium-68 somatostatin receptor PET and PET/CT in patients with thoracic and gastroenteropancreatic neuroendocrine tumours: a meta-analysis. Endocrine 2012;42(1): 80–7.
25. Lee I, Paeng JC, Lee SJ, et al. Comparison of diagnostic sensitivity and quantitative indices between 68Ga-DOTATOC PET/CT and 111In-pentetreotide SPECT/CT in neuroendocrine tumors: a preliminary report. Nucl Med Mol Imaging 2015;49(4):284–90.
26. Carrasquillo JA, Chen CC. Molecular imaging of neuroendocrine tumors. Semin Oncol 2010;37(6):662–79.
27. Sharma P, Singh H, Bal C, et al. PET/CT imaging of neuroendocrine tumors with 68Gallium-labeled somatostatin analogues: an overview and single institutional experience from India. Indian J Nucl Med 2014;29(1):2–12.
28. Wild D, Bomanji JB, Benkert P, et al. Comparison of 68Ga-DOTANOC and 68Ga-DOTATATE PET/CT within patients with gastroenteropancreatic neuroendocrine tumors. J Nucl Med 2013;54(3):364–72.
29. Sadowski SM, Neychev V, Millo C, et al. Prospective study of ^{68}Ga-DOTATATE positron emission tomography/computed tomography for detecting gastro-entero-pancreatic neuroendocrine tumors and unknown primary sites. J Clin Oncol 2016;34(6):588–96.
30. Nilica B, Waitz D, Stevanovic V, et al. Direct comparison of ^{68}Ga-DOTA-TOC and ^{18}F-FDG PET/CT in the follow-up of patients with neuroendocrine tumour treated with the first full peptide receptor radionuclide therapy cycle. Eur J Nucl Med Mol Imaging 2016;43:1585–92.
31. Yang M, Ke N, Zeng L, et al. Survival analyses for patients with surgically resected pancreatic neuroendocrine tumors by world health organization 2010 grading classifications and American Joint Committee on Cancer 2010 staging systems. Medicine 2015;94(48):e2156.
32. Ohmoto A, Rokutan H, Yachida S. Pancreatic neuroendocrine neoplasms: basic biology, current treatment strategies and prospects for the future. Int J Mol Sci 2017;18(1):143.
33. Pea A, Hruban RH, Wood LD. Genetics of pancreatic neuroendocrine tumors: implications for the clinic. Expert Rev Gastroenterol Hepatol 2015;9(11):1407–19.
34. Hayward R. Personal view: VOMIT (victims of modern imaging technology)—an acronym for our times. BMJ 2003;326:1273.
35. Roberts WC. Facts and ideas from anywhere. Proc (Bayl Univ Med Cent) 2009; 22(4):377–84.
36. Finkelstein P, Sharma R, Picado O, et al. Pancreatic neuroendocrine tumors (panNETs): analysis of overall survival of nonsurgical management versus surgical resection. J Gastrointest Surg 2017;21(5):855–66.

37. Haynes AB, Deshpande V, Ingkakul T, et al. Implications of incidentally discovered, nonfunctioning pancreatic endocrine tumors: short-term and long-term patient outcomes. Arch Surg 2011;146(5):534–8.

38. Sharpe SM, In H, Winchester DJ, et al. Surgical resection provides an overall survival benefit for patients with small pancreatic neuroendocrine tumors. J Gastrointest Surg 2014;19(1):117–23.

39. Gratian L, Pura J, Dinan M, et al. Impact of extent of surgery on survival in patients with small nonfunctional pancreatic neuroendocrine tumors in the United States. Ann Surg Oncol 2014;21(11):3515–21.

40. Oberg K, Knigge U, Kwekkeboom D, et al. Neuroendocrine gastro-enteropancreatic tumors: ESMO Clinical practice guidelines for diagnosis, treatment and follow-up. Ann Oncol 2012;23(Suppl 7):vii124–30.

41. Lee LC, Grant CS, Salomao DR, et al. Small, nonfunctioning, asymptomatic pancreatic neuroendocrine tumors (PNETs): role for nonoperative management. Surgery 2012;152(6):965–74.

42. Kelgiorgi D, Dervenis C. Pancreatic neuroendocrine tumors: the basics, the gray zone, and the target. F1000Research 2017;6:663.

43. Jung JG, Lee KT, Woo YS, et al. Behavior of small, asymptomatic, nonfunctioning pancreatic neuroendocrine tumors (NF-PNETs). Medicine 2015;94(26):e983.

44. Smith JK, Ng SC, Hill JS, et al. Complications after pancreatectomy for neuroendocrine tumors: a national study. J Surg Res 2010;163:63–8.

45. Falconi M, Bartsch DK, Eriksson B, et al. ENETS consensus guidelines for the management of patients with digestive neuroendocrine neoplasms of the digestive system: well-differentiated pancreatic non-functioning tumors. Neuroendocrinology 2012;95(2):120–34.

46. Kulke MH, Shah MH, Benson AB, et al. Neuroendocrine tumors, version 1.2015. J Natl Compr Canc Netw 2015;13(1):78–108.

47. Kishi Y, Shimada K, Nara S, et al. Basing treatment strategy for non-functional pancreatic neuroendocrine tumors on tumor size. Ann Surg Oncol 2014;21(9):2882–8.

48. Toste P, Kadera B, Tatishchev S, et al. Nonfunctional pancreatic neuroendocrine tumors <2 cm on preoperative imaging are associated with a low incidence of nodal metastasis and an excellent overall survival. J Gastrointest Surg 2013;17:2105–13.

49. Bettini R, Partelli S, Boninsegna L, et al. Tumor size correlates with malignancy in nonfunctioning pancreatic endocrine tumor. Surgery 2011;150:75–82.

50. Gaujoux S, Partelli S, Maire F, et al. Observational study of natural history of small sporadic nonfunctioning pancreatic tumors. J Clin Endocrinol Metab 2013;98(12):4784–9.

51. Jiang Y, Jin JB, Zhan Q, et al. Impact and clinical predictors of lymph node metastases in nonfunctional pancreatic neuroendocrine tumors. Chin Med J 2015;128(24):3335–44.

52. Sallinen V, Le L, Galeev S, et al. Surveillance strategy for small asymptomatic non-functional pancreatic neuroendocrine tumors–a systematic review and meta-analysis. HPB (Oxford) 2017;19(4):310–20.

53. Sallinen V, Haglund C, Seppänen H. Outcomes of resected nonfunctional pancreatic neuroendocrine tumors: do size and symptoms matter? Surgery 2015;158(6):1556–63.

54. Sadot E, Reidy-Lagunes DL, Tang LH, et al. Observation versus resection for small asymptomatic pancreatic neuroencrine tumors: a matched case–control study. Ann Surg Oncol 2016;23(4):1361–70.

55. Guo J, Zhao J, Bi X, et al. Should surgery be conducted for small nonfunctioning pancreatic neuroendocrine tumors: a systematic review. Oncotarget 2017;8(21): 35368–75.
56. Poultsides GA, Huang LC, Chen Y, et al. Pancreatic neuroendocrine tumors: radiographic calcifications correlate with grade and metastasis. Ann Surg Oncol 2012;19:2295–303.
57. Worhunsky DJ, Krampitz GW, Poullos PD, et al. Pancreatic neuroendocrine tumours: hypoenhancement on arterial phase computed tomography predicts biological aggressiveness. HPB (Oxford) 2014;16(4):304–11.
58. Pitt SC, Pitt HA, Baker MS, et al. Small pancreatic and periampullary neuroendocrine tumors: resect or enucleate? J Gastrointest Surg 2009;13:1692–8.
59. Falconi M, Zerbi A, Crippa S, et al. Parenchyma-preserving resections for small nonfunctioning pancreatic endocrine tumors. Ann Surg Oncol 2010;17:1621–7.
60. Du ZY, Chen S, Han BS, et al. Middle segmental pancreatectomy: a safe and organ-preserving option for benign and low-grade malignant lesions. World J Gastroenterol 2013;19:1458–65.

Rare Tumors and Lesions of the Pancreas

John A. Stauffer, MD, Horacio J. Asbun, MD*

KEYWORDS

- Pancreatectomy • Pancreatic neoplasm • Anaplastic carcinoma
- Adenosquamous carcinoma • Solid pseudopapillary tumor • Acinar cell carcinoma
- Primary pancreatic lymphoma • Unusual pancreas tumors

KEY POINTS

- Rare pancreatic tumors of the pancreas include adenocarcinoma variants, such as anaplastic carcinoma, adenosquamous carcinoma, colloid, hepatoid, and medullary carcinoma.
- Other neoplasms include acinar cell carcinoma, solid pseudopapillary tumor, sarcomas, or lymphomas.
- Benign solid or cystic masses, such as hamartoma, hemangioma, lymphangioma, or others also may mimic neoplastic disease.
- The pancreas may be the site of isolated metastatic disease, such as renal cell cancer, colorectal cancer, melanoma, and other carcinomas.
- Pancreatic inflammatory diseases may mimic solid neoplasms of the pancreas.

Primary pancreatic ductal adenocarcinoma (PDAC) is the most common neoplasm of the pancreas. Pancreatic neuroendocrine tumors (PNETs) are much less common but their incidence has increased over the past decade due to the increased use of cross-sectional imaging.[1] Cystic lesions, such as intraductal papillary mucinous neoplasm (IPMN), mucinous cystic neoplasms (MCN), and serous cystic neoplasms (SCN) are also relatively common. The pancreas is a complex organ that harbors a wide array of diseases. There are a variety of non-neoplastic conditions that mimic PDAC, such as groove pancreatitis (GP) and autoimmune pancreatitis (AIP).[2,3] Additionally, there are a handful of other rare neoplastic lesions infrequently found in patients with pancreatic masses that range from well known (eg, solid pseudopapillary neoplasm and acinar cell carcinoma) to less well known (eg, leiomyosarcoma and hepatoid carcinoma). Rare cystic lesions can be misdiagnosed for the more common

Disclosures: The authors have nothing to disclose.
Department of Surgery, Mayo Clinic, 4500 San Pablo Road South, Jacksonville, FL 32224, USA
* Corresponding author. Division of General Surgery, Mayo Clinic, 4500 San Pablo Road South, Jacksonville, FL 32224.
E-mail address: asbun.horacio@mayo.edu

Surg Clin N Am 98 (2018) 169–188
https://doi.org/10.1016/j.suc.2017.09.013   surgical.theclinics.com

mucinous, serous, or inflammatory pancreatic lesions. Peripancreatic solid lesions or duodenal pathology occasionally can be mistaken for pancreatic pathology as well. Finally, the pancreas is a potential site for metastatic disease, such as renal cell carcinoma (RCC), or can be involved with other diseases, such as primary pancreatic lymphoma. Any of these lesions can be mistaken for PDAC.

Contrast-enhanced computerized tomography (CT) is the most common modality to detect and diagnose pancreatic pathology. Endoscopic ultrasound (EUS) and MRI with cholangiopancreatography (MRCP) have distinct advantages in hepatopancreatobiliary imaging that may clarify the diagnosis of an unknown pancreatic mass. EUS allows gastroduodenal mucosal evaluation, and has perhaps the highest sensitivity for small lesions of the pancreas (eg, subcentimeter PNET and mural nodules within IPMN), as well as enabling direct tissue sampling with fine-needle aspiration. High-quality MRI with MRCP provides detailed anatomic information of the pancreas and ductal structures that cannot be obtained with any other modality. Additionally, with an appropriate protocol, the MRI can provide conspicuity of any liver lesions associated with pancreatic disease surpass the images of the highest-quality triple-phase CT.[4,5] Complete evaluation by an experienced team is warranted for all with pancreatic neoplasms. A multidisciplinary approach with knowledgeable surgeons, gastroenterologists, radiologists, oncologists, pathologists, and others limit misdiagnosis and/or mismanagement of the following rare pancreatic findings.

ADENOCARCINOMA VARIANTS

Ductal adenocarcinoma of the pancreas with tubular morphology accounts for more than 90% of pancreatic carcinoma. There are variants of adenocarcinoma with a different prognosis that should be distinguished from PDAC.

Anaplastic (Undifferentiated) Adenocarcinoma (Also with Osteoclastlike Giant Cells)

Anaplastic pancreatic carcinomas (APCs) are rare neoplasms that represent 2% to 7% of all exocrine pancreatic tumors. First described by Sommer and Meissner in 1954[6] they are referred to as undifferentiated carcinoma with or without osteoclastlike giant cells, carcinosarcoma, sarcomatoid carcinoma, pleomorphic carcinoma, pleomorphic giant-cell carcinoma, and pleomorphic large-cell carcinoma of the pancreas. This undifferentiated carcinoma is an aggressive epithelial neoplasm that does not display significant components of differentiated lesions. Anaplastic foci can be seen within PDAC but as a minor component. The male-to-female ratio is 3 to 1 and generally affects older men (**Fig. 1**). The lesions are distributed throughout the pancreas and are often quite large when diagnosed (average of up to 9–10 cm).[7,8] The literature focuses on histology, immunohistochemistry, electron microscopy, and gene expression of APCs. Many studies note a poor outcome after resection due to its systemic nature, but other larger studies have shown benefit to resection.[7,9] Hoshimoto and colleagues[10] reported 60 cases of APC resected in Japan with a mean age at diagnosis of 61.5 years, 63% male, and a median size of 6 cm. Nearly one-fourth required resection of adjacent organs and vascular involvement was present in (12%). Although half died within 1 year of surgery, the 5-year survival rate was 12%.[10] Strobel and colleagues[11] reported a single institutional experience of 18 patients with APC who underwent attempted resection and compared them to a similar group with PDAC. They noted a median survival of only 5.7 months, but a margin-negative resection extended survival and 17% were long-term survivors.[11] Paniccia and colleagues[12] matched 192 patients with APC from the National Cancer Data Base with 960 PDAC patients. They too noted a 1-year survival that was lower than PDAC with a similar overall long-term survival.

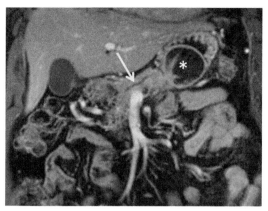

Fig. 1. Coronal MRI showing 6-cm mass in the tail of the pancreas in a 69-year-old man. Distal pancreatectomy with en bloc partial gastrectomy, splenectomy, and adrenalectomy was performed with pathology revealing anaplastic (undifferentiated) carcinoma with extensive necrosis. The tumor had focal areas (<10%) of conventional adenocarcinoma and 0/40 lymph nodes involved. The patient was alive without disease 2 years later. Asterisk indicates tumor with invasion into the posterior wall of the stomach, arrow indicates main pancreatic duct.

The presence of osteoclastlike giant cells implied a significantly better prognosis.[12] Clark and colleagues[13] evaluated the Surveillance, Epidemiology, and End Results (SEER) database over 20 years and found that the median survival of 353 APC patients was only 3 months, significantly worse than 5859 patients with PDAC (11 months). However, for those who underwent surgical resection, the overall survival was not significantly different (12% vs 24%).[13] Multiple single-center and population-based studies have confirmed the aggressive nature of APCs but operative intervention is advised when technically feasible and patient comorbidities are acceptable.

Adenosquamous Carcinoma

Adenosquamous carcinoma (ASC) is a rare and aggressive subtype of pancreatic carcinoma with glandular and squamous differentiation, the latter of which accounts for at least 30% of the neoplasm (**Fig. 2**).[8] First reported by G. Herxheimer in 1907,[14] the

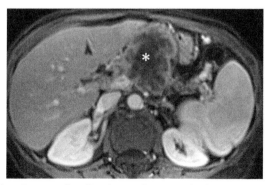

Fig. 2. Axial MRI showing 5-cm locally advanced mass in the head and body of the pancreas in an 83-year-old woman. EUS with fine needle aspiration confirmed adenosquamous carcinoma. Asterisk indicates tumor with obliteration of the superior mesenteric vein.

lesion has acquired several names, including adenoacanthoma, adenocarcinoma with squamous metaplasia, and mucoepidermoid carcinoma. This tumor is differentiated from metastatic squamous cell carcinoma to the pancreas by its glandular elements.[8] ASC has a poor prognosis and a short survival. Katz and colleagues[15] matched 95 California Cancer Registry patients over 8 years and with a similar group with PDAC. Despite a larger tumor (4.6 cm vs 3.4 cm), ASC patients were more likely to undergo surgery (33% vs 17%) Involved lymph nodes and adjuvant therapy were similar in both groups. Overall survival was equally poor with unresectable disease, but better after resection.[15] The SEER database from 1998 to 2007 was used to compare 415 ASC patients to 45,693 with PDAC. ASC was more likely to occur in the tail of the pancreas, be poorly differentiated, larger, and have more positive nodes than PDAC. Katz and colleagues[15] found that disease-specific one and 2 year survival was only 30.5% and 19.7% (median survival of 7 months) which was significantly worse than PDAC.[16] Similarly, a single-center study of 28 ASC cases by Imaoka and colleagues[17] reported that ASC had a worse survival than PDAC compared 56 matched with PDAC. Resection may improve the chance for long-term survival and is recommended when feasible.

Hepatoid Carcinoma

Hepatoid carcinomas (HCs) are malignant extrahepatic epithelial neoplasms with morphologic and immunohistologic features of hepatocellular carcinoma (HCC). Like HCC, they have elevated serum alpha-fetoprotein (AFP) and an older age at diagnosis. The main differential lesion is metastases from a liver primary.[18] Because both acinar cell and pancreatoblastoma have acinar cell differentiation that may secrete lipase, trypsin, chymotrypsin, or serum alpha-fetoprotein, lesions that must be differentiated from HC. Immunohistochemical labeling for HC is positive for hepatocyst paraffin-1, polyclonal carcinoembryonic antigen, and CD10.[8] HC lesions are often large and late stage at presentation. Marchegiani and colleagues[18] reported 22 HCs in the world literature. Only 15 patients underwent surgical resection but resected patients had a better long-term survival.[18] Systemic therapies are neither standardized nor very effective, but some report limited success with the tyrosine kinase inhibitor sorafenib.[19] Kuo and colleagues[20] reported that 40% of these tumors had other tumor components, such as PNET, PDAC, or acinar cell carcinoma (ACC) and that radical surgery was the only chance for long-term survival.

Colloid Carcinoma (Mucinous Noncystic Carcinoma)

Colloid carcinoma of the pancreas is a mucin-producing epithelial cell adenocarcinoma "floating" within large pools of extracellular mucin. The colloid generally comprises at least 80% of the neoplasm plus a tubular component, and the lesion is also known as mucinous noncystic carcinoma.[8] This is a subtype of IPMN with more indolent behavior which is attributed to 2 morphologic features of mucin overproduction. First, the mucin is secreted toward the cell-stroma interface and detaches the epithelial cells from the stroma. Second, the mucin acts as a barrier limiting the spread of neoplastic cells.[21] The differential diagnosis includes MCN and IPMN. Overall survival is as high as 70% and 57% at 2 and 5 years.[22]

Medullary Carcinoma

Medullary carcinoma of the pancreas is a rare variant of a malignant epithelial neoplasm that is characterized by poor differentiation, syncytial growth pattern, well-defined borders, and areas of focal necrosis.[8] It was first described in 1998 and often has DNA replication errors associated with wild-type K-RAS or microsatellite instability.[23] Because of this, medullary carcinoma may be a focal point for clinicians who study inherited pancreatic cancer syndromes.[24] Because of limited data, survival of medullary carcinoma compared with PDAC is unknown.

MISCELLANEOUS NEOPLASMS
Neoplastic Potential

Acinar cell carcinoma

ACC was first described in 1908 by Berner[25] as a syndrome of fever, polyarthritis, subcutaneous fat nodular necrosis, and eosinophilia. This syndrome is initiated by tumor hypersecretion of lipase. ACC tumors are very large, exophytic, well-circumscribed, and hypovascular with minimal stroma throughout the pancreas.[26] These tumors occur in older patients and are quite rare, accounting for fewer than 1% of all pancreatic tumors despite that the pancreas has more than 80% volume of acinar cells. ACC may be found in the pediatric population, where it accounts for 15% of all pediatric pancreatic neoplasms.[8] Although most acinar cell neoplasms are solid malignant tumor, rare subtypes, such as acinar cell cystadenoma, acinar cell cystadenocarcinoma, or a mixed tumor are found. A characteristic paraneoplastic process, lipase hypersecretion syndrome is found in 10% to 15% of patients, and is identified by a serum lipase >10,000 U/dL. It is characterized by multiple nodular foci of subcutaneous fat necrosis and polyarthralgia due to sclerotic bone lesions from fat necrosis. The syndrome usually resolves after tumor resection (**Fig. 3**).[27] Alternatively, in diffuse metastatic or unresectable disease, combined chemotherapy with oxaliplatin, irinotecan, and fluorouracil (FOLFIRINOX) may alleviate symptoms from lipase hypersecretion.[28]

The overall prognosis of ACC is unclear. In a recent report from China, Wang and colleagues[26] described 19 patients treated over 20 years. The predominate symptoms were abdominal pain and weight loss, and the ACC tumors were equally distributed in the head and tail. Interestingly, no patient developed jaundice despite large tumors in the head, and only 2 had elevated serum lipase. CA 19-9 was normal in all. Only 14 patients underwent an R0 resection with a median tumor size of 5.4 cm with 1 postoperative mortality. Surgical resection was associated with a longer median survival (19 vs 9 months), as was adjuvant chemotherapy. When matched to a similar group with PDAC, ACC patients were younger (54 vs 65 years), more often (84 vs 53%), with larger tumors (5.3 vs 3.1 cm), earlier stage, and a longer median survival (18 vs 4 months).[26] Matos and colleagues[29] reported a multi-institutional review of 17 ACC patients over 20 years. Four had elevated serum lipase, but none had lipase hypersecretion syndrome. Most (15) underwent resection, with a 1-year and 5-year survival rates of 88% and 50%.[29]

ACC is a rare pancreatic tumor that may be difficult to differentiate from PDAC, but is best treated by surgical resection when feasible. Long-term outcomes and prognosis are similar if not slightly better than that of PDAC.

Solid pseudopapillary neoplasm

Solid pseudopapillary neoplasms (SPNs) are a distinct, low-grade, malignant epithelial tumor first described by Frantz in 1959.[30] The lesions are distinct, a solid mass with cystic degeneration often with intracystic hemorrhage. They are also classified as papillary epithelial neoplasm, papillary cystic neoplasm, solid and papillary neoplasm, low-grade papillary neoplasm, and Hamoudi or Frantz tumor.[8] The female-to-male ratio is 10:1 and it usually presents in the second or third decade with a large mass causing abdominal symptoms, but rarely jaundice or pancreatitis despite its large size. SPNs are located throughout the pancreas, but are more frequent in the body and tail. The differential diagnosis includes PDAC, cystadenoma, cystadenocarcinoma, neuroendocrine

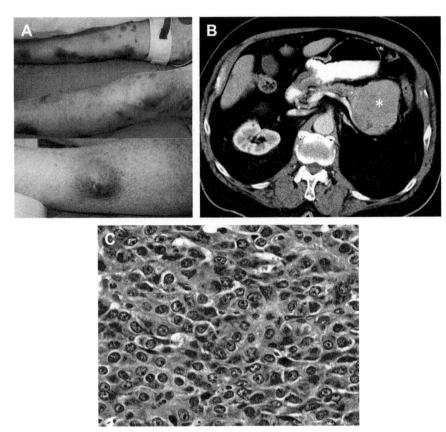

Fig. 3. (*A*) Photographs of diffuse subcutaneous nodules found on a 79-year-old man. The nodules were erythematous, firm, and cystic, with overlying epithelial exfoliation. They started on the lower extremities but spread to the whole body. Serum lipase was noted to be >13,000 U/L. (*B*) Axial CT showing 9-cm mass in the tail of the pancreas in this same patient. Asterisk indicates tumor (*C*) The serum lipase returned to normal after distal pancreatectomy. High-powered magnification of the pancreas mass showed poorly differentiated ACC. The tumor predominantly had a solid growth with a trabecular pattern. The cells had abundant basophilic cytoplasm with large nuclei and prominent nucleoli (hematoxylin-eosin, original magnification × 20).

tumor, or pancreatic cyst.[31] Usually serum tumor markers are normal and cross-sectional imaging shows a well-encapsulated complex mass containing solid and cystic components. SPNs should be suspected when hemorrhage into a nonseptated cystic mass is seen in the distal part of the pancreas in a young woman. For female patients below 40, this tumor accounts for more than 70% of pancreatic resections.

Although SPN is generally indolent, malignancy develops in up to 15% of patients. Nodal disease is rare and metastases are by local or hematogenous invasion, which most frequently involves the liver, regional lymph nodes, mesentery, omentum, and peritoneum. Vascular and/or visceral invasion is not uncommon due to their large size (**Figs. 4** and **5**).

Margin-negative surgical resection is the curative goal. Despite locally advanced or metastatic disease, the prognosis is generally quite good. Lubezky and colleagues[32] recently published their experience with 32 margin-negative SPN's. The mean tumor

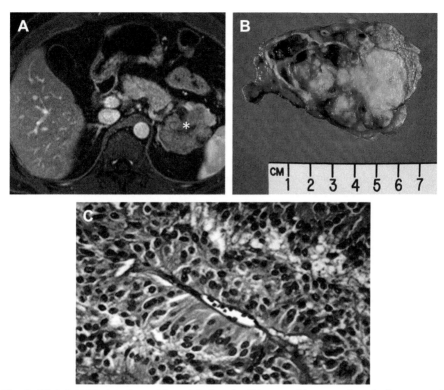

Fig. 4. (*A*) Axial MRI showing a 5.6-cm lobulated solid mass with areas of cystic changes and necrosis in the tail of the pancreas in a 39-year-old man. The splenic vessels were draped over the lesion and patent. Asterisk indicates tumor. (*B*) Distal pancreatectomy was performed and gross pathology pictures show an encapsulated, heterogeneous solid and cystic mass in the tail of the pancreas; 0/10 lymph nodes were involved. (*C*) Microscopic pictures of pseudopapillae arranged around vascular stalks indicated SPN. The tumor stained positive for synaptophysin, CD 10, and beta-catenin and negative for chromogranin and pancytokeratin (hematoxylin-eosin, original magnification × 20).

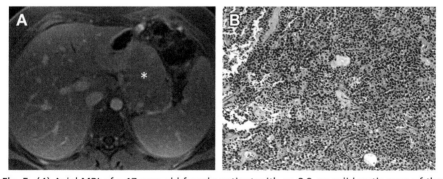

Fig. 5. (*A*) Axial MRI of a 17-year-old female patient with an 8.8-cm solid cystic mass of the tail of the pancreas. Asterisk indicates tumor. (*B*) Microscopic picture of SPN. Immunohistochemistry stains were positive for vimentin, CD 10, progesterone, beta-catenin, cytokeratin, and synaptophysin, and negative for chromogranin, E-cadherin, and trypsin (hematoxylin-eosin, original magnification × 10).

size was 5.9 cm, and 91% of the patients were women with a mean age of 28 years. The 5-year and 10-year disease-free survival was 97% and 90%. Four patients had metastatic disease, including 1 with multiple bilobar liver metastases which was stable at 37 months post resection. Three others underwent hepatectomy or observation and remained disease-free or stable in a lengthy follow-up.[32] In a recent multi-institutional report of 131 SPN patients, two with metastases underwent synchronous hepatopancreatectomy with good outcomes. Only two had recurrence 5 and 6 years after partial pancreatectomy. Disease-specific survival and disease-free survival were 98% at 5 years.[33]

Overall, SPN is a rare, indolent tumor that should be classified "malignant" only when metastatic or recurrent is evident. When indicated surgical resection is the treatment of choice for localized, metastatic, or recurrent SPN.

Pancreatoblastoma

Pancreatoblastoma is a malignant epithelial tumor that includes acinar, squamoid nests, endocrine, and ductal differentiation. They may be large at presentation and have elevated AFP levels.[8] This is the most common pancreatic neoplasm of childhood and young adults, in whom the prognosis is worse.[34] Surgical resection is indicated, although the disease often is advanced at presentation with an aggressive course and poor outcome, similar to ACC.

Schwannoma

Schwann cell tumors (Schwannoma) are mesenchymal tumors of peripheral nerve sheaths that are located throughout the body, including the pancreas. Pancreatic schwannoma are rare with fewer than 70 reported cases in the past 4 decades. Pathology shows a well-encapsulated lesion of spindle-shaped cells without atypia. Immunohistochemical staining is positive for protein S-100. The age at diagnosis is relatively young, and surgical resection is preferred.[35] These tumors are often incidental findings with an excellent overall prognosis. There are 5 reported malignant pancreatic schwannomas.[36] Degenerative changes, such as cystic formation, calcification, hemorrhage, hyalinization, or xanthomatous infiltration, are present in two-thirds of patients. Preoperative diagnosis by EUS with fine-needle aspiration will differentiate this tumor from cystic PNET, SPN, MCN, or pseudocysts.[37]

Angiosarcoma

Primary angiosarcoma of the pancreas are aggressive and extremely rare lesions, with only 5 reported cases. They present with gastrointestinal bleeding, weight loss, and abdominal pain. Surgical resection for localized disease may be curative. Risk factors for angiosarcoma include radiation, chronic lymphedema, certain familial syndromes and chemical carcinogens, but specific risk factors are not known.[38,39]

Perivascular epithelioid cell neoplasms

Perivascular epithelioid cell neoplasm (PEComa) are another mesenchymal neoplasm that arise from perivascular epithelioid cells and may occur in the pancreas. Composed of large epithelioid and spindle cells with a characteristic nuclei pattern, HMB45 immunostaining will be strongly positive. These tumors are also known as clear-cell "sugar" tumors, and angiomyolipoma (AML). AML typically occurs in the kidney.[40] Fewer than 10 cases of PEComa have been reported, including patients with local recurrence and metastatic disease after primary tumor resection. Metastatic melanoma, gastrointestinal stromal tumor (GIST), and clear-cell carcinoma are diagnostic considerations. Resection and frequent follow-up are warranted, as the prognosis is generally very good.[41–43]

Primary leiomyosarcoma

Primary pancreatic leiomyosarcoma is rare and accounts for most pancreatic sarcomas. It may mimic other rare neoplasms, such as GIST, solitary fibrous tumor, inflammatory myofibroblastic tumor, malignant schwannoma, liposarcoma, rhabdomyosarcoma, and anaplastic carcinoma. They are highly aggressive neoplasms with fewer than 40 cases in the English literature,[44,45] including 9 patients by Zhang and colleagues[46] who noted an equal male:female distribution, and a mean age and tumor size of 63 years and 1. Resection was possible in 4 (no lymph nodes were involved), but liver metastases were evident in 5 and overall mean survival was only 31 months with 5 having disease-related deaths.[46] This tumor presents late and is treated with doxorubicin-based chemotherapy with a poor response rate.[47] Surgical resection may benefit localized disease.[48]

Solitary fibrous tumor

Solitary fibrous tumor of the pancreas is a rare benign entity with fewer than 20 reported cases.[44,49,50] Most (81%) were women with a median age of 54 years, and a mean tumor size of 5.8 cm, with lesions distributed throughout the pancreas. Excision reveals a well-circumscribed encapsulated mass that is positive on immunohistochemical staining for CD34, vimentin, CD 99, and/or Bcl-2 but not CD117.

Primary pancreatic lymphoma

Primary pancreatic lymphoma (PPL) is another rare entity that can be very difficult to diagnose and is the "mimicker" of the more common PDAC. An accurate diagnosis is important because the treatment is chemotherapy and radiotherapy. Diagnostic criteria for PPL include (1) no superficial or mediastinal lymphadenopathy, (2) a normal leukocyte count, (3) a pancreatic or lymph-node mass in the peripancreatic region, and (4) absent hepatic and splenic involvement.[51] The most common pancreatic variant is diffuse large B-cell lymphoma, accounting for 80% of PPL. Common presenting symptoms are abdominal pain, jaundice, pancreatitis, small bowel obstruction, and diarrhea. Classic symptoms of fever, chills, and night sweats are uncommon.[52] Imaging characteristics include a large infiltrative mass with peripancreatic stranding and infrequent biliary, pancreatic duct, or venous obstruction. Some PPLs present as well-circumscribed tumors with infrarenal lymphadenopathy (**Fig. 6**).[53] The differential

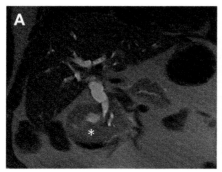

Fig. 6. (*A*) Coronal MRCP with a 7-cm mass of the head of the pancreas causing biliary and duodenal obstruction in a 64-year-old man. Asterisk indicates mass. (*B*) EUS and fine-needle aspiration showed PPL. Staining was positive for CD20, PAX-5, Bcl-6, and CD10 and negative for CD3. There was c-Myc/immunoglobulin H translocation consistent with B-cell lymphoma (hematoxylin-eosin, original magnification × 4). The patient was successfully treated with biliary stenting followed by rituximab, cyclophosphamide, vincristine, Adriamycin, and prednisone (R-CHOP).

diagnosis beside PDAC includes secondary lymphoma, pancreatitis, AIP, PNET, or ACC. Biopsy is indicated for a large bulky pancreatic mass that infiltrates beyond normal anatomic barriers, stretches local vasculature without infiltration, normal PDAC tumor markers, and elevated serum lactate dehydrogenase. This disease is treatable in all stages and endoscopic or percutaneous diagnosis is preferred.[51] Sadot and colleagues[54] reported 44 patients with PPL. Three-fourths of patients achieved complete remission, with a median overall survival of 6.1 years and a 10-year disease-specific survival of 69%. The follicular lymphoma subtype has the best prognosis, with a 100% 5-year survival. Long-term surveillance is indicated to exclude relapse.[54]

Collision/mixed tumors

Collision tumors are defined and classified by the World Health Organization as at least 2 different malignant components occurring within a tumor in the same organ or anatomic site.[55] Various combinations have been noted, including combinations of PDAC and PNET,[56] IPMN and PNET,[57,58] SPN and PNET,[59] hepatoid carcinoma and PNET,[20] mixed ACC with either PNET or PDAC,[27,60] or PDAC and biliary carcinoma.[61] For collision tumors, the possibility of metastatic disease must be ruled out, but the incidence of diagnosed dual cancers is increasing and more frequently recognized.[61]

BENIGN SOLID/CYSTIC
Hamartomas

Pancreatic hamartomas are rare with fewer than 31 reported cases. They are a malformation rather than a neoplasm and are quite benign. The median age at presentation is 50.4 years with equal sex predilection. They present as solid or solid/cystic patterns and are isolated or multiple. The average size is <5 cm and they occur anywhere within the pancreas. Most have been resected due to the uncertain nature of a pancreatic mass, but if the diagnosis is known they can and should be observed.[62–64]

Hemangioma

Pancreatic cavernous hemangioma is rare in adults. They are benign variants of vascular tumors that include lymphangioma, hemolymphangioma, hemangioendothelioma, hemangiopericytoma, hemangioblastoma, and angiosarcoma. Visceral hemangiomas are most common in the liver, but are found anywhere in the gastrointestinal tract. In a review of pancreatic hemangiomas, Mondal and colleagues[65] identified 21 cases with an average age of 48 years and male-to-female ratio of 1:3. Symptoms included abdominal pain in half. Hemangiomas occur with von Hippel-Lindau disease. They are quite benign and surgical resection should be avoided.[65] Pediatric hemangiomas may involute but adult pancreatic hemangiomas do not. They rarely obstruct or infiltrate despite large size or continued slow growth. They may be difficult to distinguish from other highly vascular tumors, especially metastatic RCC.[66] Some advise surgical resection in a pregnant patient to avoid rupture, but this is controversial and should be performed selectively.[67]

Lymphangioma

Pancreatic lymphangioma is an uncommon benign cystic tumor of the pancreas. There are 4 subtypes, dependent on the depth and size of abnormal lymph vessels: capillary lymphangioma, cavernous lymphangioma, cystic hygroma, or hemolymphangioma. They are congenital and originate from mesenchymal tissue. Less often they develop from poor lymph drainage or lymphatic injury. They are identified macroscopically as thin-walled cysts with multiple septa and variable-sized cystic cavities containing clear or hemorrhage lymph fluid. They are generally asymptomatic and are diagnosed incidentally. Surgical removal is indicated for symptomatic disease or to exclude other disease when the diagnosis is uncertain (**Fig. 7**). Incomplete resection can lead to recurrence.[68,69]

Pancreatic Lymphoepithelial Cyst

Lymphoepithelial cysts (LECs) consist of keratinized material lined by mature squamous epithelium surrounded by lymphatic tissue. Pancreatic LECs are true cystic lesions with no malignant potential and are very similar to squamoid cysts, mucinous non-neoplastic cysts, enterogenous cysts, endometrial cysts, and retention cysts or simple cysts. They account for less than 2% of pancreatectomy.[70] These cysts do not have any solid components but may occasionally have septations. The differential diagnoses of LECs includes MCN, SCN, and IPMN. EUS-guided biopsy with aspiration can be diagnostic and is recommended for all unknown cystic lesions of the pancreas. However, the clinician should be aware that a simple cyst may become complex on imaging after fine-needle aspiration with intracystic hemorrhage.[71,72]

Intrapancreatic Accessory Spleen

Intrapancreatic accessory spleen (IPAS) is a congenital anomaly caused by failure of fusion during embryology. The incidence is 10% to 15% in the general population and the tail of the pancreas is the second most common site after the hilum of the spleen.[73] They are commonly detected because of the increased frequency and sensitivity of abdominal imaging. IPASs are generally small and match the density of the spleen on all contrast phases. They can, however, be mistaken for other enhancing pancreatic lesions of the tail, including PNET, SPN, and metastatic disease. Nuclear medicine imaging can be used to confirm this diagnosis, and biopsy is rarely required.[74,75]

Plasmacytoma

Pancreatic plasmacytoma is most commonly associated with multiple myeloma and results from extramedullary plasmacytoma, which is a discrete collection of monoclonal plasmocytes arising in tissues other than bone. In the gastrointestinal tract, the liver and spleen are more commonly involved and pancreatic involvement is

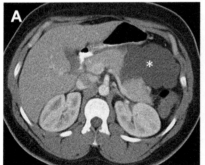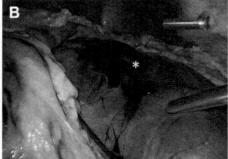

Fig. 7. (*A*) Axial CT showing a large multilobulated cystic mass in the lesser sac arising from the body of the pancreas causing abdominal pain in a 22-year-old woman. Asterisk indicates cyst. (*B*) Intraoperative picture of a cystic lesion of the tail of the pancreas. Limited pancreatic resection and excision of the mass confirmed complete resection of a 15-cm lymphangioma with resolution of the patient's symptoms. Asterisk indicates cyst.

rare.[76] Williet and colleagues[77] identified 63 reported cases of pancreatic plasmacytoma with a mean age of 58.5 years. Seventy percent presented with jaundice and only 2 cases were in the body or tail of the pancreas. Biopsy, whether percutaneous, endoscopic, or surgical, is indicated, and treatment with chemotherapy or radiotherapy resulted in 100% response rates.[77]

Pancreatic Sarcoidosis

Sarcoidosis is a granulomatous syndrome of unknown etiology that can involve all organ systems in the body, most commonly lung and lymph. Gastrointestinal involvement occurs in fewer than 1% and pancreatic sarcoidosis is rare; however, it can present with pancreatic involvement and be mistaken for pancreatitis or PDAC. Abdominal symptoms and lymphadenopathy can be seen, but high-quality imaging and tissue diagnosis will differentiate this from similar entities, and surgical intervention can be avoided.[78,79]

Pancreatic Tuberculosis

Pancreatic tuberculosis (TB) is an extremely rare presentation of abdominal TB. The retroperitoneal location and enzymatic environment of the pancreas is thought to protect it from exposure and mycobacterium invasion. However, there are reports of isolated pancreatic TB causing symptoms that mimic pancreatic malignancy. EUS with biopsy and findings of caseating necrosis, granuloma, and acid-fast bacteria have become the method of choice for the diagnosis of pancreatic TB.[80–82]

METASTATIC TUMORS
Renal Cell Carcinoma

RCC has a propensity to metastasize to the pancreas and can present as a solitary mass or multiple masses within the pancreas. It can present many years after the initial diagnosis of RCC and it should be considered in all patients with a history of RCC who present with a pancreatic mass (**Fig. 8**). Adler and colleagues[83] reported in a literature review of 399 patients who underwent pancreatectomy for metastases, that RCC was responsible for 62.6% of all operations. The prognosis is quite good for isolated RCC involvement of the pancreas after surgical resection with a 5-year survival of 70.4%. This was significantly better than for non-RCC pancreatic metastasectomies.[83]

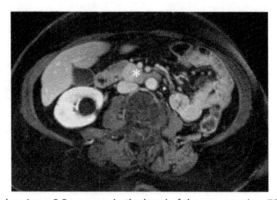

Fig. 8. Axial MRI showing a 2.3-cm mass in the head of the pancreas in a 70-year-old woman with a history of left-sided renal cell cancer 4 years prior. Pancreatic resection revealed isolated metastatic RCC. Asterisk indicates mass.

Konstantinidis and colleagues[84] reported 20 patients who underwent pancreatic resection for RCC, with most being male (65%) and a median age of 68.5 years. The right and left kidneys were the equally involved and 25% had multiple metastases in the pancreas. These lesions were equally distributed throughout the pancreas and 19 of 20 presented with metachronous disease at a median of 8.7 years after nephrectomy. Total pancreatectomy, central pancreatectomy, and enucleation were used as indicated, as well as Whipple and distal pancreatectomy. Actual 5-year survival was 61%.[84] RCC is the most common metastatic lesion to the pancreas requiring surgical resection. These tumors may mimic PNET and are generally very well circumscribed and may have cystic degeneration. For isolated RCC in the pancreas, surgical intervention is clearly indicated.[85]

Melanoma

Malignant melanoma can develop multiple distant metastases in the gastrointestinal tract; however, pancreatic involvement is rare.[86] The literature is limited regarding metastatic pancreatic melanoma and its surgical treatment. Most patients present with a symptomatic mass with or without a known previous melanoma.[86,87] The tumor is commonly discovered after cross-imaging techniques, and the diagnosis of metastatic melanoma is established by fine-needle biopsy. Goyal and colleagues[87] reported 5 patients treated with pancreatoduodenectomy and distal pancreatectomy and the median survival was only 11.4 months.

Lung Carcinoma

Common sites of lung cancer metastasis are brain, bones, liver, and adrenal with the pancreas rarely involved.[88,89] A retrospective study of 2872 patients with non–small-cell lung carcinoma revealed pancreatic disease in just 17 patients (0.59%).[90] Small-cell lung cancer is the most common histologic subtype that metastasizes to the pancreas from the lung.[88] In most cases, metachronous pancreatic metastases are found incidentally during the evaluation of patients with lung cancer, indicating stage IV disease. Lung metastases to the pancreas have poor outcomes.[88,90] There is controversy regarding attempted curative pancreatectomy for metachronous pancreatic metastasis from lung carcinoma (**Fig. 9**). A single study reported 3 resections with

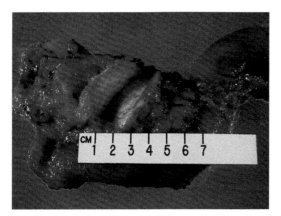

Fig. 9. Gross photograph of an isolated metastatic lung adenocarcinoma lesion within the head of the pancreas in an 84-year-old man. He remained disease-free 5 years after undergoing pancreaticoduodenectomy.

recurrence in all.[91] Others report better results and recommend resection and systemic therapy in select patients.[90,92]

Breast Carcinoma

Breast adenocarcinoma metastasis to the pancreas is extremely rare compared with other distant sites, such as kidney, lung, and colon.[93] The literature is limited to a few case reports. According to Bednar and colleagues,[94] approximately 5% of patients operated for pancreatic metastasis were found to have breast adenocarcinoma, and an autopsy series reported pancreatic involvement in 13%.[95] They present as mass lesions in the pancreas on follow-up imaging studies, and patients may have jaundice, abdominal pain, or disseminated disease.[93] Surgery relieves symptoms in select patients. In combination with chemoradiation and hormonal therapy, surgery may have a palliative role with a low perioperative mortality[95] and a 25% 5-year survival.[96]

Colorectal Cancer

Studies reporting patients with colorectal metastasis to the pancreas are also limited to single case reports or small series. Sperti and colleagues[95] reported 18 resections for metastatic disease with 9 from colorectal adenocarcinoma. Most presented with abdominal pain and jaundice, and imaging studies revealed a mass in the pancreas and a history of colorectal cancer.[93,95,97] Surgical resection or metastasectomy without other organ involvement may relieve symptoms and be adequate treatment, usually combined with other modalities.[95,96]

Other Rare Metastases from Different Sites

Three percent to 15% of resected pancreatic metastases are from the urinary bladder, ovary, and prostate.[83,93,96] Limited conclusions can be drawn due to rarity of the disease, but surgeons can apply similar reasoning to determine treatment for these lesions, Parenchyma-sparing operations, such as central pancreatectomy and enucleation can be considered when feasible.

PANCREATIC INFLAMMATORY LESIONS

Fewer than 5% of all pancreatectomies done for suspected carcinoma are benign. There are a few pancreatic inflammatory conditions, such as chronic pancreatitis, AIP, GP (**Fig. 10**), eosinophilic pancreatitis, and pyogenic abscess that mirror

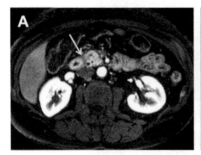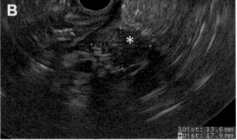

Fig. 10. (*A*) Axial MRI showing a 1-cm heterogeneous mass in a 57-year-old woman with recurrent pancreatitis (*arrow indicates mass*). (*B*) EUS of this patient confirming a 13.6 × 17.9-mm mass in the head of the pancreas. Surgical resection was performed and pathologic findings confirmed GP. The patient's recurrent pancreatitis symptoms resolved. Asterisk indicates mass.

PDAC. Clinical, biochemical, and radiographic findings may overlap, and uncertainty may infrequently require pancreatectomy for definitive diagnosis.[2,3] AIP, in particular (also known as lymphoplasmacytic sclerosing pancreatitis), now accounts for most "pseudotumors" and should be suspected if serum immunoglobulin G4 is elevated (Type I only) in younger patients with or without other autoimmune diseases. Surgical resection is not the primary treatment, and response to a short course of steroids is diagnostic.[98,99]

SUMMARY

PDAC, PNET, IPMN, mucinous cystic neoplasm, and serous cystic neoplasm account for the vast majority of solid and cystic lesions of the pancreas. However, other neoplasms may rarely involve the pancreas and require different treatment with varying prognosis. Additionally, the pancreas may be involved with other solid or cystic lesions that require pancreatectomy for diagnosis or therapy. Therefore, the clinician needs to be aware of these infrequent and rare lesions and evaluate, treat, or refer as needed.

REFERENCES

1. Liu JB, Baker MS. Surgical management of pancreatic neuroendocrine tumors. Surg Clin North Am 2016;96:1447–68.
2. Adsay NV, Basturk O, Klimstra DS, et al. Pancreatic pseudotumors: non-neoplastic solid lesions of the pancreas that clinically mimic pancreas cancer. Semin Diagn Pathol 2004;21:260–7.
3. Al-Hawary MM, Kaza RK, Azar SF, et al. Mimics of pancreatic ductal adenocarcinoma. Cancer Imaging 2013;13:342–9.
4. Feldman MK, Gandhi NS. Imaging evaluation of pancreatic cancer. Surg Clin North Am 2016;96:1235–56.
5. Singh A, Faulx AL. Endoscopic evaluation in the workup of pancreatic cancer. Surg Clin North Am 2016;96:1257–70.
6. Sommers SC, Meissner WA. Unusual carcinomas of the pancreas. AMA Arch Pathol 1954;58:101–11.
7. Paal E, Thompson LD, Frommelt RA, et al. A clinicopathologic and immunohistochemical study of 35 anaplastic carcinomas of the pancreas with a review of the literature. Ann Diagn Pathol 2001;5:129–40.
8. Hruban RH, Pitman MB, Klimstra DS. Tumors of the pancreas. Washington, DC: American Registry of Pathology in collaboration with Armed Forces Institute of Pathology; 2007.
9. Yamaguchi K, Nakamura K, Shimizu S, et al. Pleomorphic carcinoma of the pancreas: reappraisal of surgical resection. Am J Gastroenterol 1998;93:1151–5.
10. Hoshimoto S, Matsui J, Miyata R, et al. Anaplastic carcinoma of the pancreas: case report and literature review of reported cases in Japan. World J Gastroenterol 2016;22:8631–7.
11. Strobel O, Hartwig W, Bergmann F, et al. Anaplastic pancreatic cancer: presentation, surgical management, and outcome. Surgery 2011;149:200–8.
12. Paniccia A, Hosokawa PW, Schulick RD, et al. A matched-cohort analysis of 192 pancreatic anaplastic carcinomas and 960 pancreatic adenocarcinomas: a 13-year North American experience using the National Cancer Data Base (NCDB). Surgery 2016;160:281–92.
13. Clark CJ, Graham RP, Arun JS, et al. Clinical outcomes for anaplastic pancreatic cancer: a population-based study. J Am Coll Surg 2012;215:627–34.
14. Herxheimer G. Uber heterologe cancroide. Beitr Pathol Anat 1907;41:348–412.

15. Katz MH, Taylor TH, Al-Refaie WB, et al. Adenosquamous versus adenocarcinoma of the pancreas: a population-based outcomes analysis. J Gastrointest Surg 2011;15:165–74.

16. Boyd CA, Benarroch-Gampel J, Sheffield KM, et al. 415 patients with adenosquamous carcinoma of the pancreas: a population-based analysis of prognosis and survival. J Surg Res 2012;174:12–9.

17. Imaoka H, Shimizu Y, Mizuno N, et al. Clinical characteristics of adenosquamous carcinoma of the pancreas: a matched case-control study. Pancreas 2014;43:287–90.

18. Marchegiani G, Gareer H, Parisi A, et al. Pancreatic hepatoid carcinoma: a review of the literature. Dig Surg 2013;30:425–33.

19. Petrelli F, Ghilardi M, Colombo S, et al. A rare case of metastatic pancreatic hepatoid carcinoma treated with sorafenib. J Gastrointest Cancer 2012;43:97–102.

20. Kuo PC, Chen SC, Shyr YM, et al. Hepatoid carcinoma of the pancreas. World J Surg Oncol 2015;13:185.

21. Adsay NV, Merati K, Nassar H, et al. Pathogenesis of colloid (pure mucinous) carcinoma of exocrine organs: coupling of gel-forming mucin (MUC2) production with altered cell polarity and abnormal cell-stroma interaction may be the key factor in the morphogenesis and indolent behavior of colloid carcinoma in the breast and pancreas. Am J Surg Pathol 2003;27:571–8.

22. Adsay NV, Pierson C, Sarkar F, et al. Colloid (mucinous noncystic) carcinoma of the pancreas. Am J Surg Pathol 2001;25:26–42.

23. Goggins M, Offerhaus GJ, Hilgers W, et al. Pancreatic adenocarcinomas with DNA replication errors (RER+) are associated with wild-type K-ras and characteristic histopathology. Poor differentiation, a syncytial growth pattern, and pushing borders suggest RER+. Am J Pathol 1998;152:1501–7.

24. Wilentz RE, Goggins M, Redston M, et al. Genetic, immunohistochemical, and clinical features of medullary carcinoma of the pancreas: a newly described and characterized entity. Am J Pathol 2000;156:1641–51.

25. Berner O. Subkutane fettgewebsnekose. Virchow Arch Path Anat 1908;193:510–8.

26. Wang Y, Wang S, Zhou X, et al. Acinar cell carcinoma: a report of 19 cases with a brief review of the literature. World J Surg Oncol 2016;14:172.

27. Chaudhary P. Acinar cell carcinoma of the pancreas: a literature review and update. Indian J Surg 2015;77:226–31.

28. Yoshihiro T, Nio K, Tsuchihashi K, et al. Pancreatic acinar cell carcinoma presenting with panniculitis, successfully treated with FOLFIRINOX: a case report. Mol Clin Oncol 2017;6:866–70.

29. Matos JM, Schmidt CM, Turrini O, et al. Pancreatic acinar cell carcinoma: a multi-institutional study. J Gastrointest Surg 2009;13:1495–502.

30. Frantz VK. Tumors of the pancreas. Atlas of tumor pathology. Washington, DC: Armed Forces Institute of Pathology; 1959. p. 32–3.

31. Yu PF, Hu ZH, Wang XB, et al. Solid pseudopapillary tumor of the pancreas: a review of 553 cases in Chinese literature. World J Gastroenterol 2010;16:1209–14.

32. Lubezky N, Papoulas M, Lessing Y, et al. Solid pseudopapillary neoplasm of the pancreas: management and long-term outcome. Eur J Surg Oncol 2017;43:1056–60.

33. Marchegiani G, Andrianello S, Massignani M, et al. Solid pseudopapillary tumors of the pancreas: specific pathological features predict the likelihood of postoperative recurrence. J Surg Oncol 2016;114:597–601.

34. Dhebri AR, Connor S, Campbell F, et al. Diagnosis, treatment and outcome of pancreatoblastoma. Pancreatology 2004;4:441–51 [discussion: 452–3].

35. Xu SY, Sun K, Owusu-Ansah KG, et al. Central pancreatectomy for pancreatic schwannoma: a case report and literature review. World J Gastroenterol 2016; 22:8439–46.

36. Moriya T, Kimura W, Hirai I, et al. Pancreatic schwannoma: case report and an updated 30-year review of the literature yielding 47 cases. World J Gastroenterol 2012;18:1538–44.

37. Nishikawa T, Shimura K, Tsuyuguchi T, et al. Contrast-enhanced harmonic EUS of pancreatic schwannoma. Gastrointest Endosc 2016;83:463–4.

38. Meeks M, Grace S, Veerapong J, et al. Primary angiosarcoma of the pancreas. J Gastrointest Cancer 2016. [Epub ahead of print].

39. Worth PJ, Turner M, Hammill CW. Incidental angiosarcoma of the pancreas: a case report of a rare, asymptomatic tumor. J Pancreat Cancer 2017;3:24–7.

40. Heywood G, Smyrk TC, Donohue JH. Primary angiomyolipoma of the pancreas. Pancreas 2004;28:443–5.

41. Nagata S, Yuki M, Tomoeda M, et al. Perivascular epithelioid cell neoplasm (PE-Coma) originating from the pancreas and metastasizing to the liver. Pancreas 2011;40:1155–7.

42. Mourra N, Lazure T, Colas C, et al. Perivascular epithelioid cell tumor: the first malignant case report in the pancreas. Appl Immunohistochem Mol Morphol 2013; 21:e1–4.

43. Mizuuchi Y, Nishihara K, Hayashi A, et al. Perivascular epithelial cell tumor (PE-Coma) of the pancreas: a case report and review of previous literature. Surg Case Rep 2016;2:59.

44. Kim JY, Song JS, Park H, et al. Primary mesenchymal tumors of the pancreas: single-center experience over 16 years. Pancreas 2014;43:959–68.

45. Soreide JA, Undersrud ES, Al-Saiddi MS, et al. Primary leiomyosarcoma of the pancreas—a case report and a comprehensive review. J Gastrointest Cancer 2016;47:358–65.

46. Zhang H, Jensen MH, Farnell MB, et al. Primary leiomyosarcoma of the pancreas: study of 9 cases and review of literature. Am J Surg Pathol 2010;34:1849–56.

47. ESMO/European Sarcoma Network Working Group. Soft tissue and visceral sarcomas: ESMO clinical practice guidelines for diagnosis, treatment and follow-up. Ann Oncol 2012;23(Suppl 7):vii92–9.

48. Aihara H, Kawamura YJ, Toyama N, et al. A small leiomyosarcoma of the pancreas treated by local excision. HPB (Oxford) 2002;4:145–8.

49. Paramythiotis D, Kofina K, Bangeas P, et al. Solitary fibrous tumor of the pancreas: case report and review of the literature. World J Gastrointest Surg 2016;8:461–6.

50. D'Amico FE, Ruffolo C, Romano M, et al. Rare neoplasm mimicking neuoroendocrine pancreatic tumor: a case report of solitary fibrous tumor with review of the literature. Anticancer Res 2017;37:3093–7.

51. Saif MW. Primary pancreatic lymphomas. JOP 2006;7:262–73.

52. Anand D, Lall C, Bhosale P, et al. Current update on primary pancreatic lymphoma. Abdom Radiol (NY) 2016;41:347–55.

53. Yu L, Chen Y, Xing L. Primary pancreatic lymphoma: two case reports and a literature review. Onco Targets Ther 2017;10:1687–94.

54. Sadot E, Yahalom J, Do RK, et al. Clinical features and outcome of primary pancreatic lymphoma. Ann Surg Oncol 2015;22:1176–84.

55. Kloppel G, Hruban RH, Longnecker DS, et al. Ductal adenocarcinoma of the pancreas. In: Hamilton SR, Aaltonen LA, editors. World Health Organization classification of tumours. Pathology and genetics of tumours of the digestive system. Lyon (France): International Agency for Research on Cancer; 2000. p. 221–30.

56. Serafini S, Da Dalt G, Pozza G, et al. Collision of ductal adenocarcinoma and neuroendocrine tumor of the pancreas: a case report and review of the literature. World J Surg Oncol 2017;15:93.

57. Tewari N, Zaitoun AM, Lindsay D, et al. Three cases of concomitant intraductal papillary mucinous neoplasm and pancreatic neuroendocrine tumour. JOP 2013;14:423–7.

58. Ishida M, Shiomi H, Naka S, et al. Concomitant intraductal papillary mucinous neoplasm and neuroendocrine tumor of the pancreas. Oncol Lett 2013;5:63–7.

59. Yan SX, Adair CF, Balani J, et al. Solid pseudopapillary neoplasm collides with a well-differentiated pancreatic endocrine neoplasm in an adult man: case report and review of histogenesis. Am J Clin Pathol 2015;143:283–7.

60. Jakobsen M, Kloppel G, Detlefsen S. Mixed acinar-neuroendocrine carcinoma of the pancreas: a case report and a review. Histol Histopathol 2016;31:1381–8.

61. Izumi H, Furukawa D, Yazawa N, et al. A case study of a collision tumor composed of cancers of the bile duct and pancreas. Surg Case Reps 2015;1:40.

62. Matsushita D, Kurahara H, Mataki Y, et al. Pancreatic hamartoma: a case report and literature review. BMC Gastroenterol 2016;16:3.

63. Zhang J, Wang H, Tang X, et al. Pancreatic hamartoma, a rare benign disease of the pancreas: a case report. Oncol Lett 2016;11:3925–8.

64. Kawakami F, Shimizu M, Yamaguchi H, et al. Multiple solid pancreatic hamartomas: a case report and review of the literature. World J Gastrointest Oncol 2012;4:202–6.

65. Mondal U, Henkes N, Henkes D, et al. Cavernous hemangioma of adult pancreas: a case report and literature review. World J Gastroenterol 2015;21:9793–802.

66. Kim SH, Kim JY, Choi JY, et al. Incidental detection of pancreatic hemangioma mimicking a metastatic tumor of renal cell carcinoma. Korean J Hepatobiliary Pancreat Surg 2016;20:93–6.

67. Soreide JA, Greve OJ, Gudlaugsson E. Adult pancreatic hemangioma in pregnancy–concerns and considerations of a rare case. BMC Surg 2015;15:119.

68. Figueroa RM, Lopez GJ, Servin TE, et al. Pancreatic hemolymphangioma. JOP 2014;15:399–402.

69. Chung JC, Kim HC, Chu CW, et al. Huge cystic lymphangioma of the pancreas. Can J Surg 2009;52:E303–5.

70. Assifi MM, Nguyen PD, Agrawal N, et al. Non-neoplastic epithelial cysts of the pancreas: a rare, benign entity. J Gastrointest Surg 2014;18:523–31.

71. Oh Y, Choi Y, Son SM, et al. Pancreatic lymphoepithelial cysts diagnosed with endosonography-guided fine needle aspiration. Korean J Gastroenterol 2017;69:253–8.

72. Terakawa H, Makino I, Nakagawara H, et al. Clinical and radiological feature of lymphoepithelial cyst of the pancreas. World J Gastroenterol 2014;20:17247–53.

73. Rodriguez E, Netto G, Li QK. Intrapancreatic accessory spleen: a case report and review of literature. Diagn Cytopathol 2013;41:466–9.

74. Spencer LA, Spizarny DL, Williams TR. Imaging features of intrapancreatic accessory spleen. Br J Radiol 2010;83:668–73.

75. Guo W, Han W, Liu J, et al. Intrapancreatic accessory spleen: a case report and review of the literature. World J Gastroenterol 2009;15:1141–3.

76. Miljkovic M, Senadhi V. Use of endoscopic ultrasound in diagnosing plasmacytoma of the pancreas. JOP 2012;13:26–9.

77. Williet N, Kassir R, Cuilleron M, et al. Difficult endoscopic diagnosis of a pancreatic plasmacytoma: case report and review of literature. World J Clin Oncol 2017; 8:91–5.

78. Mony S, Patil PD, English R, et al. A rare presentation of sarcoidosis as a pancreatic head mass. Case Rep Pulmonol 2017;2017:7037162.

79. Kersting S, Janot MS, Munding J, et al. Rare solid tumors of the pancreas as differential diagnosis of pancreatic adenocarcinoma. JOP 2012;13:268–77.

80. Gupta D, Patel J, Rathi C, et al. Primary pancreatic head tuberculosis: great masquerader of pancreatic adenocarcinoma. Gastroenterol Res 2015;8:193–6.

81. Kaur M, Dalal V, Bhatnagar A, et al. Pancreatic tuberculosis with markedly elevated CA 19-9 levels: a diagnostic pitfall. Oman Med J 2016;31:446–9.

82. Waintraub DJ, D'Souza LS, Madrigal E, et al. A rare case of isolated pancreatic tuberculosis. ACG Case Rep J 2016;3:e91.

83. Adler H, Redmond CE, Heneghan HM, et al. Pancreatectomy for metastatic disease: a systematic review. Eur J Surg Oncol 2014;40:379–86.

84. Konstantinidis IT, Dursun A, Zheng H, et al. Metastatic tumors in the pancreas in the modern era. J Am Coll Surg 2010;211:749–53.

85. Hung JH, Wang SE, Shyr YM, et al. Resection for secondary malignancy of the pancreas. Pancreas 2012;41:121–9.

86. De Moura DT, Chacon DA, Tanigawa R, et al. Pancreatic metastases from ocular malignant melanoma: the use of endoscopic ultrasound-guided fine-needle aspiration to establish a definitive cytologic diagnosis: a case report. J Med Case Rep 2016;10:332.

87. Goyal J, Lipson EJ, Rezaee N, et al. Surgical resection of malignant melanoma metastatic to the pancreas: case series and review of literature. J Gastrointest Cancer 2012;43:431–6.

88. Sperti C, Moletta L, Patane G. Metastatic tumors to the pancreas: the role of surgery. World J Gastrointest Oncol 2014;6:381–92.

89. Mokhtar Pour A, Masir N, Isa MR. Obstructive jaundice in small cell lung carcinoma. Malays J Pathol 2015;37:149–52.

90. Niu FY, Zhou Q, Yang JJ, et al. Distribution and prognosis of uncommon metastases from non-small cell lung cancer. BMC Cancer 2016;16:149.

91. Hiotis SP, Klimstra DS, Conlon KC, et al. Results after pancreatic resection for metastatic lesions. Ann Surg Oncol 2002;9:675–9.

92. Mourra N, Arrive L, Balladur P, et al. Isolated metastatic tumors to the pancreas: Hopital St-Antoine experience. Pancreas 2010;39:577–80.

93. Pan B, Lee Y, Rodriguez T, et al. Secondary tumors of the pancreas: a case series. Anticancer Res 2012;32:1449–52.

94. Bednar F, Scheiman JM, McKenna BJ, et al. Breast cancer metastases to the pancreas. J Gastrointest Surg 2013;17:1826–31.

95. Sperti C, Pasquali C, Berselli M, et al. Metastasis to the pancreas from colorectal cancer: is there a place for pancreatic resection? Dis Colon Rectum 2009;52: 1154–9.

96. Reddy S, Wolfgang CL. The role of surgery in the management of isolated metastases to the pancreas. Lancet Oncol 2009;10:287–93.

97. Matsubara N, Baba H, Okamoto A, et al. Rectal cancer metastasis to the head of the pancreas treated with pancreaticoduodenectomy. J Hepatobiliary Pancreat Surg 2007;14:590–4.

98. Farris AB 3rd, Basturk O, Adsay NV. Pancreatitis, other inflammatory lesions, and pancreatic pseudotumors. Surg Pathol Clin 2011;4:625–50.

99. Asbun H, Conlon K, Fernandez-Cruz L, et al, International Study Group of Pancreatic Surgery. When to perform a pancreatoduodenectomy in the absence of positive histology? A consensus statement by the International Study Group of Pancreatic Surgery. Surgery 2014;155(5):887–92.

Ex Vivo Resection and Autotransplantation for Pancreatic Neoplasms

Peter Liou, MD, Tomoaki Kato, MD, MBA*

KEYWORDS

- Pancreas • Pancreatic tumors • Ex vivo resection • Autotransplantation
- Mesenteric root involvement • SMA involvement

KEY POINTS

- Ex vivo resection and autotransplantation is a technique derived from multivisceral and intestinal transplantation whereby tumor-infiltrated organs are removed en bloc and preserved in the cold, followed by tumor resection and reimplantation of the remaining viscera.
- Advantages of ex vivo resection include tumor removal in a bloodless field while minimizing the risk of ischemic injury to the involved organs.
- Access to the mesenteric root is greatly facilitated with ex vivo resection, and allows for safe reconstruction of major vasculature while preserving visceral integrity.
- Certain low-grade, non-adenocarcinomatous pancreatic neoplasms involving the mesenteric vessels where aggressive surgical resection would be warranted, may benefit from ex vivo resection.
- Although ex vivo resections have been performed for pancreatic adenocarcinomas with major arterial involvement, the associated morbidity is significant and benefit remains unclear.

INTRODUCTION

Pancreatic neoplasms are a heterogeneous group of tumors arising from the pancreas with distinct and varied clinical profiles.[1] Although pancreatic adenocarcinoma remains by far the most common and deadliest of these, there are several low-grade or benign neoplasms that may benefit from aggressive, curative resection.[2,3] Due to the proximity of the pancreas to major abdominal vasculature, these tumors can sometimes infiltrate these vessels and preclude complete or safe resection by conventional surgical technique. Ex vivo resection and autotransplantation, whereby

Financial Disclosures: The authors have nothing to disclose.
Department of Surgery, Columbia University Medical Center, 622 West 168 Street PH14-105, New York, NY 10032, USA
* Corresponding author.
E-mail address: TK2388@cumc.columbia.edu

tumor-laden viscera are explanted and reimplanted following tumor removal in cold preservation, allows the possibility of complete resection and vascular reconstruction while minimizing organ injury and obviating the need for allotransplantation.[4]

Ex vivo surgery was first described in 1963 for the reimplantation of a kidney following a high ureteral injury.[5] In 1988, Rudolf Pichlmayr and colleagues[6] successfully described the first ex vivo tumor resection for large liver neoplasms located at the confluence of the hepatic veins. Although radical pancreatectomy with vascular reconstruction had been previously performed for tumors invading the mesenteric vessels,[7] further experience in multivisceral transplantation led to the first successful description of ex vivo resection and intestinal autotransplantation for a large fibroma located in the head of the pancreas invading the mesenteric root by Andreas Tzakis and colleagues.[8] Since then, more than 40 cases of ex vivo tumor resection and intestinal autotransplantation have been reported worldwide for tumors involving the superior mesenteric vessels, and 32 of these involved pancreatic neoplasms.[9] Additionally, our institution has reported 2 multivisceral ex vivo resections with combined liver, intestinal, and pancreas autotransplantation for pancreatic tumors involving both the superior mesenteric artery (SMA) and the celiac axis.[10]

The technique of ex vivo surgery, which involves the explantation of all tumor-associated organs and tumor removal in cold preservation, allows for safe and complete resection or separation of critical vascular structures while minimizing ischemic organ injury. Exposure to these mesenteric vessels is also significantly improved in a bloodless field, where the organ bloc can be flipped over and easily manipulated.[11] Most importantly, ex vivo surgery can help facilitate the safe reconstruction of critical vasculature while ensuring visceral preservation. For certain pancreatic tumors, this technique could help prevent the need for allotransplantation and its associated morbidities.[12]

The ideal candidate for ex vivo surgery is a patient with a low-grade or benign yet symptomatic mass involving the mesenteric vessels that is not feasible with conventional surgical or vascular reconstructive techniques. Symptoms are often nonspecific, but patients can present with abdominal pain, difficulty eating, and signs of intestinal or biliary obstruction, or of portal hypertension. Several pancreatic tumor types have been successfully resected using ex vivo techniques with excellent long-term outcomes, including pancreatic fibromas,[8] desmoid tumors of the pancreas,[8] solid pseudopapillary tumors,[9] pancreatic neuroendocrine tumors,[9] ganglioneuromas,[13] serous cystadenocarcinomas,[14] inflammatory myofibroblastic tumors, and hemangioendotheliomas.[10]

Most of these tumors are located at the head of the pancreas and therefore amenable for pancreaticoduodenectomy. A few occur diffusely throughout the entire gland, and require total pancreatectomy to achieve complete resection.[10]

The benefit of ex vivo resection in patients with pancreatic adenocarcinoma involving the SMA is unclear.[14–16] Although surgical resection of all gross disease has traditionally been the best hope for long-term survival, aggressive surgery for disease that has already spread to encase the mesenteric arteries is controversial. In a meta-analysis by Mollberg and colleagues,[17] patients who underwent arterial reconstruction during pancreatectomy exhibited higher perioperative mortality and poorer 1-year and 3-year survival compared with patients who underwent pancreatectomy without vascular reconstruction or with venous reconstruction only. However, patients who underwent arterial reconstruction were associated with longer survival than patients with locally advanced disease who did not undergo pancreatectomy altogether.

For patients with locally advanced pancreatic adenocarcinoma, ex vivo resection can theoretically provide a means to completely resect all gross disease, including the involved vasculature. But due to the high likelihood of micrometastatic disease at the time of diagnosis, tumors that have already encased the SMA would almost invariably recur despite the degree of resection.[1] This is supported by data available for patients who have undergone ex vivo resection for adenocarcinoma with limited long-term survival.[9] We currently do not advocate for the routine use of ex vivo techniques for patients with pancreatic adenocarcinoma. For younger patients with stable disease involving the SMA despite neoadjuvant therapy who still wish to pursue surgery, discussions must be held weighing the benefits and risks of major surgery for an incurable disease, and the potential for significant life-long morbidity.

PREOPERATIVE EVALUATION

Patients with pancreatic neoplasms amenable for ex vivo resection will require a complete medical evaluation before surgery. Every patient should be evaluated by a multidisciplinary team experienced in both autotransplantation and allotransplantation. Specialists should include a surgeon, medical oncologist, gastroenterologist, nutritionist, nurse coordinator, physical therapist, and a social worker. Comorbidities, exercise tolerance, cardiopulmonary status, and availability of psychosocial support must all be considered when evaluating a candidate for ex vivo resection.

Management of the patient's specific tumor type also should be discussed in the multidisciplinary setting. Preoperative tissue biopsies can usually be obtained using minimally invasive techniques, and are valuable in establishing a diagnosis and guiding chemotherapeutic options.

Neoadjuvant chemoradiation should be considered before ex vivo surgical resection as appropriate. Preoperative procedures, such as biliary stenting or transjugular intrahepatic portosystemic shunting also should be considered.

High-quality cross-sectional imaging with computed tomography angiography is necessary for surgical planning. The tumor can be assessed in relation to adjacent vessels, which is critical in guiding the strategy for vascular reconstruction. Positron emission (PET) and Magnetic resonance imaging (MRI) may be helpful in further delineating tumor anatomy and ruling out distant metastases unclear on computed tomography imaging.

SURGICAL TECHNIQUE

Due to the heterogeneity and anatomic variability of pancreatic tumors requiring ex vivo resection techniques, specific surgical techniques have not been standardized. Careful and meticulous planning with high-quality cross-sectional imaging is always necessary to modify the surgical approach to each tumor.

Pancreaticoduodenectomy with Ex Vivo Intestinal Resection and Autotransplantation

Pancreaticoduodenectomy with intestinal autotransplantation is generally reserved for pancreatic tumors that encase the SMA, or involve the distal superior mesenteric vein (SMV) branches. The general approach and technical considerations are described as follows.

Abdominal exploration and mobilization

The initial exploration and mobilization of the abdominal contents is similar to the standard open pancreaticoduodenectomy.[18] A vertical midline incision from the xiphoid process to below the umbilicus with a right subcostal extension will usually facilitate generous exposure of the abdominal cavity. The entire peritoneum is thoroughly explored to assess for evidence of tumor spread. The liver surface is first examined and palpated to check for abnormal lesions. Although modern cross-sectional imaging is highly sensitive in detecting liver metastases, intraoperative ultrasound can be used to assess the liver parenchyma for questionable imaging findings and biopsied if necessary. If there is evidence of hepatic disease in the setting of certain neoplasms (ie, nonfunctional pancreatic neuroendocrine tumors), the lesions are again assessed for resectability. In circumstances in which there is high preoperative concern for metastatic spread precluding surgical resection, staging laparoscopy can be performed before laparotomy. In addition, the omentum and bowel are checked for disease spread.

Once the decision is made to proceed with resection, a full right medial visceral rotation is performed, mobilizing the right colon off its peritoneal attachments and exposing the retroperitoneal contents, part of the duodenum, and pancreatic head. Often there are extensive adhesions from prior surgeries or radiation and must be carefully taken down. The lesser sac is opened to further expose the head of the pancreas and tumor. The transverse colon is transected to form the distal end of the intestinal autograft and dissected off the duodenum to complete the exposure of the mesenteric vessels as they run posteriorly behind the pancreas.

The hepatoduodenal ligament is then dissected in the usual fashion, exposing the common bile duct, common hepatic artery, and gastroduodenal artery (GDA). After confirmation of normal hepatic arterial anatomy, the GDA is test clamped and divided, revealing the portal vein beneath. A traditional cholecystectomy is then performed and the common bile duct is transected and gently clamped. The antrum of the stomach is divided, forming the proximal end of the organ bloc for removal. The pancreas is then assessed for resection. Often because of extensive mesenteric vessel involvement, it may be difficult or impossible to create a tunnel between the pancreas and SMV. The pancreas is transected and margins are sent for frozen pathologic analysis in the appropriate setting (**Fig. 1**). If the entire pancreas is to be removed, the spleen is

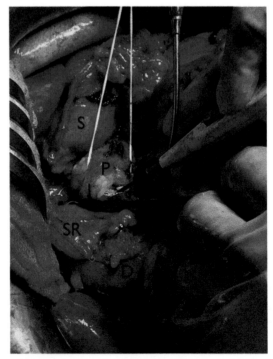

Fig. 1. Transection of the pancreas before small bowel explant. D, duodenum; P, pancreas; S, stomach; SR, stomach remnant.

concomitantly mobilized and splenic artery and vein identified for ligation. The SMA is now identified and encircled. With the remaining attachments taken down, the entire tumor-multivisceral bloc is mobilized and suspended by the 2 mesenteric vessels (**Fig. 2**). The artery and vein are then clamped and divided, and the viscera are removed and immediately flushed with organ preservation solution via the SMA. For certain tumors involving the portomesenteric junction, proximal transection of the portal vein necessitates reconstruction of the splenic vein either with creation of a splenorenal shunt, or via anastomosis to an interposition autologous vein graft.

An alternative approach to intestinal autotransplantation is the isolation of a segment of small bowel in the manner of the living donor intestinal transplant procurement.[19] At the time of exploration, a segment of uninvolved small bowel (usually midjejunum or distal ileum) is isolated on a single vascular pedicle distal to the tumor region. The vessels are preserved and its associated bowel and mesentery are transected. This segment is removed first and flushed in cold preservation solution as a means of ensuring a usable portion of healthy small bowel for autotransplantation, without risk of injury during tumor resection. Isolation of a single vascular pedicle often limits the length of small bowel preserved to approximately 200 cm, although segments greater than 100 cm are probably enough to safely sustain the patient without the need for long-term parenteral nutrition.

Back-table resection and reconstruction
After the tumor-multivisceral bloc is preserved on ice (**Fig. 3**), the mesenteric vasculature is examined in relation to the tumor and resection is performed while carefully preserving the uninvolved vessels and its associated bowel. The SMA is traced distally, identifying the first jejunal branches, which may need to be removed if involved with tumor. The ileocolic artery is also identified and preserved if possible.

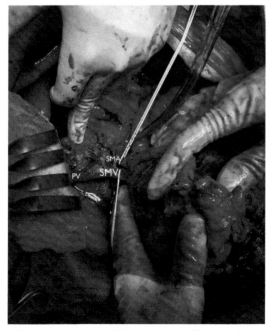

Fig. 2. Skeletonizing the mesenteric vessels in preparation for bowel explant. PV, portal vein; SMA, superior mesenteric artery; SMV, superior mesenteric vein.

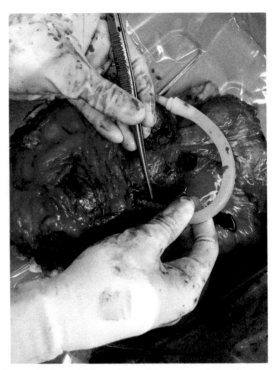

Fig. 3. Flushing the multivisceral bloc with cold preservation solution for ex vivo tumor resection.

If additional length on the artery is required for implantation, a segment of internal iliac artery may be harvested. The SMV is similarly traced and resected to obtain a tumor-free margin. Occasionally, 2 or more segments of mesenteric vein branches may need to be reconstructed to form a new venous outflow tract. The left internal jugular vein may be harvested to facilitate this reconstruction. Once vascular reconstruction is complete, the vessels are carefully checked for leaks to minimize bleeding after reperfusion, and the autograft is flushed with albumin and brought back to the operating field (**Fig. 4**). During back-table resection and preparation of the autograft, a second "recipient" team performs hemostasis, completion lymphadenectomy, vascular shunting, or intraoperative radiation, as appropriate (**Fig. 5**).

Reimplantation and Reconstruction

Once the autograft is brought to the field, it is checked for vessel orientation and positioned without any mesenteric twisting. Heparin is administered and the arterial anastomosis is performed with graft implantation onto the SMA stump or infrarenal aorta. Subsequently, the reconstructed venous conduit is anastomosed to the portal vein or directly onto the vena cava. The graft is then reperfused and hemostasis performed (**Fig. 6**). Intestinal viability is evaluated visually or with indocyanine green fluorescence angiography and additional bowel resected if perfusion is inadequate.

The gastrointestinal tract is reestablished in a manner similar to the standard pancreaticoduodenectomy. The proximal jejunal limb is brought up and a pancreaticojejunostomy, hepaticojejunostomy, and gastrojejunostomy are created in the usual fashion. An alternative to the pancreaticojejunostomy is the pancreaticogastrostomy, which may be the preferred reconstructive method in this procedure, as it avoids

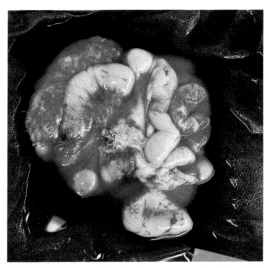

Fig. 4. The prepared intestinal autograft after tumor resection. The SMA and SMV are seen here and used for implantation.

anastomosing pancreas to reperfused bowel.[20] Distally, the ileum or ascending colon, depending on the remaining length of the autograft, is reconnected to the left colon. If an ileocolonic anastomosis is created, a Santulli-type "chimney" ileostomy is performed proximal to the side-to-end anastomosis. Otherwise, a standard loop ileostomy can be brought up if a colocolonic anastomosis is formed. A gastrostomy tube is placed if long-term enteral nutritional support is anticipated.

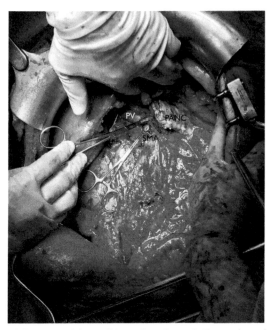

Fig. 5. The "empty abdomen" with small bowel explanted. Clamps have been placed on the SMA and SMV stumps. The pancreatic tail is seen. PANC, pancreas.

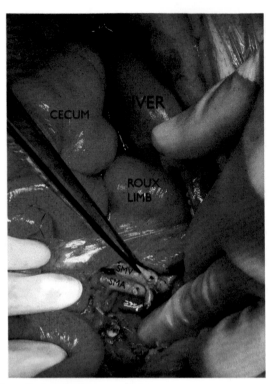

Fig. 6. Completed anastomoses after reperfusion.

If there is concern for inadequate graft perfusion or the patient is hemodynamically unstable, the abdomen can be temporarily closed and brought back for a second-look laparotomy with completion of the gastrointestinal reconstruction at that time. As an alternative, the distal end of the autograft can be brought up as a terminal enterostomy, leaving a long colonic Hartmann-type stump that can be reversed after full recovery.

Pancreaticoduodenectomy with Ex Vivo Liver Resection and Autotransplantation

For low-grade or benign tumors of the pancreatic head invading the hepatic hilum, pancreaticoduodenectomy with ex vivo resection and reconstruction of the hilum with liver autotransplantation can be performed (**Fig. 7**). We have previously described a case of a pancreatic head ganglioneuroma diffusely infiltrating the hepatoduodenal structures, causing complete portal vein, SMV, and splenic vein thrombosis and bile duct obstruction that was removed using this technique.[13]

Due to massive venous collaterals from mesenteric thrombosis, a mesocaval shunt with an autologous jugular vein graft, as well as a distal splenorenal shunt, were first created to decompress the portal system. The liver was then completely dissected off the vena cava and pancreaticoduodenal mobilization performed with stomach, jejunum, and pancreas transections. After the division of the common hepatic artery and the hepatic veins, the entire multivisceral bloc was flushed and preserved in the cold via the portal vein.

The tumor was carefully dissected off the hepatic hilum ex vivo in a bloodless field. The left hepatic artery was completely encased with tumor, so a left lateral

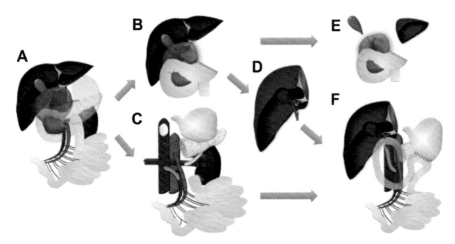

Fig. 7. Diagram of pancreaticoduodenectomy with liver ex vivo tumor resection. (*A*) The visceral bloc containing the pancreatic tumor invading the hepatic hilum. (*B*) The liver, pancreatic head and duodenum are removed and preserved in cold preservation leaving the intestines in situ (*C*). (*D*) The tumor is resected (*E*), leaving only part of the liver behind for implantation. (*F*) The tumor-free lobe of the liver is reimplanted. (*From* Matsuoka N, Weiner JI, Griesemer AD, et al. Ex vivo pancreaticoduodenectomy and liver autotransplantation for pancreatic head tumor with extensive involvement of the hepatoduodenal ligament. Liver Transpl 2015;21(12):1554; with permission.)

hepatectomy was performed at this time. The patient remained stable during this anhepatic phase, supported with the mesocaval and splenorenal shunts.

Once the tumor was completely removed, the right lobe was reimplanted by taking down the mesocaval shunt and connecting it to the portal vein. The right hepatic artery was anastomosed to the common hepatic artery stump and the liver was reperfused. The gastrointestinal tract was then reestablished with a pancreaticojejunostomy, hepaticojejunostomy, and gastrojejunostomy.

Pancreatectomy with Multivisceral Ex Vivo Resection and Combined Liver/Intestine Autotransplantation

Certain pancreatic tumors encasing both the celiac artery and SMA may be amenable to ex vivo tumor resection and autotransplantation of the liver and intestine. We have previously described this multivisceral ex vivo procedure for an inflammatory myofibroblastic tumor involving most of the pancreas, as well as a hemangioendothelioma of the pancreatic head, both encasing the celiac artery and SMA.[10] The techniques of this complex procedure are developed from experience performing multivisceral transplantations. Strategies for vascular and gastrointestinal reconstruction are highly dependent on tumor size, location, and involvement of adjacent structures, and must be individualized with careful preoperative planning.

At the time of exploration, the abdominal viscera are fully mobilized as previously described to expose the tumor and its involvements. The gastrointestinal tract is divided at the gastroesophageal junction and at the transverse colon. The kidneys are usually left in situ, unless there is tumor involvement. Using techniques similar to that of multivisceral transplant procurement, the stomach, pancreas, spleen, small bowel, and proximal colon are mobilized en bloc. The liver is dissected off the vena cava to the level of the major hepatic veins, and the entire multivisceral bloc is lifted out after the ligation of the SMA and celiac arteries. If portions of the vena cava or aorta are involved with tumor, segments of these great vessels can be removed as well with the organs and reconstructed with synthetic graft. In these cases, venovenous or venoarterial bypass should be considered but is usually not necessary.

Because of both SMA and celiac arterial involvement, total pancreatectomy generally must be performed. Depending on the level of tumor invasion and parenchymal sparing, islet cells potentially could be harvested for autotransplantation. If the distal pancreas is spared from tumor, it is possible to reimplant the pancreatic tail and spleen in the groin with drainage into the bladder.

After flushing the organ bloc with preservation fluid via the SMA and celiac artery, the tumor is resected ex vivo. The strategy of tumor removal is highly variable and dependent on its vessel and organ involvement. Organs deemed unsalvageable are removed, and can include the stomach, spleen, pancreas, segments of small bowel, and segments of the liver. Vascular reconstruction poses a significant challenge and often relies on the use of both autologous grafts from the jugular and saphenous veins, as well as synthetic grafts. With some creativity, the splenic and gastric vessels also can be used for hepatic arterial reconstruction, especially in the setting of variant anatomy.

Owing to the general location of pancreatic tumors requiring multivisceral ex vivo resection, the organs are usually detached and implanted separately. The liver is implanted first, with reconnection to the vena cava or synthetic conduit. A renoportal anastomosis is created to establish portal flow via a jugular vein graft, before the small bowel is autotransplanted. The reconstructed hepatic artery is then reconnected to the existing celiac artery stump or the synthetic aortic graft. Once the liver is perfused, the small bowel is brought to the field and implanted, with the reconstructed mesenteric artery connected to the aorta and mesenteric vein to the side of the renoportal anastomosis. As previously mentioned, a spared distal pancreas and spleen is amenable for implantation. In our experience, the splenic artery and vein can be anastomosed to the iliac vessels in the pelvis and the pancreas is connected to the bladder. Once the organs are reperfused, intestinal continuity is restored with an esophagojejunostomy, hepaticojejunostomy, and ileocolostomy.

POSTOPERATIVE MANAGEMENT

Due to the complex and invasive nature of these procedures, multidisciplinary management in the postoperative phase is crucial. Patients are transferred to the intensive care unit for hemodynamic monitoring. They typically remain intubated, especially if a second-look laparotomy is planned. Laboratory values and hemodynamic parameters are carefully trended with a low threshold for reexploration if there is concern for inadequate graft perfusion. Doppler ultrasound is performed postoperatively to examine the patency of the hepatic and mesenteric vasculature.

Once the hematocrit has stabilized or there is low concern for bleeding, a heparin drip is initiated. Although there is no standardization for timing of initiation, we typically start a low-dose heparin drip intraoperatively if the field appears hemostatic, and uptitrate over the next 24 to 48 hours. Sublingual aspirin is usually started as well, particularly when synthetic grafts are used. Insulin is administered as needed, especially in the setting of total pancreatectomy. Total parenteral nutrition is begun 3 to 4 days after surgery and continued until the patient can be supported entirely on enteral nutrition. Intra-abdominal drains are left in place until output is minimal and a pancreatic or bile leak has effectively been ruled out. Intestinal output is generally higher with shorter intestinal autografts and may require parenteral hydration and the use of antimotility agents. When the patient is tolerating enteral feeding without need for parenteral nutrition, the stoma can be evaluated for closure, usually within 2 to 3 months.

COMPLICATIONS

Ex vivo resection for pancreatic tumors is associated with significant morbidity and is subject to the same complications as pancreaticoduodenectomy, including pancreatic fistulae, bile leak, significant bleeding, intra-abdominal infection, delayed gastric emptying, and wound complications. The most devastating complications specific to intestinal or multivisceral autotransplantation relate to loss of the autograft from vessel thrombosis or dissection. Early suspicion of graft loss and prompt surgical exploration is necessary to prevent irreversible ischemia of the autograft. Doppler ultrasound and close laboratory and clinical monitoring can aid in the detection of these complications. There is no proven method for prevention, but until more evidence becomes available, we routinely anticoagulate all patients after autotransplantation and use autologous vessel grafts for reconstruction when possible. Postoperative arterial anastomotic disruption causing massive hemorrhage is another serious complication after autotransplantation and is likely related to a concomitant pancreatic fistula. It is our preference to perform a pancreaticogastrostomy when possible, as limited evidence supports lower fistula rates when compared with a pancreaticojejunostomy. In addition, we would avoid performing this anastomosis on reperfused bowel. Long-term complications of the vascular reconstruction relate to vessel stenosis and venous thrombosis, which may be amenable to endovascular intervention.

Other major complications relate to delayed graft function, especially in shorter intestinal autografts. During ex vivo resection, every effort is made to preserve an adequate length of bowel to support sufficient enteral absorption. The recovery process becomes more challenging with shorter autografts, as intestinal absorption is decreased, leading to higher rates of dehydration and a longer dependence on parenteral nutrition. Due to the neoplastic tendencies of teduglutide, its use in managing short-bowel syndrome in these patients is not currently recommended. Patients who are unable to be weaned off parenteral nutrition should be considered for intestinal allotransplantation in the appropriate setting.

SUMMARY

There are several low-grade pancreatic tumors whose biology permits the use of aggressive surgery to achieve a curative resection. Tumors that are deemed unresectable by conventional techniques due to mesenteric vessel involvement may benefit from ex vivo tumor resection and autotransplantation to allow complete resection while minimizing ischemic organ injury. Ex vivo techniques also facilitate wide exposure of the major vessels and allow for complex vascular reconstruction. Despite the excellent oncologic outcomes when used for these neoplasms, the procedure carries substantial morbidity and a high complication rate. But for patients who were otherwise offered total enterectomy and allotransplantation or told that their tumor was unresectable, ex vivo resection may offer them a hope for cure.

REFERENCES

1. Wolfgang CL, Herman JM, Laheru DA, et al. Recent progress in pancreatic cancer. CA Cancer J Clin 2013;63(5):318–48.
2. Norton JA, Harris EJ, Chen Y, et al. Pancreatic endocrine tumors with major vascular abutment, involvement, or encasement and indication for resection. Arch Surg 2011;146(6):724–32.

3. Haugvik SP, Labori KJ, Waage A, et al. Pancreatic surgery with vascular reconstruction in patients with locally advanced pancreatic neuroendocrine tumors. J Gastrointest Surg 2013;17(7):1224–32.

4. Tzakis AG, Pararas NB, Tekin A, et al. Intestinal and multivisceral autotransplantation for tumors of the root of the mesentery: long-term follow-up. Surgery 2012; 152(1):82–9.

5. Hardy JD. High ureteral injuries. Management by autotransplantation of the kidney. JAMA 1963;184:97–101.

6. Pichlmayr R, Weimann A, Oldhafer KJ, et al. Role of liver transplantation in the treatment of unresectable liver cancer. World J Surg 1995;19(6):807–13.

7. Lai DT, Chu KM, Thompson JF, et al. Islet cell carcinoma treated by induction regional chemotherapy and radical total pancreatectomy with liver revascularization and small bowel autotransplantation. Surgery 1996;119(1):112–4.

8. Tzakis AG, De Faria W, Angelis M, et al. Partial abdominal exenteration, ex vivo resection of a large mesenteric fibroma, and successful orthotopic intestinal autotransplantation. Surgery 2000;128(3):486–9.

9. Wu G. Intestinal autotransplantation. Gastr Report 2017;1–8.

10. Kato T, Lobritto SJ, Tzakis A, et al. Multivisceral ex vivo surgery for tumors involving celiac and superior mesenteric arteries. Am J Transplant 2012;12(5): 1323–8.

11. Tzakis AG, Kato T, Mittal N, et al. Intestinal autotransplantation for the treatment of pathologic lesions at the root of the mesentery. Transplant Proc 2002;34(3):908–9.

12. Moon JI, Selvaggi G, Nishida S, et al. Intestinal transplantation for the treatment of neoplastic disease. J Surg Oncol 2005;92(4):284–91.

13. Matsuoka N, Weiner JI, Griesemer AD, et al. Ex vivo pancreaticoduodenectomy and liver autotransplantation for pancreatic head tumor with extensive involvement of the hepatoduodenal ligament. Liver Transpl 2015;21(12):1553–6.

14. Wu G, Zhao Q, Wang W, et al. Clinical and nutritional outcomes after intestinal autotransplantation. Surgery 2016;159(6):1668–76.

15. Quintini C, Di Benedetto F, Diago T, et al. Intestinal autotransplantation for adenocarcinoma of pancreas involving the mesenteric root: our experience and literature review. Pancreas 2007;34(2):266–8.

16. Nikeghbalian S, Aliakbarian M, Kazemi K, et al. Ex-vivo resection and small-bowel auto-transplantation for the treatment of tumors at the root of the mesentery. Int J Organ Transplant Med 2014;5(3):120–4.

17. Mollberg N, Rahbari NN, Koch M, et al. Arterial resection during pancreatectomy for pancreatic cancer: a systematic review and meta-analysis. Ann Surg 2011; 254(6):882–93.

18. Griffin JF, Pork KE. The management of periampullary cancer. In: Cameron J, editor. Current surgical therapy. 12th edition. Philadelphia: Elsevier; 2016. p. 538–48.

19. Selvaggi G, Levi DM, Kato T, et al. Expanded use of transplantation techniques: abdominal wall transplantation and intestinal autotransplantation. Transplant Proc 2004;36(5):1561–3.

20. Menahem B, Guittet L, Mulliri A, et al. Pancreaticogastrostomy is superior to pancreaticojejunostomy for prevention of pancreatic fistula after pancreaticoduodenectomy: an updated meta-analysis of randomized controlled trials. Ann Surg 2015;261(5):882–7.

Moving?

Make sure your subscription moves with you!

To notify us of your new address, find your **Clinics Account Number** (located on your mailing label above your name), and contact customer service at:

Email: journalscustomerservice-usa@elsevier.com

800-654-2452 (subscribers in the U.S. & Canada)
314-447-8871 (subscribers outside of the U.S. & Canada)

Fax number: 314-447-8029

Elsevier Health Sciences Division
Subscription Customer Service
3251 Riverport Lane
Maryland Heights, MO 63043

ELSEVIER

Printed and bound by CPI Group (UK) Ltd, Croydon, CR0 4YY

03/10/2024

01040397-0002